Clinical Consultant

Jo Anne Kirk, MSN, RN
Clinical Instructor
University of Texas at Tyler
Tyler, Texas

P9-CPY-652

Preface

The Pocket Guide for Nursing Health Assessment: A Best Practice Approach was designed to work as a clinical handbook and up-to-date reference for nurses when interviewing patients of all age groups and cultural backgrounds, taking health histories, promoting health, and performing physical assessments. The content derives from and has been developed in conjunction with *Nursing Health Assessment: A Best Practice Approach* and serves to both review the core content provided in the textbook as well as help students apply their foundational learning through reinforcement and streamlined presentation.

The content focuses on key questions in the area of health promotion, reviewing important risk factors and outlining essential teaching points for risk assessment and intervention. It includes essential questions to review common and concerning signs and symptoms for each health assessment topic. The chapters review the key techniques of examination, outlining normal and unexpected findings. Finally, tables of findings provide a quick reference by which students can compare and contrast results to assist with eventual nursing and medical diagnoses.

Key Features

Key features include the following:

- Abundant full-color illustrations and photos throughout highlighting essential anatomy and physiology, techniques of physical assessment, and normal and abnormal physiologic findings
- Inclusion of health promotion content throughout, which focuses on the nurse's key role in patient education and advocacy and disease prevention
- Safety alerts, which call attention to areas of concern that require special techniques or adaptations to protect or preserve the health of patients or caregivers
- Samples of documentation that assist students to remember how to record their findings

- Lifespan and Cultural Considerations that remind students of variations according to age or background that may influence findings
- Spiral binding that allows the pocket guide to remain open on any flat surface, which is especially useful in clinical settings

Organization

This book is organized into four units. The first two chapters (Unit I) focus on the basic foundations of nursing health assessment, reviewing essential concepts of interviewing/history taking and physical assessment. Unit II contains chapters that review assessments pertinent to all patients in all circumstances: general survey, vital signs, pain, nutrition, and mental health. Unit III reviews the health assessment of each body system, from skin through the genital/rectal examinations. Finally, Unit IV contains assessments for patients at every stage of the lifespan.

Contents

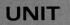

Basic
Assessment
Concepts

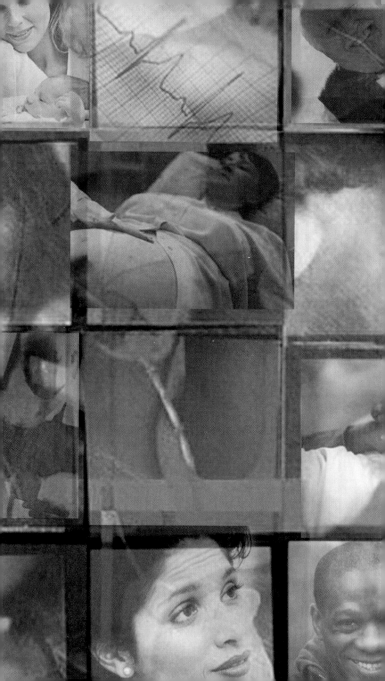

Interview and Health History

The nursing role focuses on promoting health, screening for problems, and intervening to restore or improve health or function as optimally as possible. The health history forms the foundation for care as patterns emerge and problems are identified. It provides context for the current situation and a more complete picture of how issues are related. During history taking and interviewing, the nurse establishes trust with patients. Through therapeutic communication, the patient and the nurse work together to resolve problems through collaborative solutions. As the nurse develops and refines interviewing capabilities, conversation with patients becomes more comfortable, with smooth transitions between questions. Each nurse develops a style of communication that suits his or her personality and values, blending the professional and the personal.

Interviewing and Therapeutic Communication

All nursing practice revolves around the **nurse–patient relationship**. Unlike personal and social relationships, the nurse–patient relationship is based on the therapeutic use of self through verbal and nonverbal communication skills. The nurse has a privileged role as a respected care provider. In some situations, patients disclose information to nurses not even shared with family members. Within the nurse–patient relationship, the nurse learns wide-ranging things about patients—from minute physical details to deep-seated feelings about spirituality, culture, and psychosocial concerns.

Therapeutic communication is a basic nursing tool in which the nurse ensures that the interaction focuses on the patient and the patient's concerns. Key elements include caring and empathy. **Caring** is the ability to connect with the patient and demonstrate compassion, sensitivity, and patient-centered care. **Empathy** means the ability to

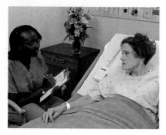

Figure 1.1 The nurse uses caring and empathy in the therapeutic relationship to see and feel the situation from the patient's perspective, not the nurse's.

perceive, reason, and communicate understanding of another person's feelings without criticism. It is being able to see and feel the situation from the patient's perspective, not the nurse's (Fig. 1-1).

Nonverbal Communication Skills

During interviewing and history taking with patients, nonverbal communication is equally as, if not more, important than verbal communication. The nurse's physical appearance, facial expression, posture and positioning in relation to the patient, gestures, eye contact, voice, and use of touch are all important components. The nurse should not assume that touch is culturally acceptable. Permission to touch the patient is a courtesy.

Verbal Communication Skills

Effective interviewing skills evolve through practice and repetition. They encourage patients to further expand initial brief answers and also help redirect patients who wander from topic.

- **Active listening** is the ability to focus on patients and their perspectives. It requires the nurse to constantly decode messages, including thoughts, words, opinions, and emotions.
- **Restatement** relates to the content of communication. The nurse makes a simple statement, usually using the same words of patients. The purpose is to ask patients to elaborate.
- **Reflection** is similar to restatement; however, instead of simply echoing the patient's comments, the nurse summarizes the main themes. Patients, thus, gain a better understanding of underlying issues, which helps to identify their feelings.
- **Encouraging elaboration (facilitation)** assists patients to more completely describe problems. Responses encourage patients to

say more, continue the conversation, and show patients that the nurse is interested.

- **Purposeful silence** allows patients time to gather their thoughts and provide accurate answers. Silence can be therapeutic, communicating nonverbal concern. It gives patients a chance to decide how much information to disclose.
- **Focusing** helps when patients stray from topic and need redirection. It allows the nurse to address areas of concern related to current problems.
- **Clarification** is important when the patient's word choice or ideas are unclear.
- **Summarizing** happens at the end of the interview, when the nurse reviews and condenses important information into two or three of the most important findings. Doing so also helps to reassure the patient that he or she has been heard accurately.

Nontherapeutic Responses

Often in social situations, people use nontherapeutic casual responses that are inappropriate in the nurse–patient relationship:

- **False reassurance** helps to minimize uncomfortable feelings but may mislead a patient into minimizing a health concern or neglecting to perform a needed health-promoting activity.
- **Sympathy** is feeling what a patient feels from the viewpoint of the nurse, not of the patient.
- **Unwanted advice**, although common in social situations, is nontherapeutic, because it usually is from the nurse's perspective, not the patient's.
- **Biased (leading) questions** impose judgment and lead patients to respond in the way they think the nurse wants.
- **Changing the subject** may happen when a situation is uncomfortable for a nurse because of personal experiences or coping mechanisms.
- **Environmental distractions** contribute to nontherapeutic communication.
- **Too many technical terms** or **too much information** can overwhelm patients. As she or he develops medical vocabulary and knowledge, the beginning nurse must practice translating from medical terminology to lay language.
- **Talking too much** and **interrupting** are nontherapeutic. The professional nurse listens more than talks.

Professional Expectations

Learning when to use the various techniques of therapeutic communication is part of both the science and art of nursing. Because it is easy to overidentify with some patients, establishing clear professional boundaries is important. **Nonprofessional involvement** occurs when the nurse develops social, personal, or economic ties with patients, all of which are inappropriate. **Sexual boundary violation**, the clearest example of nonprofessional involvement, is never acceptable within the therapeutic nurse–patient relationship.

Phases of the Interview Process

Preinteraction Phase

Before meeting with the patient, the nurse collects data from the medical record and reviews the patient's history of medical illnesses or surgeries, current medication list, and problem list.

Beginning Phase

The nurse initially introduces herself or himself by name, states the purpose of the interview, and asks the patient his or her preferred name (Fig. 1-2). The nurse shakes hands if that seems comfortable with the patient and is appropriate for culture and setting. The beginning phase may continue with discussion of neutral topics (eg, the weather) if the patient seems anxious. Ensuring privacy within the specific health care setting by pulling drapes, closing doors, or moving to a remote area before proceeding is essential, especially considering confidentiality guidelines.

Working Phase

The nurse asks specific questions, two types of which are closed ended and open ended. Each has a purpose, which the nurse chooses to elicit appropriate responses:

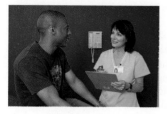

Figure 1.2 During the beginning phase, the nurse introduces herself by name, states the purpose of the interview, and asks the patient his or her preferred name.

- **Closed-ended (direct) questions** yield "yes" or "no" answers. An example is "Do you have a family history of heart disease?" They are important in emergencies or when a nurse needs to establish basic facts.
- **Open-ended questions** require patients to elaborate. They are broad and provide responses in the patient's own words. They are key to understanding symptoms, health practices, and areas requiring intervention.

Closing Phase

The nurse ends the interview by summarizing and stating what the two to three most important patterns or problems might be, as well as asking patients if they would like to mention or need anything else. The nurse also thanks patients and family members for taking the time to provide information.

🌐 Intercultural Communication

During **intercultural communication**, the sender of an intended message belongs to one culture, while the receiver is from another. Cultural differences may exist related to group or ethnicity, region, age, degree of acculturation into Western society, or a combination of these factors. The nurse must individualize care to the specific patient's practices and always use principles of **communication etiquette** (good manners that show respect for others) when working with those from various cultures, ethnicities, and religions.

Patients with **limited English** often identify frustrating language barriers when navigating the health care system. If possible, an interpreter is used; however, interpreters cannot be involved continuously throughout a patient's care. Thus, the nurse must use other communication tools, such as short phrases, communication sheets, and picture boards.

Gender and Sexual Orientation Issues

Communication styles vary between and within each gender group. Men may prefer more information and facts, whereas women might appreciate more social and emotional interactions.

The nurse must be aware of societal biases about sexual preference when working with gay, transgender, lesbian, or bisexual patients. She or he takes care to treat all patients with respect and to provide pertinent information, such as safe-sex practices for all patients.

Special Situations

Fears about illness, results from tests, interactions with health care professionals, and other factors may cause patients to have emotional responses, such as crying, anxiety, or anger. Sometimes, problems arise related to sexual aggression or the crossing of professional boundaries. Other patients have special situations that require altering the usual approach to interviewing.

Hearing Impairment

The nurse who suspects that patients have new or previously unsubstantiated hearing loss asks, "Just to be sure that you understand, please repeat what I said." For patients using hearing aids, the nurse makes sure that such devices are turned on and working. Gentle touch and visual signals can verify that patients are paying attention. Closing the door limits background noise. The nurse gives thorough explanations, provides diagrams and pictures, supplies written information, and asks open-ended questions.

Many deaf patients use several communication methods (eg, signing, writing, using speech, moving the lips). They may pantomime or use facial expressions to communicate. The nurse sits closer to patients to facilitate lip reading. He or she uses regular speech volume and lip movement but may speak slightly more slowly. If a patient does not understand, the nurse uses other wording because the sounds involved may be better decoded.

Low Level of Consciousness

Patients with a low level of consciousness may be unable to provide interview answers. In this case, the nurse needs to rely on family members and previous documentation.

Cognitive Impairment

Patients with dementia often have word-finding difficulties. They may substitute sound-alike words and sounds, making conversation difficult to track. Allowing these patients time to process as much as possible to avoid a one-sided conversation is essential.

Mental Health Issues

Patients with mental health issues may have difficulty attending to and sequencing communication. The nurse should observe patients for behaviors that indicate distraction, such as looking around the room or appearing to hear noises.

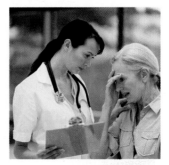

Figure 1.3 When sensitive or sad health issues arise during interviewing and history taking, the nurse stops posing questions and instead employs therapeutic verbal and nonverbal communication skills to assist the patient.

Anxiety. Anxiety is an expected response to a threat to well-being. Behaviors that indicate anxiety are nail-biting, foot tapping, sweating, and pacing. The nurse should use active listening, honesty, and a calm and unhurried manner to reduce anxiety. If patients have severe anxiety, the nurse teaches breathing and relaxation exercises and provides structure so that patients know they will remain safe.

Crying. Health issues are sensitive and sometimes pose sad situations for both patients and the nurse (Fig. 1-3). When sensitive issues arise, the nurse uses therapeutic communication techniques rather than progressing with additional interview questions.

Anger. When patients are angry, the nurse listens for associated themes and avoids becoming defensive or personalizing the situation. The beginning nurse may think that she or he did something wrong, but usually anger from patients does not directly relate to one specific nurse. Such emotion usually is a response to a situation in which patients have lost control and feel helpless.

Alcohol or Drug Use. Patients with chemical impairment have difficulty answering complex questions, so the nurse uses direct and simple questions instead. Interview questions include the type of drug, amount ingested, and date and time of the last drink or use.

Personal Questions

When interviewing patients, the nurse asks questions within the nursing role. Some patients do not understand the boundaries that define the nurse–patient relationship and ask personal questions of the nurse. The nurse must choose how much (if anything) to disclose and provide a brief response or redirect the conversation.

Sexual Aggression

Sexual aggression includes inappropriate jokes, flirtatious comments, sexual suggestions, or sexual advances. Patients with low self-esteem may flaunt their sexual prowess to increase feelings of self-worth. The nurse listens for these themes to understand why patients are acting this way and, most importantly, set limits on these behaviors.

Health History: Subjective Data Collection

Interviewing is the method by which health care providers take health histories and gather subjective data. Information discussed allows the nurse to assess the patient's health status and to provide therapeutic communication when indicated. The following sections review the elements of a complete comprehensive health history.

Sources

The individual patient is considered the **primary data** source. Charts and family members are considered **secondary data** sources. A **reliable historian** provides comprehensive information consistent with existing records. If information differs from past descriptions or details change each time, the patient may be unreliable or considered an **inaccurate historian**.

Components

Demographical Data

Demographical data include name, address, billing information, employment, and insurance details. They also encompass environmental data about exposure to contagious diseases, travel to high-risk areas, and concerns about exposure to pollution, hazards, and allergens. For hospitalized patients, the nurse assesses housing information to identify the level of independence and support needed following discharge, number of stairs at home, and any concerning structural barriers. Further occupational information helps to establish the ability of patients to return to work, work safely, avoid occupational hazards, and have access to personal protective equipment, handicapped access, and adaptive devices.

Reason for Seeking Care

This brief statement, usually in the patient's own words, establishes why he or she is making the visit. The nurse asks, "Tell me why you came to the clinic today" or "What happened that brought you to the hospital?" and records responses in the subjective part of documentation or puts the statement in quotes.

History of Present Illness

The nurse begins with open-ended questions and asks patients to explain symptoms. A complete description of the present illness is essential. Questions about **symptoms** (subjective sensations or feelings of patients) in six to eight categories assist patients to be more specific and complete: location, duration, intensity, description, aggravating factors, alleviating factors, pain goal, and functional impairment.

Common mnemonics used to remember the key elements of the presenting symptom(s) are **OLDCARTS** (**O**nset, **L**ocation, **D**uration, **C**haracter, **A**ssociated/**A**ggravating factors, **R**elieving factors, **T**iming, **S**everity) and **PQRSTU** (**P**rovocative/**P**alliative, **Q**uality, **R**egion, **S**everity, **T**iming, **U**nderstanding patient perception).

Past Health History

The past health history includes the patient's history of medical and surgical problems along with treatments and outcomes. Some problems are acute, others resolve, and others are chronic.

Current Medications and Indications

The nurse asks about current medications including names, doses, and routes; purpose of each; and any over-the-counter medications, supplements, or herbal remedies uses. If confusion about any medication exists, the nurse may ask patients or their family members to bring in pill bottles. For hospitalized patients, the nurse must reconcile all medication lists with medications taken regularly at home so that patients continue using the correct drugs.

The nurse verifies allergies with patients and compares findings against legal records. The nurse notes the type of allergic response (eg, rash, throat swelling, anaphylaxis) and differentiates allergies from side effects or adverse reactions to medications.

Family History

Questions about the health of parents, grandparents, siblings, and children help identify those diseases for which patients may be at risk and enable nurses to provide health teaching. Important familial conditions include high blood pressure, coronary artery disease, high cholesterol, stroke, cancer, diabetes mellitus, obesity, alcohol or drug addiction, mental illness, and genetic conditions.

Functional Health Assessment
Functional health patterns, especially important to nursing, focus on the effects of health or illness on quality of life. By using this approach, the nurse can assess the strengths of patients as well as areas needing improvement. See Table 1-1 for descriptions.

During functional health screening, the nurse assesses overall psychosocial well-being, including self-perception/self-concept, role/relationships, and coping/stress tolerance. Spirituality and belief systems arise during the functional health screening questions related to values/beliefs. Additionally, the nurse explores specific spiritual or religious preferences, rituals, and practices that improve health status as needed. This information can support the patient when he or she needs hope and guidance. Religious preference helps the nurse initiate referrals to pastoral care as the patient desires.

▲ Growth and Development
With children and adolescents, the nurse observes growth, physical activities, fine and gross motor skills, and speech. Developmental assessment is especially important to determine achievement of milestones, gain awareness of deficits, and facilitate any needed early intervention and management.

For all age groups, psychosocial development is part of assessment. Even some adults have delays and do not progress as expected (eg, patients with addictions that interfere with relationships, employment, and housing). The nurse also carefully evaluates cognitive stage for all patients to ensure there are no signs of dementia or other impairments.

Review of Systems
The **review of systems** is a series of questions about all body systems that helps to reveal concerns or problems. In clinic settings, patients usually fill out forms that give pertinent information, and then the nurse reviews answers during the interview. Some nurses ask questions related to each body system (eg, cough in the respiratory system) systematically before proceeding to the physical assessment. Others integrate questions while physically examining each region (eg, chest pain when assessing the heart). Sequence and format vary with setting, urgency of the problem, and style of the nurse.

Table 1.1 Gordon's Functional Health Patterns

Functional Health Pattern and Description	Sample Questions
Health perception/health management: Perceived health and well-being and how health is managed	How has your general health been? What things do you do to stay healthy?
Nutrition/metabolic: Food to metabolic need and indicators of local nutrient supply	How does your current nutritional status influence your health?
Elimination: Excretory function (bowel, bladder, and skin)	Do your patterns of bowel or bladder habits affect the types of activities that you do?
Activity/exercise: Exercise, activity, leisure, and recreation	Do you have sufficient energy for completing desired/required activities?
Cognition/perception: Sensory perceptions and thought patterns	Have you made any changes in your environment because of vision, hearing, or memory decrease?
Sleep/rest: Sleep, rest, and relaxation	Are you generally rested and ready for activities after sleeping?
Self-perception/self-concept: Self-concept, body comfort, body image, and feeling state	How would you describe yourself? Are there any changes in the way that you feel about yourself/your body?
Role/relationship: Role engagements and relationships	Are there any family problems that you have difficulty handling? How has your illness affected your family?
Sexuality/reproductive: Satisfaction and dissatisfaction with sexuality and reproductive patterns	Have you had changes in sexual relations that you are concerned about? How has this illness affected your sexual relationship?

(table continues on page 14)

Table 1.1   Gordon's Functional Health Patterns *(continued)*

Functional Health Pattern and Description	Sample Questions
Coping/stress tolerance: General coping pattern and effectiveness in terms of handling stress	Have you had any major changes in the past year? How do you usually deal with stress? Is it effective?
Values/beliefs: Values, beliefs (including spiritual), or goals that guide choices or decisions	What are the most important things to you in life? What gives you hope when times are troubled?

Questions are not mutually exclusive. For example, weight gain or loss is part of the general health state, but it also provides information about fluid balance, edema, and appetite. The nurse adapts questions to the patient, directs comfortable and logical conversation, omits questions that do not apply, and adds questions that seem pertinent.

General Health State. Weight gain or loss, fatigue, weakness, malaise, pain, usual activity, fever, chills.

Nutrition and Hydration. Conditions that increase risk of malnutrition or obesity. Nausea, vomiting. Normal daily intake, weight and weight change, dehydration, dry skin, fluid excess with shortness of breath or edema in the feet and legs. Diet practices to promote health.

Skin, Hair, and Nails. History of skin, hair, or nail disease. Rash, itching, pigmentation or texture change, lesions, sweating, dry skin, hair loss or change in texture, brittle or thin nails, thick or yellow nails.

Head and Neck. History of high or low thyroid level. Headaches, syncope, dizziness, sinus pain.

Eyes. History of poor vision or vision problems, glaucoma, cataracts, hearing loss, ear infections. Use of contact lenses or glasses, change in vision, blurring, diplopia, light sensitivity, burning, redness, discharge. Last eye examination.

Ears. History of ear or hearing problems. Ear pain, change in hearing, tinnitus, vertigo. Last hearing evaluation, ear protection.

Nose, Mouth, and Throat. History of mouth or throat cancer. Colds, sore throat, nasal obstruction, nosebleeds, cold sores, bleeding or swollen gums, tooth pain, dental caries, ulcers, enlarged tonsils, dry mouth or lips. Difficulty chewing or swallowing, change in voice. Last dental cleaning.

Thorax and Lungs. History of emphysema, asthma, or lung cancer. Wheezing, cough, sputum, dyspnea, last chest x-ray, last tuberculin skin test.

Heart and Neck Vessels. History of congenital heart problems, myocardial infarction, heart surgery, heart failure, arrhythmia, murmur. Chest pain or discomfort, palpitations, exercise tolerance. Results of last screening for cholesterol and triglycerides.

Peripheral Vascular. History of high blood pressure, peripheral vascular disease, thrombophlebitis. Peripheral edema, ulcers, circulation, claudication, redness, pain, tenderness.

Breasts. History of breast cancer or cystic breast condition. For adolescents, concerns about breast changes. Pain, tenderness, discharge, lumps, last mammogram, frequency, and date of last self-examination.

Abdominal-Gastrointestinal. History of colon cancer, gastrointestinal bleeding, cholelithiasis, liver failure, hepatitis, pancreatitis, colitis, ulcer or gastric reflux. Appetite, nausea, vomiting, diarrhea. Food intolerance or allergy, constipation, diarrhea, change in stool color, blood in stool. Last sigmoidoscopy, colonoscopy, stool for occult blood.

Abdominal-Urinary. Renal failure, polycystic kidney disease, urinary tract infection, nephrolithiasis. Pain, change in urine, dysuria, urgency, frequency, nocturia, incontinence. For children, toilet training, bed-wetting.

Musculoskeletal. History of injury, arthritis. Joint stiffness, pain, swelling, restricted movement, deformity, change in gait or coordination, strength. Pain, cramps, weakness.

Neurological. History of head or brain injury, stroke, seizures. Tremors, memory loss, numbness or tingling, loss of sensation or coordination.

Male Genitalia. History of undescended testicle, hernia, testicular cancer. Pain, burning, lesions, discharge, swelling. Change in penis or scrotum, protection against pregnancy and sexually transmitted infections. Testicular self-examination.

Female Genitalia. History of ovarian or uterine cancer, ovarian cyst, endometriosis, number of pregnancies and children. Pain, burning, lesions, discharge, itching, rash. Menstrual and physical changes, protection against pregnancy and sexually transmitted infections. Last Pap smear.

Anus, Rectum, and Prostate. History of hemorrhoids, prostate cancer, benign prostatic hyperplasia. Urinary incontinence, pain, burning, itching. For men, hesitancy, dribbling, loss in force of urine stream.

Endocrine and Hematologic Systems. History of diabetes mellitus, high or low thyroid levels, anemia. Polydipsia, polyuria, unexplained weight gain or loss, changes in body hair and body fat distribution, intolerance to heat or cold, excessive bruising, lymph node swelling. Result of last blood glucose.

Psychosocial and Lifestyle Factors

The nurse reserves psychosocial and lifestyle factors for the end of the interview, because these issues may naturally arise during the review of systems. Because of the personal nature of the questions, the nurse also saves them for the end after the relationship and trust are established.

Mental Health Concerns. If patients are anxious, depressed, or illogical, or if an association exists between current physical status and psychiatric concerns, mental health requires closer examination. The nurse assesses alcohol and drug use by direct questioning and also observation of behaviors that indicate impairment such as slurred speech, nodding off, and unstable gait.

Human Violence. Because of the high prevalence of physical abuse in children and women, especially during pregnancy, many nurses routinely question patients about this sensitive topic. They pose questions so that the patient feels comfortable talking.

Sexual History and Orientation. The comprehensive history includes sexual history and orientation to establish a baseline for behaviors and identify the need for health education.

▲ Lifespan Considerations

Pregnant Women

The comprehensive health history is performed at the first prenatal visit. The nurse obtains details about the current pregnancy, any previous pregnancies, obstetrical/gynecological history, the family, and psychosocial profile. He or she also collects history on nutrition, genetically inherited diseases, social networks, occupation, and violence. Patients may be accompanied by family members or their partners. The nurse builds a relationship with support people as part of the process if patients give permission.

Newborn, Children, and Adolescents

Health history for infants and children is provided by parents or other adult caregivers. As children move into adolescence, the nurse may interview both the parent and the teen. The relationship between the adolescent and the parent determines how the nurse collects data. It may be more comfortable and reliable to ask questions directly of the teen regarding sexual activity and recreational drug use with the parent stepping out of the room for a moment.

Older Adult

Increased risk for sensory deficits (eg, vision or hearing loss) might alter history taking with older adults. These patients may have more complex histories because of their increased prevalence of disease. It is important to identify the pattern of the illnesses and recognize how they might be related. In addition to the increased risk of illness because of family history, lifestyle choices also begin to influence health later in life.

◉ Cultural and Environmental Considerations

As previously discussed, the nurse considers religious and spiritual, social, political, economic, and educational factors that influence beliefs and care decisions. The nurse is also aware of illnesses that are more common among groups of patients, such as diabetes or genetically inherited diseases. Questions regarding the patient's environment might include safety in the home, transportation issues, or community involvement. An exposure history includes the agent, length of exposure, and type of exposure. The nurse can use this information to make a referral for further evaluation and follow-up if necessary.

Overview of Physical Examination

Infection Control and Related Issues

Health care environments contain a multitude of threatening organisms. Multidrug-resistant organisms and Gram-negative bacilli are becoming more prevalent, and the treatment of such pathogens is becoming increasingly difficult. Nurses must follow infection-control principles before, during, and after physical assessments. Practices include, but are not limited to, diligent hand hygiene and use of standard precautions.

Hand Hygiene

The single most important action to prevent infection is hand hygiene (Fig. 2-1). Contact transmission from the hands of all health care providers to patients is the most common mode of transmission, because microorganisms from one patient are then spread to others.

Proper technique for using alcohol-based hand rubs is necessary for effectiveness. Apply at least two pumps of the gel to the palm of one hand, rub both hands together, and make sure to cover all surfaces of the fingers and hands until they are dry.

Soap and water are necessary for visibly soiled hands and when *Clostridium difficile*, a spore-forming bacterium, is in the environment. When washing the hands

1. Wet them
2. Apply soap
3. Scrub the hands together vigorously for 15 seconds
4. Rinse
5. Turn off the faucet with a paper towel

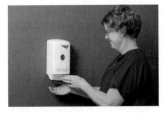

Figure 2.1 Hand hygiene.

Nails must be trimmed to ¼ inch or shorter; use of artificial nails is not recommended.

Gloves are used when nurses touch blood, body fluids, secretions, excretions, and contaminated items. Clean gloves are donned just before touching the mucous membranes or nonintact skin of patients, or when a nurse anticipates general contact with any "wet" body secretion. Changing of gloves occurs between tasks and procedures on the same patient after contact with material that contains a high concentration of microorganisms and when going from a contaminated to a cleaner area. Prompt removal of gloves is necessary after use, before touching non-contaminated items and surfaces, and before going to another patient.

⚠ *SAFETY ALERT 2-1*

Health care personnel should never wear gloves from the room into the hallway. They must wash hands immediately after glove removal to avoid transfer of microorganisms to other patients or environments.

Standard Precautions

Standard precautions help reduce the transmission of pathogens. Their intention is to prevent disease transmission when health care providers are in contact with the nonintact skin, mucous membranes, body substances, and blood-borne contacts (eg, needle-stick injury) of patients. Because many patients are unaware they have infections, standard precautions facilitate equal treatment of all patients.

Those with symptoms of a respiratory infection should cover their mouths/noses when coughing or sneezing. Additional infection-control measures are the prompt disposal of tissues directly into receptacles and the performance of hand hygiene after hands have been in contact with respiratory secretions.

The Centers for Disease Control and Prevention has developed transmission-based precautions for airborne, droplet, and contact routes. Health care providers combine the use of these specific precautions with standard precautions. The general guideline is for health care providers to wear personal protective equipment whenever they are at risk for coming into contact with body secretions from patients, such as droplet exposure during coughing with tracheal suctioning. See also Table 2-1.

Table 2.1	Recommendations for Standard Precautions
Device	**Standard Precautions**
Mask, eye protection, face shield	Wear a mask and eye protection or a face shield to protect mucous membranes of the eyes, nose, and mouth during procedures and activities that are likely to generate splashes or sprays of blood, body fluids, secretions, and excretions.
Gown	Wear a gown (a clean, nonsterile gown is adequate) to protect skin and to prevent soiling of clothes during procedures and activities that are likely to generate splashes or sprays of blood, body fluids, secretions, or excretions. Remove a soiled gown as promptly as possible and wash hands to avoid transfer of microorganisms to other patients or environments.
Patient care equipment	Ensure that reusable equipment is not used for the care of another patient until it has been cleaned and reprocessed appropriately. Ensure the proper discarding of single-use items.
Environmental control	Ensure that the facility has adequate procedures for the routine care, cleaning, and disinfection of environmental surfaces, beds, bedrails, bedside equipment, and other frequently touched surfaces.
Linen	Handle, transport, and process used linen soiled with blood, body fluids, secretions, and excretions in a manner that prevents skin exposures and contamination of clothing and that avoids transfer of microorganisms to other patients and environments.

Table 2.1 Recommendations for Standard Precautions (continued)

Device	Standard Precautions
Occupational health and blood-borne pathogens	Never recap used needles. Do not remove used needles from disposable syringes by hand; do not bend, break, or otherwise manipulate used needles by hand. Place used disposable syringes and needles, scalpel blades, and other sharp items in appropriate puncture-resistant containers. Use mouthpieces, resuscitation bags, or other ventilation devices as an alternative to mouth-to-mouth resuscitation methods in areas where the need for resuscitation is predictable.
Patient placement	Place a patient who contaminates the environment or who does not (or cannot be expected to) assist in maintaining appropriate hygiene or environmental control in a private room.

Source: CDC. (2009). *Standard precautions excerpt from the guideline for isolation precautions: Preventing transmission of infectious agents in health care settings 2007*. Retrieved April 16, 2009, from: http://www.cdc.gov/ncidod/dhqp/gl_isolation_standard.html

Latex Allergy and Skin Reactions

Latex allergy can result from repeated exposures through skin contact or inhalation to proteins in latex. Reactions usually begin within minutes of exposure, but they can occur hours later with various symptoms. Nurses are more likely to have latex allergy than the general population. Patients also can develop latex allergy, especially those who are frequently hospitalized. Preventive actions include avoiding contact with latex when possible, establishing latex-free zones for patients and staff, preventing the transfer of latex substances into such zones, and substituting powder-free, low-allergen gloves and latex-free gloves for latex gloves when possible.

Nurses have an increased rate of skin reactions because of their increased frequency of hand hygiene. Some health care facilities provide less irritating hand-hygiene products. Additional measures for reducing exposure to skin irritants include applying moisturizer, using hand gel instead of soap and water in disinfection procedures when the hands are not visibly dirty, and using gloves for "wet" activities (eg, bathing patients) to prevent the hands from becoming wet and visibly dirty.

Cardinal Techniques of Physical Assessment

The four techniques of inspection, palpation, percussion, and auscultation form the basis for physical assessment.

- **Inspection** means conscious observation of the patient for general appearance; physical characteristics and behavior; odors; and any specific details related to the body system, region, or condition under examination.
- **Palpation** involves use of the hands to feel the firmness of body parts, such as the abdomen.
- **Percussion** is using tapping motions with the hands to produce sounds that indicate solid or air-filled spaces over the lungs and other areas.
- **Auscultation** involves use of a stethoscope to hear movements of air or fluid in the body over the lungs and abdomen.

Inspection

Inspection is the first technique of the overall general survey and for each body part because it provides so much information. It is the only technique performed for every body system. Initial inspections focus on overall characteristics such as age, gender, level of alertness, body size and shape, skin color, hygiene, posture, and level of discomfort or anxiety. This **general survey** is intentional and conscious for beginners (see Chapter 3). Data during this initial phase help nurses to form an overall impression of the situation and its acuity. Cues from patient during inspection might indicate a problem that needs further assessment. Inspection of specific body systems and areas follows completion of the general survey.

During inspection, adequate exposure of each body part is necessary. Concurrently, the privacy of patients can be maintained with appropriate draping, especially over the breasts in women and genitalia in both men and women. Adequate lighting is essential to observe color, texture, and mobility. Nurse should ask patients for permission to examine body areas, especially when assessments involve compromising modesty.

Palpation

Palpation employs touch to assess texture, temperature, moisture, size, shape, location, position, vibration, crepitus, tenderness, pain, and edema. Palpation should begin with a gentle and slow technique. The patient's face can serve as a reliable nonverbal indicator of discomfort such as furrowed brows or grimacing.

The finger pads facilitate fine discrimination, because they are the most mobile parts of the hand. The palmar surface of the fingers and joints are best for assessing firmness, contour, position, size, pain, and tenderness. The back of the hand (dorsal) is most sensitive to temperature. Vibratory tremors can sometimes be felt on the chest as the patient speaks; these are best felt with the ulnar, or outside, surface of the hand.

Light Palpation

Light palpation allows the patient to become accustomed to the touch. Tender or painful areas should not be palpated until the end. Helpful measures before beginning include ensuring correct draping and alerting the patient about what will happen and gaining his or her permission to proceed. It may be necessary to warm the hands under running water or to gently rub them together. Short and smooth nails also are necessary to avoid causing discomfort.

Palpation is difficult when patients' muscles are tense. A gentle, calm, and easy touch can assist patients to relax. Light palpation is appropriate for the assessment of surface characteristics, such as texture, surface lesions or lumps, or inflamed areas of skin. The nurse places the finger pads of the dominant hand on the patient's skin and slowly moves the fingers in circular areas of approximately 1 cm in depth (Fig. 2-2). Intermittent palpation using this technique is more effective than a single continuous palpation.

Moderate to Deep Palpation

Moderate palpation facilitates the assessment of the size, shape, and consistency of abdominal organs, as well as any abnormal findings of pain, tenderness, or pulsations. The same gentle circular motion of light palpation is appropriate but with the palmar surfaces of the

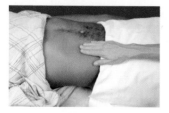

Figure 2.2 Technique for light palpation.

fingers instead of the finger pads. Pressure is firm enough to depress approximately 1 to 2 cm.

Deep palpation involves pressure from both hands. The examiner places the extended fingers of the nondominant hand over the dominant hand and uses the same circular motion to palpate 2 to 4 cm.

Percussion

The third technique of physical assessment is **percussion** to produce sound or elicit tenderness by tapping the fingers on the patient, similar to that of a drumstick on a drum. The vibrations that the fingers produce create percussion tones conducted into the patient's body. If the vibrations travel through dense tissue, the percussion tones are quiet; if they travel through air, the tones are loud. The loudest tones are over the lungs and hollow stomach; the quietest are over bone.

Direct percussion involves tapping the fingers directly on the patient's skin (Fig. 2-3). With **indirect percussion,** the examiner's

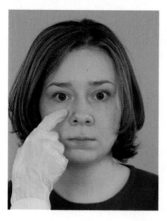

Figure 2.3 Direct percussion of the sinuses.

BOX 2.1 HELPFUL HINTS WHEN LEARNING PERCUSSION

- Most of the nondominant finger should be touching the patient or the sound transmission will be decreased.
- The motion of the striking finger should be quick, forceful, and snappy. The snapping finger must be brisk for a loud sound.
- Because you must use the tip of the finger, nails must be short and smooth to avoid tenderness and to facilitate good contact. Using the pad of the finger dampens the sound.
- The downward motion of the striking hand should be from the wrist, not the finger, elbow, or arm.
- To avoid dampening the sound, immediately withdraw the snapping finger once the nondominant finger is struck.
- The person with small hands and fingers needs to strike more forcefully than the person with large hands.

nondominant hand serves as a barrier between the dominant hand and patient. He or she places the nondominant palm on the patient and initiates a quick moderately strong tap with the dominant hand. The ulnar surface of the fist is used to percuss the kidneys, gallbladder, or liver for tenderness. See Box 2-1 for helpful tips when using percussion.

Four percussion tones in the body have different characteristics:

1. **Intensity (loudness)** refers to how soft or loud the sound is. The louder the sound, the louder the intensity and the easier it is to hear. If air fills the structure, there is more ability to vibrate and the sound is louder.
2. **Pitch (frequency)** depends on how quickly the vibration oscillates, similar to music. If the frequency of the sound is fast, the pitch is high; if the frequency of the sound is slow, the pitch is low. Although both the lungs and hollow stomach are loud, the lungs are low pitched and the stomach is high pitched.
3. **Duration** refers to how long the sounds last once elicited. A sound that is freer to vibrate, such as over air-filled spaces, has a longer duration
4. **Quality** means the subjective description of the percussion sound, such as a low-pitched thud of short duration versus a drum-like sound with high pitch and long duration.

See Table 2-2 for a review of the percussion tones and their characteristics.

Table 2.2	Percussion Sounds
Sound	**Characteristics**
Hyperresonant	**Intensity:** Very loud **Pitch:** Low **Duration:** Long **Quality:** Boom-like **Location:** Emphysematous lungs
Resonant	**Intensity:** Loud **Pitch:** Low **Duration:** Long **Quality:** Hollow **Location:** Healthy lungs
Tympanic	**Intensity:** Loud **Pitch:** High **Duration:** Moderate **Quality:** Drumlike **Location:** Gastric bubble (stomach)
Dull	**Intensity:** Moderate **Pitch:** High **Duration:** Moderate **Quality:** Thud **Location:** Liver
Flat	**Intensity:** Soft **Pitch:** High **Duration:** Short **Quality:** Dull **Location:** Bone

Auscultation

Auscultation reveals the sounds produced by the body, usually from movement of organs and tissues. Descriptors vary depending on the body part auscultated. Characteristics of sounds for auscultation are the same as for percussion: intensity, pitch, duration, and quality. Descriptors for quality are different with auscultation. See Table 2-3.

The stethoscope conducts sound from the patient's body to the listener and also blocks environmental noise to more clearly pinpoint the patient's body movements (Fig. 2-4). The stethoscope

Table 2.3 Comparison of Auscultation Sounds

Sound	Characteristics
Blood pressure	**Intensity:** Soft to loud **Pitch:** High **Duration:** 60–100/min **Quality:** Swooshing or knocking **Location:** Arm
Abdominal sounds	**Intensity:** Soft to loud **Pitch:** High **Duration:** 5–35/min **Quality:** Gurgly, intermittent **Location:** Abdomen
Heart sounds	**Intensity:** Moderate **Pitch:** Low **Duration:** 60–100/min **Quality:** Lub-dub, rhythmic **Location:** Anterior thorax
Lung sounds vesicular	**Intensity:** Soft **Pitch:** Low **Duration:** Inspiration > expiration, 12–20/min **Quality:** Rustling, wispy **Location:** Anterior and posterior thorax

includes the eartips, earpiece, flexible tubing, and chestpiece. To be effective, the eartips must fit into the ear canal snugly but comfortably. They are tilted slightly forward so that the point on the earpiece is forward in the same direction as the nose.

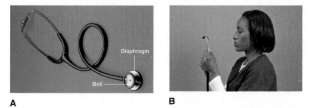

A   B

Figure 2.4 (A) The stethoscope. **(B)** Correct positioning of the stethoscope to direct sound toward the tympanic membrane.

Most stethoscopes have a diaphragm and bell on the chestpiece. The bell is used with light skin contact to hear low-frequency sounds, while the diaphragm is used with firm skin contact to hear high-frequency sounds.

Disinfection of the stethoscope between patients is necessary.

Equipment

All equipment needed for the physical assessment should be gathered and in place before the examiner enters the room to avoid interruption and to increase the patient's trust. Appropriate equipment depends on the type of examination. See Box 2-2.

Frequently used equipment for more advanced assessments are as follows:

- The **ophthalmoscope** is a hand-held system of lenses, lights, and mirrors. It enables visualization of the interior structures of the eye. See Chapter 8 for further discussion.
- The **otoscope** directs light into the ear to visualize the ear canal and tympanic membrane. The otoscope head and body connect and are activated in the same way as with the ophthalmoscope. A proper-sized speculum is required, based on the largest size

---

BOX 2.2   EQUIPMENT FOR PHYSICAL ASSESSMENT

Comprehensive Physical Examination (Including Papanicolaou Test for Women)

Platform scale with height measure	Tongue depressor
Thermometer	Snellen chart
Blood pressure cuff/machine	Tape measure
Watch with second hand	Reflex hammer
Stethoscope	Cotton swab
Clean gloves	Tuning fork: low pitched
Flashlight or penlight	Coin, paper clip, key, or pen
Ophthalmoscope	Gloves
Otoscope	Bivalve vaginal speculum
Tuning fork: high pitched	Materials for cytological study
Nasal speculum	Lubricant
	Fecal occult blood materials

that fits most comfortably into the patient's ear. See Chapter 9 for further discussion.

- The **tuning fork** is used with two body systems: to determine conductive versus sensorineural hearing loss in the ears (see Chapter 9) and to determine vibration sense in the neuromuscular system (see Chapter 17). Depending on their design, tuning forks create vibrations that produce sound waves of low- and high-pitched frequency. The tuning fork for hearing loss produces a high-pitched tone of 512 to 1,024 Hz, within the range of human hearing. The tuning fork for vibration is at a lower frequency of 128 to 256 Hz.

Lifespan Considerations

Pregnant Women

Most pregnant women provide a urine sample during each visit, so they can empty their bladder before undergoing the abdominal and vaginal examination. They may be uncomfortable while lying flat. Most components of the physical examination can be done with the patient sitting. The lithotomy position is necessary for vaginal examination. See also Chapters 20 and 21.

Newborns and Infants

Positioning of newborns and infants for physical assessment can be either on an examination table or held against a parent's chest. Extra attention to physical and visual contact with infants is vital if the assessment is on the examination table. Newborns and infants are comfortable without clothing in a warm environment; however, leaving their diapers on as long as possible is preferable, especially with boys, to avoid contamination of the nurse with urine or feces.

Once infants can sit, most of the examination can occur with the infant sitting in a caregiver's lap. For sleeping infants, first listen to the heart, lung, and bowel sounds. The most uncomfortable assessments are at the end of the examination, to prevent an infant's crying from compromising the quality of assessment findings. See also Chapter 22.

Children and Adolescents

Active toddlers may be afraid or shy. Parents can assist by holding or positioning their children as needed. Young children may hesitate to have body parts exposed. An alternative is for a parent to partially undress a child and then cover each body part after it is examined. Many toddlers automatically say "no" to any question asked. To prevent negativism from prolonging the examination, choices should be specific, such as "Would you like to sit on the table or on your grandmother's lap while I listen to your heart?" Games also become prominent. Children may better participate in activities such as "blowing out" the ophthalmoscope light or listening to their own heart and lungs.

Adolescents are aware of their rapidly changing bodies and may have increased feelings of modesty or self-consciousness. Draping is especially important for these patients. Additionally, adolescents appreciate explanations of the rationale for assessments, especially any related to or that can affect body image or developmental stage.

Older Adults

Older adults may chill more easily than younger patients, so they may benefit from an additional blanket or drape. Because they may also fatigue quickly, the most important assessments are done at the beginning. When positioning older adults, slight elevation of the head of the bed or examination table may help facilitate breathing.

Cultural Considerations

Each assessment must be individualized according to the patient's cultural, religious, and social beliefs. Anxious patients may be afraid to disclose private or uncomfortable information, embarrassed about being touched or looked at, or worried about abnormal findings. Before starting the physical assessment, patients should be asked about their preferences, such as having a family member or same-gender examiner in the room. Less invasive assessments should be done first, with the most personal assessments at the end.

2

General
Health
Assessments

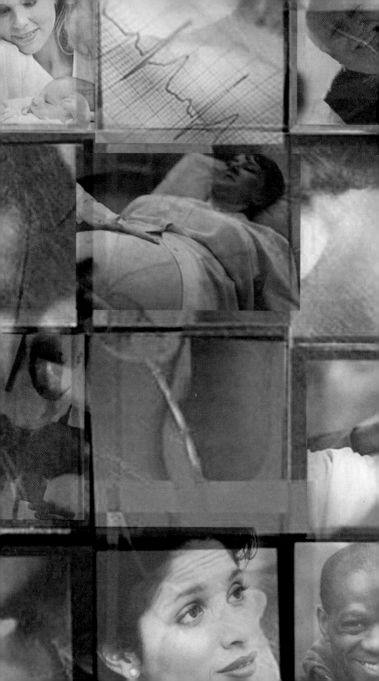

General Survey, Vital Signs, and Pain Assessment

The general survey begins during the interviewing and history taking (see Chapter 1). While collecting subjective data, nurses observe patients, develop initial impressions, and formulate plans for collecting objective physical data. Vital signs, encompassing temperature, pulse, respirations, and blood pressure (BP), are important indicators of the patient's physiological status and response to the environment. The fifth vital sign is pain.

Acute Assessment

Indicators of an acute situation are extreme anxiety, acute distress, pallor, cyanosis, and change in mental status. In such cases, the nurse begins interventions while continuing assessment. He or she obtains all vital signs and requests help. The nurse may call a rapid response team if he or she intuitively senses that something is going wrong or if the patient displays

- Stridor
- Respirations less than 10 breaths/min or greater than 32 breaths/min
- Increased effort to breathe
- Oxygen saturation less than 92%
- Pulse less than 55 beats/min or greater than 120 beats/min
- Systolic BP less than 100 or greater than 170
- Temperature less than 35°C or greater than 39.5°C
- New onset of chest pain
- Agitation or restlessness

Objective Data Collection

Equipment

- Scale
- Height bar
- Stethoscope
- Thermometer
- Watch with second hand
- Sphygmomanometer
- Pulse oximeter
- Tape measure (for infants)

General Survey

General survey is the first component of assessment. Mental notes of the patient's overall behavior, physical appearance, and mobility help form a global impression of the person. Some general things to note when first meeting the patient are as follows:

- What is your first impression? Are there any outstanding features?
- State the patient's name. Does the patient respond immediately?
- Is the patient's hand moist? Did the patient extend the arm completely? Assess temperature and texture of the skin on the hand. Note muscle strength. Assess for edema, clubbing, malformations, or enlarged joints.
- Observe the patient interacting with others. Can he or she participate in conversation? Does the patient look healthy or ill?

Technique and Normal Findings	Abnormal Findings
Physical Appearance Overall Appearance. Does the patient appear the stated age? Is appearance consistent with chronological age? Are face and body symmetrical? Any obvious deformities? Does the patient look well, ill, or in distress? *Patient appears stated age. Facial features, movements, and body are symmetrical.*	Deficiencies in growth hormones may cause patients to appear younger than stated. Severe or chronic illness, prolonged sun exposure, or various genetic syndromes may contribute to premature aging. Facial asymmetry may indicate *Bell's palsy* or cerebral vascular ischemia. Obvious deformities may indicate fractures or displacements.
Hygiene and Dress. Observe clothes, hair, nails, and skin. What is the patient wearing?	Ill-fitting clothes may indicate weight changes. Bad breath can be from poor hygiene,

Technique and Normal Findings	Abnormal Findings
Is it appropriate for age, gender, culture, and weather? Is it clean and neat? Does it fit? Any breath or body odors? Look for the odor of alcohol or urine. Is the skin clean and dry? Are nails and hair well kept and clean? *Dress is appropriate for age, gender, culture, and weather. Patient is clean and well kempt. No odors are noted.*	*allergic rhinitis*, or respiratory infection. Sweet-smelling breath may indicate *diabetic ketoacidosis*. Body odor may be from poor hygiene or increased sweat-gland activity (as with some hormonal disorders). Previously well-groomed and now-disheveled patients may have *depression*. Eccentric makeup or dress may indicate *mania*. Worn clothes may indicate inadequate finances or self-care.
Skin Color. Observe skin tones and symmetry. Note any redness, pallor, cyanosis, or jaundice. Observe for any lesions or variations in pigmentation. Note amount, texture, quality, and distribution of hair. *Skin color is even, with pigmentation appropriate to genetic background and no obvious lesions or color variations. Hair is smooth, thick, and evenly distributed.*	Pallor, erythema, cyanosis, jaundice, and lesions can indicate disease states (see Chapter 6).
Body Structure and Development. Is physical and sexual development consistent with stated age? Is the patient obese or lean? How tall is the patient? Are body parts symmetrical? Is the patient barrel chested? Note fingertips. Are there any joint abnormalities? *Physical and sexual development is appropriate for age, culture, and gender. No joint abnormalities.*	Delayed puberty or markedly short or tall stature may indicate problems with growth hormones. Disproportionate height and weight, obesity, or emaciation can indicate *eating disorders* or hormonal dysfunction.
Behavior. Is the patient cooperative? Is affect animated or flat? Does the patient appear anxious? *Patient is cooperative and interacts pleasantly.*	Uncooperative behavior, flat affect, or unusual elation may indicate a psychiatric disorder (see Chapter 4).

(text continues on page 36)

Technique and Normal Findings	Abnormal Findings
Facial Expressions. Assess the face for symmetry. Note expressions while the patient is at rest and during speech. Are movements symmetrical? Does the patient maintain eye contact appropriate to culture? *Facial expression is relaxed, symmetrical, and appropriate for setting and circumstances. Patient maintains appropriate eye contact.*	Inappropriate affect, inattentiveness, impaired memory, and inability to perform activities of daily living (ADLs) may indicate a cognitive disorder. Flat or mask-like expression may be *Parkinson's disease* or *depression*. Facial drooping on one side may be *transient ischemic attack* or *cerebral vascular accident*. Exophthalmos (protruding eyes) may indicate *hyperthyroidism*.
Level of Consciousness. Can the patient state name, location, date, month, season, and time? Is he or she awake, alert, and oriented? Any agitation, lethargy, or inattentiveness? *Patient is awake, alert, and oriented to person, place, and time (A&O × 3). He or she attends and responds to questions.*	Confusion, agitation, drowsiness, or lethargy may indicate hypoxia, decreased cerebral perfusion, or a psychiatric disorder.
Speech. Listen to the speech pattern. How quick is it? Is speech clear and articulate? Are words appropriate? Vocabulary and sentence structure may offer clues to education. Assess for fluency in language and need for an interpreter. *Patient responds quickly and easily. Volume, pitch, rate, and word choice are appropriate. Speech is clear and articulate, flowing smoothly.*	Slow, slurred speech can indicate *alcohol intoxication* or *cerebral vascular ischemia*. Rapid speech may indicate *hyperthyroidism, anxiety,* or *mania*. Difficulty finding words or using words inappropriately may indicate *cerebral vascular ischemia* or a psychiatric disorder. Loud speech may indicate hearing difficulties.
Mobility **Posture.** Note how the patient sits and stands. Is the patient sitting upright? When standing, is the body straight and aligned? *Posture is upright while sitting, with limbs and trunk proportional to body height.*	Slumping or hunching may indicate pain, *depression,* fatigue, or *osteoporosis*. Long limbs may indicate *Marfan's syndrome*. A tripod position when sitting can indicate respiratory disease. If the patient is in bed, note the

Technique and Normal Findings	Abnormal Findings
Patient stands erect with no signs of discomfort, and arms relaxed at the sides.	position of the head of the bed or if the patient is lying on the left or right side.
Range of Motion. Can the patient move all limbs equally? Are there limitations? *Patient moves freely in the environment.*	Asymmetrical motion occurs in *stroke*; paralysis may be present with a spinal cord injury. Limited range of motion might be present with injuries or degenerative disease.
Gait. For the ambulatory patient, observe movements around the room. Are they coordinated? Note any tremors or tics, as well as body parts that do not move. Does the patient use assistive devices? *Gait is steady and balanced, with even heel-to-toe foot placement and smooth movements. Other movements are smooth, purposeful, effortless, and symmetrical.*	Tics, paralysis, ataxia, tremors, or uncontrolled movements may indicate *neurological disease*. Patients with *Parkinson's disease* may display a shuffling gait. *Arthritis* may result in a slow, unsteady gait. For patients in bed, note their ability to move and reposition themselves in bed, turn side to side, and sit up.

▲Lifespan Considerations

Infants/Children. General survey considerations are similar to those for adults, with the examiner always remaining aware of the patient's developmental level and ability to interact. An additional consideration is the interaction between parent and child. Do they mutually respond? Are they warm and affectionate?

Older Adults. By the eighth or ninth decade, physical appearance changes, with sharper body contours and more angular facial features. Posture tends to have a general flexion, and gait tends to have a wider base of support. Steps tend to be shorter and uneven. Patients may need to use the arms to help aid in balance. Observe normal changes of aging. Assess for any decreasing abilities to function and care for self. Note any changes in mental status.

Anthropometric Measurements ——————

Anthropometric measurements are the various measurements of the human body, including height and weight. They provide critical information about health, nutritional status, fluid gain or loss, medication dosages, and, for children, growth patterns (see Chapter 22). Taking baseline height and weight provides a reference point for weight changes and body mass index (BMI). The BMI is considered a more reliable indicator of health than weight measurement alone (see Chapter 4). For accurate height and weight, the patient should remove shoes and heavy clothing (eg, winter coat).

Technique and Normal Findings	Abnormal Findings
Height. A patient older than 2 years should stand and place the heels against a height bar. Feet should be together, with knees straight and the patient looking forward. Lower the horizontal bar until it touches the top of the patient's head. Read and record the measurement on the height bar (Fig. 3-1).	*Chronic malnutrition* or *osteoporosis* may result in decreased height. Hormonal abnormalities may cause excessive growth. Deficiency in growth hormone may be seen in *dwarfism*. See Table 3-1 at the end of the chapter.

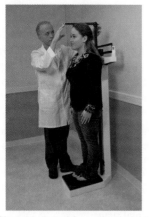

Figure 3.1 Measuring height in an adult.

Technique and Normal Findings	Abnormal Findings
Some patients cannot stand up straight for height measurement. Estimate by measuring "wing-span." The patient holds both arms straight from the sides of the body. Measure from the tip of one middle finger to the tip of the other. This distance is approximately the same as the patient's height.	The patient with muscle weakness, *scoliosis*, or neurological disorders may not be able to stand.
Weight. Primary care facilities may use a calibrated balance-beam scale. Prior to starting, balance the scale by sliding both weight bars to zero. Have the patient stand on the scale. Slide the lower weight bar to the right until the arm drops to the bottom of the gauge. Slide the weight bar one notch back. Move the upper weight bar to the right until the arrow is balanced in the center of the gauge. The patient's weight is the total of these readings. These scales must be calibrated, or "zeroed," prior to use. See Fig. 3-2.	Excessive unexplained weight loss may be from nutritional deficiencies, decreased intake or absorption, or increased metabolism. Other causes are endocrine, neoplastic, gastrointestinal, psychiatric, infectious, or neurological. Chronic disease also may contribute. Excessive weight gain results when a person consumes more calories than the body requires, endocrine disorders, genetics, or emotional factors.

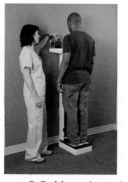

Figure 3.2 Measuring weight in an adult.

(text continues on page 40)

Technique and Normal Findings	Abnormal Findings
To obtain the most accurate readings when a series of weights is required, weigh the patient at the same time of day in similar clothing each time.	
Calculate BMI by dividing weight in kilograms by height in meters squared (or weight in pounds divided by height in inches squared and then multiply by 703).	Underweight is BMI < 18.5 kg/ m²; overweight is BMI of 25 to 29.9 kg/m²; obesity is BMI > 30 kg/m²; extreme obesity is BMI > 40 kg/m².

▲Lifespan Considerations

Infants and Children. Measurements for this age group are essential to assess health status. Values are plotted on growth charts and compared to same-age children. For detailed information on measurements for infants and children, see Chapter 22.

Older Adults. People in their 80s and 90s may be shorter than in their 70s from thinning of vertebral discs and postural changes. The long bones do not shorten, but the trunk does. After age 70 years, body weight decreases from muscle shrinkage and fat distribution changes. Subcutaneous fat is lost from the face and periphery even with adequate nutrition.

Vital Signs

Vital signs reflect health status, cardiopulmonary function, and overall body function. They are main indicators of physiological state and response to physical, environmental, and psychological stress. Changes in vital signs often indicate changes in health. Their assessment helps nurses establish a baseline, monitor a patient's condition, evaluate responses to treatment, identify problems, and monitor risks for alterations in health.

Initial vital signs provide a baseline. A series of readings is more informative than a single value because the series provides information about trends over time. Many variables may affect vital signs (Box 3-1). It is imperative that nurses measure vital signs correctly and accurately, understand the data, and communicate appropriately.

BOX 3.1 FREQUENCY OF VITAL SIGNS

*N*urses should take a patient's vital signs
• Upon admission to a facility
• Before and after any surgical procedure
• Before, during, and after administration of medications that affect vital signs
• As per the institution's policy or physician orders
• Any time the patient's condition changes
• Before and after any procedure affecting vital signs

Technique and Normal Findings	Abnormal Findings
Temperature	
Oral. Wait 15 to 30 minutes after a patient has had anything hot or cold to eat or drink, smoked, or chewed gum. Turn on the device. Cover the tip of the probe with a protector. Gloves are unnecessary unless you expect contact with body secretions. Place the thermometer in the sublingual area at the base of the tongue. Instruct the patient to keep the lips closed tightly and to breathe through the nose. Hold the probe until it beeps, then remove it. Note reading and directly dispose of the cover into a wastebasket. *Oral temperature ranges from 35.8°C to 37.3°C (96.4°F to 99.1°F).*	**Hypothermia** is temperature less than 35°C (95°F) and may be caused by prolonged exposure to cold or induced purposefully during surgery. **Hyperthermia**, also known as *pyrexia* or *fever*, is body temperature exceeding 38.5°C (101.5°F) orally. It occurs during infections caused by toxic bacterial secretions called pyrogens. Another cause is tissue breakdown, as seen in trauma, surgery, *myocardial infarction*, and *malignancy*. Certain neurological disorders, such as *cerebral vascular accident*, *cerebral edema*, *tumor*, or cerebral trauma, can affect the thermoregulation of the brain.
Axillary. Follow the procedure above, except place the electronic thermometer in the axillary fold and have the patient lower the arm. Hold it in place until it reads the temperature. Stay with the patient to ensure correct placement. *Axillary temperature is 36.5°C (97.4°F) or approximately 1°C lower than oral.*	Axillary temperature is the least accurate, so if there are discrepancies, recheck temperature with another route.

(text continues on page 42)

Technique and Normal Findings	Abnormal Findings

Tympanic. Turn the unit on and wait for the signal. Place a disposable single-use cover on the probe tip. Place the tip gently in the ear canal, angling the thermometer toward the patient's jaw. In an adult, pull the pinna up and back to straighten the ear (Fig. 3-3). Do not force the probe or occlude the ear canal. Push the trigger and note the reading. *Tympanic temperature is 37.5°C (99°F) or approximately equal to oral.*

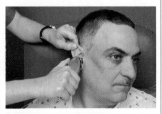

Figure 3.3 Tympanic temperature assessment.

Temporal. Position the probe directly on the skin above the eyebrow. Activate the thermometer by depressing and holding the scan bottom. Move the probe slowly from the forehead, across the temporal artery to level with the top of the ear (Fig. 3-4). Continue to hold the scan button while moving the probe to behind the earlobe. The process requires 5 to 7 seconds. *Temporal temperature is 37°C (98.6°F) or approximately equal to oral.*

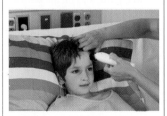

Figure 3.4 Temporal temperature assessment.

Rectal. Ensure that the correct rectal tip is in place. Turn on the unit. Don gloves and cover the probe with a protector. Lubricate the rectal thermometer, and insert the probe 2 to 3 cm (1 inch) into the adult rectum. Hold the thermometer in place and stay with the patient until the temperature is read. *Rectal temperature is 37.5°C (99°F) or approximately 1°C warmer than oral.*

Avoid placing the probe directly into stool, which may cause an inaccurate reading. The probe should be in contact with the rectal mucosa.

Technique and Normal Findings	Abnormal Findings
Pulse. Contraction of the heart causes blood to flow forward, which creates a pressure wave known as a **pulse**. The number of pulses in 1 minute is the heart (pulse) rate. To assess pulse, palpate one of the patient's arterial pulse points (usually the radial), noting rate, rhythm, and strength (amplitude) of the pulse. Also, note elasticity of the vessel.	
Rate. Normal heart rates vary with age. Infants and children have a faster heart rate than adults (see Chapter 22). Gender, activity, pain, stimulants, emotions, medications, and diseases also can affect heart rate. *Heart rate for an adult is 60 to 100 beats/min (bpm).*	**Tachycardia** (adult heart rate > 100 beats/min) can be from trauma, *anemia*, blood loss, infection, fear, fever, pain, shock, anxiety, or *hyperthyroidism*). With cardiac disease, tachycardia may indicate *congestive heart failure, myocardial ischemia,* or *dysrhythmia*. **Bradycardia** (adult heart rate < 60 beats/min) may be from medications, *myocardial infarction, hypothyroidism, increased intracranial pressure*, and eye surgery. **Asystole** (no pulse) signifies *cardiac arrest, hypovolemia, pneumothorax, cardiac tamponade*, and *acidosis*.
Rhythm. Pulse rhythm refers to the interval between beats and is regular or irregular. A regular pulse occurs at evenly spaced intervals. An irregular pulse has varied intervals. If a pulse is irregular, auscultate an apical pulse for one full minute.	Rhythm may vary with respirations, speeding up during inspiration and slowing with expiration. This is common in children and young adults, and it is called a **sinus dysrhythmia** or **sinus arrhythmia**.
A **pulse deficit** (difference between apical and radial pulse rates) provides an indirect	Pulse deficits are frequently associated with *dysrhythmias*.

(text continues on page 44)

Technique and Normal Findings	Abnormal Findings
measure of the ability of each heart contraction to eject blood into the peripheral circulation. Two nurses at the same time assess peripheral and apical pulse rates and compare measurements.	
Amplitude. Strength of the pulse indicates the volume of blood flowing through the vessel. It is described on a scale of 0 to 4+ (Box 3-2). *Strength is 2+*.	*Heart failure, hypovolemia, shock,* and *dysrhythmias* can decrease pulse strength. Bounding pulses are noted with early septic shock, exercise, fever, and anxiety.

BOX 3.2 SCALE FOR MEASURING PULSE

- 0 = Nonpalpable or absent
- 1+ = Weak, diminished, barely palpable
- 2+ = Normal, expected
- 3+ = Full, increased
- 4+ = Bounding

Technique and Normal Findings	Abnormal Findings
Elasticity. The normal artery feels smooth, straight, and resilient. This is known as elasticity of the pulse.	Vessels become less elastic with increasing age.
Any artery may be used to assess pulse rate, but the radial and apical arteries are the most common sites because of their accessibility (Fig. 3-5).	If a peripheral pulse is diminished or absent, the tissue below may have an inadequate blood supply.

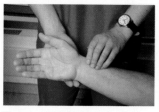

Figure 3.5 Taking a radial pulse.

Use the pads of your index and middle fingers. Do not use the thumb, which has pulsations that may interfere with accuracy. Press the artery gently against the underlying bone or muscle until you feel a pulsation. If the pulse is regular, count the beats for 30 seconds and then multiply by two to obtain beats per minute. If the rhythm is irregular, auscultate the apical pulse for one full minute and assess for a pulse deficit. Assess the pulse for one full minute when obtaining a baseline value. When counting, begin with "0" to avoid double counting beats at both beginning and end.

To assess apical pulse, place the diaphragm of a stethoscope at the left, fifth intercostal space, midclavicular line and auscultate for one full minute. *Apical pulse is 60 to 100 beats/min and regular.*

***Respirations.* Respiration** (breathing) supplies oxygen to the body and eliminates carbon dioxide. **Inspiration** occurs when the intercostal muscles and diaphragm contract and expand the pleural cavity, creating a negative pressure for air to flow actively into the lungs. During **expiration**, the intercostal muscles and diaphragm relax, decreasing the space in the pleural cavity and passively pushing air out of the lungs.

△ *SAFETY ALERT 3-1*
Sudden changes in pulse rates or pulse rates > 120 beats/min or < 55 beats/min may indicate life-threatening emergencies requiring immediate attention.

△ *SAFETY ALERT 3-2*
Absent pulse indicates a need for further assessment. In combination with pain, pallor, or paresthesia, the viability of a limb may be threatened.

Clinical Significance 3-1

Assess patients with dyspnea (difficulty breathing) in the position of greatest comfort to them. Repositioning may increase the work of breathing, which will alter the respiratory rate.

(text continues on page 46)

Technique and Normal Findings	Abnormal Findings
Rate and depth of respiration change with the body's demands. Factors that influence respirations include exercise, anxiety, pain, smoking, neurological injury, positioning, medications, and hemoglobin level.	
Observe both inspiration and expiration discretely. Most patients are not aware of their breathing. Increased awareness may alter normal respiratory pattern. *Respirations are relaxed, smooth, effortless, and silent.*	⚠ *SAFETY ALERT 3-3* *Get help if the respiratory rate is <10 or >32 breaths/min. Such findings may indicate acute distress and prompt the need for a rapid response.*
Respiratory rate is a count of each full inspiration and expiration cycle in one minute. Count for 30 seconds and multiply by two to obtain breaths per minute. *Respiratory rates for adults are 12 to 20 breaths/min and regular.*	**Tachypnea** (rapid, persistent adult respiratory rate > 20 breaths/min) may be from fever, exercise, *anemia*, or anxiety. **Bradypnea** (persistent adult respiratory rate < 12 breaths/min) accompanies *increased intracranial pressure*, neurological disease, and sedation. **Dyspnea** is a term used for difficult breathing. Resting respiration that is deeper and more rapid than normal is **hyperpnea**. **Apnea** is the absence of spontaneous respirations for more than 10 seconds.
In addition to rate, observe for rhythm, depth, and quality of respiration. *Normal respiratory rate, rhythm, and effort are called **eupnea**.*	**Hyperventilation** is deep, rapid respirations that result from hypoxia, *anxiety*, exercise, or *metabolic acidosis*. **Hypoventilation** is shallow, slow respiration related to sedation or *increased intracranial pressure*. Use of accessory muscles to breathe may indicate *respiratory distress*. Note cyanosis, retractions, or audible sounds of wheezing or congestion.
⚠ *SAFETY ALERT 3-4* *High-pitched crowing sounds from tracheal or laryngeal spasm, called stridor, may indicate a life-threatening emergency. Any periods of apnea, tachypnea, bradypnea, or irregular respiratory pattern are indications of underlying disease and warrant further assessment.*	

Technique and Normal Findings	Abnormal Findings

Oxygen Saturation. Pulse oximetry is a noninvasive technique to measure **oxygen saturation** (the percent to which hemoglobin is filled with oxygen) of arterial blood. It does not replace measurement of arterial blood gases for assessment of abnormalities, but it does indicate abnormal gas exchange.

Assess capillary refill and strength of the pulse in the extremity to be used for measuring oxygen saturation. Typically a finger is used to obtain a reading.

Potential errors may result from abnormal hemoglobin value, hypotension, skin breakdown, hypothermia, or patient movement. Falsely low readings may be from cold extremities, hypothermia, and hypovolemia. Falsely high readings are associated with carbon monoxide poisoning and anemia. *Pulse oximetry is SpO$_2$ of 92% to 100%.*

SpO$_2$ of 85% to 89% may be acceptable for patients with chronic conditions such as emphysema. Conditions that decrease arterial blood flow may compromise the accuracy of readings. Patients with *anemia* may have a falsely elevated pulse oximetry reading from circulating hemoglobin containing sufficient oxygen but inadequate hemoglobin to carry adequate oxygen.

Blood Pressure. Blood pressure (BP) is the measurement of the force exerted by the flow of blood against the arterial walls, which changes during contraction and relaxation of the heart. Maximum pressure is exerted on the arterial walls with contraction of the left ventricle at the start of systole (**systolic blood pressure,** SBP). Lowest pressure (**diastolic blood pressure,** DBP) occurs when the left ventricle relaxes between beats. A series of measurements gives more information than a single measurement.

(text continues on page 48)

Technique and Normal Findings	Abnormal Findings
BP is measured using a stethoscope and **sphygmomanometer**, which consists of an aneroid or mercury gauge and an inflatable rubber bladder in a cloth covering called the *cuff*. Cuffs are available in various sizes, from very small for newborns to extra-large thigh cuffs. The correct size is necessary for accurate readings. Cuff width equals 40% of the length of the patient's arm. Bladder length equals 80% of limb circumference.	If a large cuff is not available for a patient with morbid obesity, BP can be measured on the forearm. The cuff can be placed midway between the elbow and the wrist.
Arm BP. Be sure the patient is calm and relaxed and has not eaten, smoked, or exercised for 30 minutes prior to measurement. Allow the patient to rest for at least 5 minutes prior to beginning. Measure initial BP in both arms for comparison. *A variation of 5 to 10 mm Hg between arms is normal.* If values differ, use the higher value but record both.	A difference of 10 to 15 mm Hg or more between the two arms may indicate arterial obstruction on the side with the lower value.
The patient may be supine or sitting. Support the bare arm at heart level with palm upward. When sitting, the patient's feet are flat on the floor. Support the back.	The patient should not hold up the arm. Muscle tension can elevate SBP. Elevating the arm above the heart may result in a false low measurement.
Assess the extremity to be used for BP assessment. Do not use an extremity with a shunt, on the same side as a mastectomy, or with an intravenous infusion. Choose the correct size cuff.	
Palpate the brachial artery above the antecubital fossa and medial to the biceps tendon. Center the deflated cuff approximately 2.5 cm (1 inch) above the	

Technique and Normal Findings	Abnormal Findings
brachial artery. Line up the arrow on the cuff with the brachial artery. Tuck the Velcro end of the cuff under so that the cuff is snugly fastened around the arm.	
Estimate SBP by palpating the brachial or radial artery and inflating the cuff until the pulsation disappears. Hold the bulb in your dominant hand. Close the valve on the bulb by turning it away from you but make sure that it will easily release. To control the bulb, it is easiest to brace your fingers against the metal of the valve. Squeeze the bulb to pump air into the bladder. Continue feeling the pulse, and identify when it disappears. Pump the cuff to 20 mm Hg above where the pulse stopped.	Estimating SBP will prevent missing an **auscultatory gap**, a period in which there are no Korotkoff sounds during auscultation.
Slowly open the valve by turning it toward you to deflate the cuff. Feel for the pulse, noting the number when the pulsation is palpable again. Then quickly deflate the cuff completely. This is the estimated SBP. Wait 15 to 30 seconds before reinflating the cuff to allow trapped blood in the veins to dissipate.	
Position the earpieces of the stethoscope in your ears and place the diaphragm or bell of the stethoscope over the brachial artery, using a light touch (Fig. 3-6). Position yourself so that you can avoid bumping the tubing and can easily see the gauge. Note that you will not hear the tapping of the pulse until the cuff is inflated.	The bell is designed to pick up low-pitched sounds, such as the turbulent blood flow caused by the BP cuff partially occluding the brachial artery. Some studies have shown that the bell and diaphragm are equally effective.

(text continues on page 50)

Technique and Normal Findings	Abnormal Findings

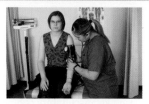

Figure 3.6 Note placement of the earpieces of the stethoscope in the nurse's ears as she auscultates over the brachial artery.

Inflate the cuff around the extremity alters the flow of blood through the artery, which generates Korotkoff sounds (Fig. 3-7). The sounds are audible with a stethoscope at a pulse site distal to the cuff. You will hear sounds only during the period of partial occlusion, and not at the top or bottom.

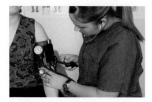

Figure 3.7 Inflating the BP cuff around the arm alters arterial blood flow.

Quickly inflate the cuff to 20 to 30 mm Hg above estimated SBP. Then deflate the cuff slowly, approximately 2 to 3 mm Hg per second, while listening for Korotkoff sounds (Box 3-3).

Hypertension is not diagnosed on one BP reading alone but on an average of two or more readings taken on subsequent visits.

Note the number when you hear the first Korotkoff sound, which coincides with the patient's SBP.

Hypotension is SBP < 90 mm Hg. Some adults have a normal low BP, but in most adults, low BP

BOX 3.3 KOROTKOFF SOUNDS

- I: Characterized by the first appearance of faint but clear tapping sounds that gradually increase in intensity; the first tapping sound is the systolic pressure
- II: Characterized by muffled or swishing sounds; these sounds may temporarily disappear, especially in people with hypertension; the disappearance of the sound during the latter part of phase I and during phase II is called the *auscultatory gap* and may cover a range of as much as 40 mm Hg; failing to recognize this gap may cause serious errors of underestimating systolic pressure or overestimating diastolic pressure
- III: Characterized by distinct, loud sounds as the blood flows relatively freely through an increasingly open artery
- IV: Characterized by a distinct, abrupt, muffling sound with a soft, blowing quality; in adults, onset of this phase is considered the first diastolic sound
- V: The last sound heard before a period of continuous silence; the pressure at which the last sound is heard is the second diastolic measurement

*From Taylor, C., Lillis, C., LeMone, P., & Lynn, P. (2011). *Fundamentals of nursing: The art and science of nursing care* (7th ed.). Philadelphia, PA: Wolters Kluwer Health/Lippincott Williams & Wilkins.

Technique and Normal Findings	Abnormal Findings
Be aware of the tendency to round to zero and make sure to read the gauge accurately. Continue deflating the cuff, noting the point of the last pulse sound (Korotkoff IV) and when it disappears (Korotkoff V, which is used to define DPB).	indicates illness. See Table 3-2 at the end of this chapter.
Record BP in even numbers as a fraction, with SBP as the numerator and DBP as the denominator. Also, record the patient's position, arm used, and cuff size if different from the standard cuff. Slow or frequent cuff inflations can cause venous congestion. Be sure to deflate the cuff completely after each measurement and wait at least 2 minutes between measurements.	⚠ *SAFETY ALERT 3-5* *Sudden change in BP may be an emergency. SBP < 90 mm Hg or 30 mm Hg below baseline needs immediate attention. Sudden drop in BP can signify blood loss or a cardiovascular, respiratory, neurological, or metabolic disorder. Sudden, severe rise in BP (above 200/120 mm Hg) is a life-threatening hypertensive crisis.*

(text continues on page 52)

Technique and Normal Findings	Abnormal Findings
The **pulse pressure** is the difference between SBP and DBP and reflects stroke volume. *Normal pulse pressure is approximately 40 mm Hg.* The **mean arterial pressure** is calculated by adding one third of SBP and two thirds of DBP. *A mean pressure of 60 mm Hg is needed to perfuse the vital organs.*	Decreased elasticity of the arterial walls, as well as increased intracranial pressure, can cause pulse pressure to increase. This is called a *widened pulse pressure*. Patients with *hypovolemia*, *shock*, or *heart failure* may exhibit narrowed pulse pressure. DBP is weighted more heavily because two thirds of the cardiac cycle is spent in diastole.
Thigh BP. Compare a thigh BP with an arm BP if the arm BP is extremely high, particularly in young adults and adolescents, to assess for coarctation of the aorta. Position the patient prone if possible. Place a large cuff around the lower third of the thigh, centered over the popliteal artery. *Thigh SBP is 10 to 40 mm Hg higher than arm SBP, while DBP is similar for both.*	A thigh or calf may also be used if the patient's arms are unavailable, such as in those with bilateral burns or IVs. *Coarctation of the aorta* produces high arm BP and lower thigh BP as a result of restricted blood supply below the narrowing.
Orthostatic (Postural) Vital Signs. Orthostatic blood pressure means a drop in BP and change in heart rate with position changes. When a healthy patient changes position, blood vessels in the extremities constrict and heart rate increases to maintain adequate BP for perfusion to the heart and brain.	Orthostatic changes may indicate blood volume depletion. Some medications can have a side effect of orthostatic hypotension. Additionally, conditions that cause the arterial system to become less responsive, such as immobility or spinal cord injury, can cause orthostatic changes.
Assess BP and heart rate with the patient supine, sitting, and then standing. The patient should rest supine for at least 2 minutes prior to assessment of the baseline reading. Repeat measurements with the patient sitting and standing, waiting 1 to 2 minutes after each position change to assess the readings. *A drop in SBP of less than 15 mm Hg is considered normal.*	Drop in SBP of 15 mm Hg or greater, drop in DBP of 10 mm Hg or greater, or increased heart rate indicates **orthostatic hypotension** and possibly intravascular volume depletion. Affected patients may exhibit dizziness, lightheadedness, or syncope. *Hypovolemia*, medications, *Parkinson's disease*, and prolonged bed rest may be causes.

▲Lifespan Considerations

Infants and Children. When assessing vital signs in young children, assess respiratory rate first, then pulse, and then temperature. (This will minimize elevations of respiratory and heart rates that accompany crying.

Respirations. Count respirations as with adults, but with an infant, watch the abdomen for respiratory movement. Assess rate for one full minute. Young children have a more rapid respiratory rate than that of adults.

Pulse. For those younger than 2 years, assess the apical pulse at the point of maximum intensity (PMI), which for infants is located at the third to fourth intercostal space just above and lateral to the nipple. The PMI moves to a more medial and slightly lower area (fourth or fifth intercostal space, midclavicular line) at approximately 7 years. In children older than 2 years, use a radial pulse for assessment.

Temperature. Tympanic and temporal methods are useful with young children. The inguinal route is safer than the rectal route. To assess here, abduct the infant's leg and palpate for the femoral pulse. Place the tip of the thermometer lateral to the pulse site and adduct the leg to create a seal. Axillary temperature assessments are safer than rectal temperatures, but accuracy in children has been questioned. Axillary temperature is commonly assessed in healthy newborns to avoid the risk of perforating the rectum with the thermometer. Place the thermometer well into the axilla and hold the child's arm close to the body.

Oral temperatures are contraindicated in children younger than 4 years, sometimes even older, and should be used only when a child can keep the mouth closed around and not bite the thermometer. Rectal temperature is used in infants and other children when other routes are not practical. The child is supine or side-lying with knees flexed. The lubricated thermometer is placed no further than 2.5 cm (1 inch) and held securely.

Blood Pressure. BP is assessed annually in healthy children 3 years or older; it is not part of routine assessment for children younger than 3 years. BP measurement is generally the same for children as for adults, but the procedure will go more smoothly if children are prepared for what to expect. Cuff width must cover two thirds of the upper arm, and the bladder must encompass the whole arm. Auscultate using a pediatric end piece on the stethoscope.

Older Adults. Temperature is at the lower end of the normal range. Because of changes in the body's regulatory mechanisms and decreased subcutaneous fat, fevers are less likely, but risk for hypothermia increases.

Normal range for pulse is 60 to 100 beats/min. Variation in rhythm may develop. The radial artery may stiffen from peripheral vascular disease. Pulse rate takes longer to rise to meet sudden increases in demand and longer to return to resting state. Resting heart rate tends to be lower.

Respirations may be shallower and more rapid than that of younger adults, with a normal respiratory rate of 16 to 25 breaths/ min. Decreased efficiency of respiratory muscles results in breathlessness at lower activity levels.

Special attention to correct cuff size is necessary when assessing BP because of loss of upper arm mass, obesity, and decreased arm size. BP tends to increase from atherosclerosis.

Pain

Assessment of pain, considered the fifth vital sign, is always subjective. For verbal patients, self-report is the gold standard for assessing pain. Nurses also assess additional pain behaviors, such as grimacing, rocking, or guarding. Increased heart rate and BP are indicators of the physiological response to pain.

In a basic pain assessment, the nurse asks the patient to rate pain intensity using a simple one-dimensional scale. An example is the numeric pain intensity scale with 10 numbers ranked from 0 (no pain) to 10 (worst possible pain) to indicate pain severity. The higher the number that patient selects, the more severe is the pain.

Questions to Assess Symptoms	Rationales/Abnormal Findings
Location. Where is the pain? Point to the painful area. (If more than one area hurts, have the patient rate each separately, and note which is most painful.)	Note any pain that radiates from the affected area (eg, down the leg with low back pain). Such radiation may affect treatment choices.
Duration. When did you first become aware of the pain? How long have you had it?	Pain lasting more than 6 months is chronic or persistent pain.

Questions to Assess Symptoms	Rationales/Abnormal Findings
Intensity. How much pain do you have on a 0 to 10 scale (0 being none and 10 the worst you can imagine? • Is the pain worse or better at different times of the day? • Does current pain medication decrease the intensity?	If the patient cannot use a numeric rating scale to describe the intensity, ask the patient if the pain is mild, moderate, or severe.
Quality/Description. What does your pain feel like? Describe it in your own words.)	Descriptors such as burning, numb, or tingling may alert the nurse to a neuropathic source for the pain.
Alleviating/Aggravating Factors. What makes the pain better? What makes it worse? • What have you used to manage it? • Does applying heat make pain better or worse? • Does a cold pack help? • Does activity increase the pain? • Does sitting make it better?	Patients may try to treat their own pain before they seek health care.
Pain Management Goal. What level of pain would be acceptable for you?	Most patients are willing to tolerate some discomfort.
Functional Goal. What would you like to be able to do that you can't do because of the pain? (This question is most often used for patients with chronic, persistent pain.) • How does the pain interfere with your ADLs? • How far can you walk? • Can you care for yourself at home? • What does the pain mean to you?	Setting a functional goal allows the nurse to measure the efficacy of pain interventions and adjust treatment accordingly. Some patients believe that pain is a punishment or worsening of disease.

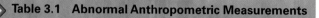

Table 3.1   Abnormal Anthropometric Measurements

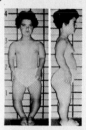

Achondroplastic Dwarfism
Characteristics of this genetic disorder include short stature, short limbs, and a relatively large head. Note the thoracic kyphosis and lumbar lordosis.

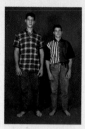

Gigantism Excessive growth hormone secretion in childhood causes increased height and weight with delayed sexual development. Note the differences in these same-age individuals, one of whom has gigantism.

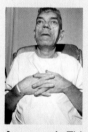

Acromegaly This condition results from excessive growth hormone secretion during adulthood, after completion of body growth. Overgrowth of bone causes changes in the size of the head, face, hands, feet, and internal organs; height is not affected.

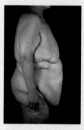

Obesity Excessive body fat results when calories continually exceed body requirements. It can result from overeating, genetics, endocrine or hormonal disorders, lifestyle issues, or a combination of factors.

Table 3.1 Abnormal Anthropometric Measurements (*continued*)

Anorexia Nervosa Severe caloric restriction and disturbed body image contribute to this psychiatric disorder. Affected patients are clearly emaciated and display other physical findings, such as brittle hair and nails, absent menstruation, delayed puberty, sunken eyes, dry skin, and other manifestations.

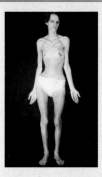

Table 3.2 Abnormal Blood Pressure in Adults (mm Hg)

Category	Systolic	Diastolic
Hypotension	<90	<60
Normal	<120 and	<80
Prehypertension	120–139 or	80–90
Stage 1 hypertension	140–159 or	90–99
Stage 2 hypertension	>160 or	>100

Nutrition Assessment

Key Topics and Questions for Health Promotion

Key Questions	Rationales/Abnormal Findings
Medical History. Do you have a medical condition, such as diabetes or hypertension?	Medical conditions, increased metabolic demand, and malabsorption increase risk for nutritional deficits.
Do you have, or have you recently had, fever, sepsis, thermal injuries, skin breakdown, cancer, AIDS, major surgery, or trauma?	These conditions increase nutritional needs.
Do you have, or have you recently had, malabsorption or certain renal diseases?	These conditions lead to loss of nutrients; special attention to increased nutritional requirements is necessary.
Weight History. Do you have a history of any problems related to nutrition or weight?	Being underweight, overweight, or obese influences self-perception of health. Such perception may be distorted or inaccurate, but it is important to know it to address it.
Appetite and Taste Changes • Have you noticed any changes in your ability to smell odors? In the taste of food? If so, what are the changes? • How would you rate your appetite? • How does food taste to you?	Senses of taste and smell decrease with aging. Additionally, some medications alter taste and smell.

Key Questions	Rationales/Abnormal Findings
Gastrointestinal Symptoms. Have you ever been diagnosed with a gastrointestinal or other disease that affects nutrition (eg, anorexia, heartburn, nausea, diarrhea, vomiting, pain)?	Gastrointestinal diseases may impair appetite and also reduce absorption of nutrients.
Food Allergy or Intolerance. Have you ever been diagnosed with a food intolerance or allergy?	These must also be considered when evaluating risk factors for malnutrition because they affect food choices.
Family History. Do you have a family history of gastrointestinal or other diseases that influence your nutrition? • Who had the illness? • What was the illness? • When did the person have it? • How was the illness treated? • What were the outcomes?	Family history of problems such as *Crohn's disease, type 2 diabetes, cystic fibrosis,* or *anemia* should be included. Consideration must be given to respecting cultural food patterns and preferences.
Food and Fluid Intake Patterns **Eating Patterns.** Describe a typical day's eating (content and amount of meals, meal times, snacking patterns). • Are you on a special diet? If so, please describe. • Are there times of the day when you feel hungry? If so, when? What is satisfying? Are there particular foods that you like? Dislike? If so, please describe. • Are any foods or food habits important to you? If so, please describe. • Who shares your mealtimes?	Food habits and intake patterns may vary according to culture, religion, and region.
Fluid Intake Patterns • How much fluid do you drink each day? (Glasses and approximate size of glass) • Are there fluids that you like? Dislike?	Fluid intake may be in excess of needs, causing fluid volume excess. Low fluid intake may cause a fluid volume deficit or dehydration. *(text continues on page 60)*

Key Questions	Rationales/Abnormal Findings
• Are there certain times of the day when you drink or refrain from drinking fluids? • How much coffee, tea, chocolate, or caffeinated beverages do you drink in a day? If you don't have any caffeine for a few days, how do you feel (eg, headache, nausea, other sensations)?	Large consumption of unfiltered coffee such as through a French press may increase LDL levels and risk for miscarriage.
Psychosocial Profile **Habits** • Does stress affect your eating or drinking habits? Is so, please describe. • Does smoking affect your appetite? If so, describe.	Some patients gain weight with stress, while others lose weight. Smoking impairs both senses of smell and taste.
Cooking Ability • Who does your food shopping? • Do you have a food budget? Describe. • How often do you eat out? Who prepares your food? • Does food preparation provide enjoyment for you? • Describe your food preparation facilities?	Functional limitations influence ability to obtain or prepare food.
Dietary Lifestyle Changes • Do environmental or social factors affect your ability to make dietary changes? • Do you feel you have sufficient resources to support healthy nutrition?	Many social functions revolve around food. If signs, symptoms, or treatments disrupt such functions, social isolation can be a consequence.
Medications and Supplements **Medication Schedule** • What system(s) have you developed to ensure an accurate medication schedule? • Are particular reminders or methods helpful for you? Please describe.	Medication history is included because diet and food intake affect medications.
Barriers to Accuracy. Have you experienced any difficulty getting or taking medicines as prescribed? If so, please describe.	Remembering to take medications requires intact memory and cognitive skills.

Key Questions	Rationales/Abnormal Findings
Adverse Effects. When do you tend to report any adverse effects of your medicines?	Patterns of health-seeking be-havior vary widely.
Resources for Medication-Related Information • From whom have you received most of your medication information? • Do you ask questions about your medicines? Do you expect that people helping you with medicines will give you needed information?	Nurses can provide patients with resources for answers.
Supplements. Do you take any vitamin, mineral, or other nutritional supplements? If so, describe substance, amount, and frequency.	Approximately one third of patients use some type of supplement.
Alcohol and Drug Use • How much alcohol do you drink? • Do you feel that you are a "normal" drinker? (Normal meaning that you drink less than, or as much as, others). • (If person does drink): How-much did you drink yesterday? Is that usual for you? When did you take your last drink (date and hour)? What is your usual pattern for alcohol intake? • Could you tell me about your drug use? (ask about substance and quantity)	Alcohol intake can affect the metabolism of nutrients, as well as alter the overall nutrient density of the diet.

Health-Promotion Teaching

Food Pyramid. Nurses can teach about the Food Pyramid, increasing fruits and vegetables, and decreasing intake of foods with low nutrient density. Visit www.mypyramid.gov for more information.

Food Labels. Patients can be taught to read food labels, especially when intake of a nutrient is limited because of dietary restrictions, such as a low-salt diet.

Key Topics and Questions for Common Symptoms —

For each symptom, be sure to review characteristics, duration, accompanying symptoms, treatment, and the patient's view of the problem.

Common Symptoms of Altered Nutrition

- Sudden or gradual changes in body weight
- Change in eating habits
- Changes in skin, hair, or nails
- Decreased energy level

Questions to Assess Symptoms	Rationales/Abnormal Findings
Weight Changes. What is your present height and weight? How do these compare with 5 years ago? Have there been any weight changes in the past year? If so, please describe. How do you feel about your present weight?	Weight can change or remain stable with illness.
Change in Eating Habits. Have you experienced a change in a regular diet pattern (number, size, contents of meals)?	If yes, investigate potential causes (eg, change in appetite, mental status, or mood; ability to prepare meals, chew, or swallow; nausea or vomiting).
Symptoms of Malnutrition • Have you noticed any changes in your hair, nails, and skin? If so, describe. • Would you say that you heal well? Poorly? Other? Do you have any difficulty tolerating hot or cold weather? • How much energy would you say that you have? • Has your energy level changed recently (past year)? If so, describe.	Skin, hair, and nails are indicators of nutritional status because these cells turn over rapidly. Thin or brittle hair, thin skin, skin that bruises easily or flakes, and weak or brittle nails are typical symptoms. A malnourished person lacks energy.

Objective Data Collection

Equipment Needed

- Scale
- Measuring tape
- Growth charts (for children)
- Skin calipers

Technique and Normal Findings	Abnormal Findings
Body Type Observe body type. Note as small, average, or large build.	Abnormal findings are *obesity*, lack of subcutaneous fat with prominent bones, abdominal *ascites*, and *pitting edema*. Amenorrhea is a cardinal symptom of *eating disorders*. **Cachexia** means a highly catabolic state with accelerated muscle loss and a chronic inflammatory response.
General Appearance Observe general appearance. *A healthy adult appears energetic, alert, and erect. Skin, hair, and nails look healthy.*	Clinical findings of malnutrition can occur throughout the body (see Box 4-1 and Table 4-1).

(text continues on page 64)

BOX 4.1 PHYSICAL SIGNS AND SYMPTOMS SUGGESTIVE OF MALNUTRITION

- Hair that is dull, brittle, dry, or falls out easily
- Swollen glands of the neck and cheeks
- Dry, rough, or spotty skin that may have a sandpaper feel
- Poor or delayed wound healing or sores
- Thin appearance with lack of subcutaneous fat
- Muscle wasting (decreased size and strength)
- Edema of the lower extremities
- Weakened hand grasp
- Depressed mood
- Abnormal heart rate, heart rhythm, or blood pressure
- Enlarged liver or spleen
- Loss of balance and coordination

From Dudek, S. G. (2010). *Nutrition essentials for nursing practice* (6th ed.). Philadelphia, PA: Wolters Kluwer Health/Lippincott Williams & Wilkins.

Table 4.1 Overweight and Obesity by BMI, Waist Circumference, and Associated Disease Risks

| | BMI (kg/m^2) | Disease Risk* Relative to Normal Weight and Waist Circumference | |
		Men 102 cm (40 inches) or less / Women 88 cm (35 inches) or less	Men > 102 cm (40 inches) / Women > 88 cm (35 inches)
Underweight	<18.5	—	—
Normal	18.5–24.9	—	—
Overweight	25.0–29.9	Increased	High
Obesity (Class I)	30.0–34.9	High	Very high
Obesity (Class II)	35.0–39.9	Very high	Very high
Extreme obesity (Class III)	40.0+	Extremely high	Extremely high

*Disease risk for type 2 diabetes, hypertension, and CVD.

(+) Increased waist circumference can also be a marker for increased risk even in persons of normal weight.

Adapted from NHLBI. (2009). *Classification of overweight and obesity by BMI, waist circumference, and associated disease risks.* Retrieved May 8, 2009, from http://www.nhlbi.nih.gov/health/public/heart/obesity/lose_wt/bmi_dis.htm

Technique and Normal Findings	Abnormal Findings
Swallowing Observe the patient's ability to swallow.	Difficulty swallowing is common in *stroke* and *neuromuscular diseases.*
Elimination Inspect urine, emesis, and stool.	Describe and measure any emesis (vomited contents from the gastrointestinal tract).

Table 4.2 Calculations and Analysis of Weight for Height

1. "Ideal" weight based on height:
Men: 106 lbs for the first 5 ft of height and 6 lbs for each additional inch
Women: 100 lbs for the first 5 ft of height and 5 lbs or each additional inch
Add or subtract 10%, depending on body frame size
2. Use current weight and "ideal" weight to determine percent ideal body weight:

$$\text{Percentage of ideal body weight} = \frac{\text{current weight}}{\text{ideal weight}} \times 100$$

>200%	Morbid obesity
120%–199%	Obese
110%–119%	Overweight
90%–110%	Within normal range
89%–90%	Mild malnutrition
70%–79%	Moderate malnutrition
<69%	Severe malnutrition

From Dudek, S. G. (2010). *Nutrition essentials for nursing practice* (6th ed.). Philadelphia, PA: Wolters Kluwer Health/Lippincott Williams & Wilkins.

Technique and Normal Findings	Abnormal Findings
Body Mass Index (BMI) BMI is a guide for maintaining ideal weight for height. Calculate BMI as follows: $$BMI = \frac{\text{weight in kilograms OR weight in pounds}}{\text{height in meters square OR height in inches square}} \times 703.$$ *BMI of 18.5 to 24.9 is healthy or normal.*	BMI < 18.5 or > 24.9 is abnormal and a health risk (see Table 4-2). *(text continues on page 66)*

Technique and Normal Findings	Abnormal Findings

Weight Calculations

Percentage of Ideal Body Weight.
This percentage is based on ideal and current weights:

$$\text{Percentage of ideal body weight} = \frac{\text{current weight}}{\text{body height}} \times 100$$

Mild malnutrition: 80% to 90% of ideal weight

Moderate malnutrition: 70% to 80% of ideal weight

Severe malnutrition: <70% of ideal weight

Recent Weight Change.
Carefully assess circumstances surrounding any change in weight to determine causes. Cluster with other data to analyze if the change is from fluid, muscle mass, or fat stores. After collecting usual weight from the history and current weight on a scale, calculate the percent weight change (loss of usual weight) as follows:

$$\frac{\text{usual weight} - \text{present weight}}{\text{usual weight}} \times 100$$

The following guidelines indicate significant weight loss:

- 1% to 2% in 1 week
- 5% in 1 month
- 7.5% in 3 months
- 10% in 6 months

Unintentional weight gain or loss is a significant finding.

Percent Usual Body Weight.
Another calculation can be made based on the current and usual weight. The percentage of usual weight is calculated as follows:

$$\text{Percentage of usual body weight} = \frac{\text{current weight}}{\text{usual height}} \times 100$$

Mild malnutrition: 85% to 95% of usual body weight

Moderate malnutrition: 75% to 84% of usual body weight

Severe malnutrition: <75% of usual body weight

Waist Circumference

Where fat is deposited on the body is a more reliable indicator

Waist circumference > 40 inches (102 cm) in men or > 35 inches

Technique and Normal Findings	Abnormal Findings
of disease risk than the amount of fat deposited in the body. Use waist circumference to evaluate the amount of abdominal fat in men and women.	(88 cm) in women increases risk for chronic illness associated with adiposity.

Mid Upper Arm Muscle Circumference

The **mid upper arm muscle circumference** is an indirect measure of bone, muscle area, and fat reserves. Measure around the arm, midway between the elbow and shoulder (Fig. 4-1).

Findings below the 10th percentile are abnormal, indicating loss of muscle. Trends that decrease over time are also significant.

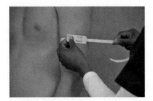

Figure 4.1 Measuring mid upper arm muscle circumference.

Derived Measures (MAC and TSF)

The **mid upper arm muscle circumference (MAMC)** and the **mid upper arm muscle area (MAMA)** are indicators of muscle and body protein reserves.
$$MAMC = MAC - (\pi \times TSF)....$$
$$MAMA = (MAC - MAMC)^2 \div 4\pi$$
A higher number indicates more muscle.

Findings below the 10th percentile are abnormal, indicating loss of muscle. Trends that decrease over time are also significant.

Documentation of Normal Findings

Patient denies changes in body weight or eating habits. Denies bruising or flaking of skin. Hair thick and healthy. Nails strong. States that energy level is adequate. Height 5′3″, weight 130 lbs, BMI 23.

Common Associated Nursing Diagnoses, Outcomes, and Interventions

Diagnosis	Nursing Interventions
Imbalanced nutrition, less than body requirements	Weigh patient daily. Monitor intake. Provide nutritional supplement. Offer food frequently.
Imbalanced nutrition, more than body requirements	Keep a food diary and record every food and drink. Teach reading of food labels. Weigh twice a week. Teach increased intake of vegetables and fruits.
Fluid volume excess	Monitor intake and output. Weigh daily at the same time of the day. Evaluate serum sodium, creatinine, and hematocrit.
Deficient fluid volume	Monitor intake and output. Weigh daily. Provide fluids every 2 hours. Treat causes including nausea, vomiting, or diarrhea.*

*Collaborative interventions.

▲ Lifespan Considerations

Pregnant Women

Pregnant and lactating women need an extra 300 to 500 cal/day, with emphasis on protein sources to boost tissue building. Whole foods offer the best sources of vitamins and minerals; certain circumstances may necessitate vitamin and mineral supplementation, especially to ensure that daily needs are met for vitamins A and C, folate, iron, calcium, and zinc.

Women who skip meals or have a high intake of empty calories may benefit from nutritional counseling by a Registered Dietician. Because of financial concerns, some women may qualify for assistance (eg, Special Supplemental Food Program for Women, Infants, and Children [WIC]).

The main measure of nutritional health is prepregnancy BMI. Prepregnancy body weight and weight gain are associated with both the infant's birth weight and length of term. Recommendations for pregnancy weight gain are as follows:

- 12.5 to 18 kg for underweight women—BMI < 19.8 kg/m²
- 11.5 to 16 kg for normal weight women—BMI 19.9 to 26.0 kg/m²
- 7 to 11.5 kg for overweight women—BMI 26.0 to 29.0 kg/m²
- At least 6.8 kg for obese women—BMI > 29.0 kg/m²

Infants, Children, and Adolescents

Children need more protein for tissue building in periods of rapid growth (eg, adolescence), tissue damage occurs, or during prolonged illness. Infants, children, and teens require different nutrients based on developmental and growth factors. For example, because fat intake is crucial to brain development in infants and young toddlers, whole milk is recommended for those younger than 2 years.

Growth charts are commonly used to indicate nutritional status. One set for those from birth to 36 months includes length, weight, and head circumference. Another set for children 2 to 18 years includes height and weight. Children who need a more complete nutritional assessment include those whose height-for-age is less than the 10th percentile, weight-for-height is less than the 15th percentile, or BMI is greater than the 85th percentile.

Obesity in children is a growing and concerning problem. Obese children and teens are at increased risk for factors associated with cardiovascular disease. Obesity and malnutrition are not mutually exclusive. Children with high-fat, high-carbohydrate diets may lack sufficient fruits and vegetables to meet daily requirements for other nutrients such as vitamins.

Older Adults

Older adults may compensate for diminished taste by adding sugar and salt to their diet at a time when their caloric needs are significantly reduced, and they are at increased risk for diabetes, hypertension, and heart disease. They may need increased intake of fortified milk and dairy products, fatty fish, and fortified cereals as well as vitamin D supplementation because of changes in nutrient metabolism, particularly when exposure to sunlight is reduced. Other nutrients that may be deficient include calcium, folate, vitamin B_{12}, and riboflavin.

Reduced thirst may increase risk for dehydration. Social isolation poses additional risks for malnutrition. Eating alone is particularly problematic for people with reduced mobility, receiving social assistance, or both. Financial constraints and poor dentition may compromise intake. Community programs (eg, Meals on Wheels) offer food services to those who qualify.

In older adults, BMI and weight change are the simplest screening measures. Weight loss in older adults, especially unintentional, is associated with an increased risk of death. It may be difficult to obtain an accurate weight in an older adult. A chair or bed scale that is regularly calibrated may be needed for patients who cannot stand on a scale.

⚠ Cultural Considerations

Some cultural groups believe in the healing properties of foods, while others follow food restrictions during illness. It is important for nurses working with patients from different cultures to assess dietary habits. The nurse who recognizes that each culture has its own food standards, determining what is edible and what is not, how foods are prepared and when they are eaten, as well as what role foods play in treating illness, is not likely to be ethnocentric when assessing nutritional status. Food preferences are learned, yet they vary depending on tradition, geography, education, income, and employment outside the home. Major U.S. cultural subgroups are Hispanics, Africans, Asians, and Middle Easterners. While each group shares certain eating practices, food choices vary widely within cultural subgroups. Additionally, food practices may be based on religious beliefs, such as fasting or abstaining from eating certain foods.

⚠ **Table 4.3 Abnormal Findings: Physical Signs of Nutritional Deficiency**

	Signs
Hair	Alopecia, brittle, color change, dryness, easy pluckability

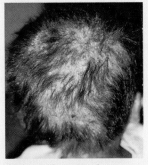

Alopecia (hair loss)

Skin	Acneiform lesions, follicular keratosis, xerosis (dry skin), ecchymosis, intradermal petechia, erythema, hyperpigmentation, scrotal dermatitis, angular palpebritis

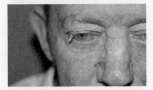

Follicular keratosis

Eyes	Bitot's spots, conjunctival xerosis

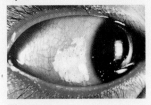

Bitot's spots

(table continues on page 72)

	Signs
Mouth 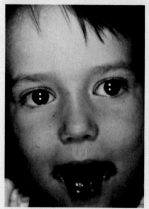 Magenta tongue	Angular stomatitis, atrophic papillae, bleeding gums, cheilosis, glossitis, magenta tongue
Extremities 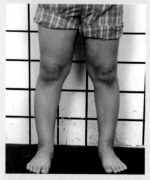 Genu varum	Genu valgum or varum; loss of deep tendon reflexes of the lower extremities

Source: Adapted from Bernard, M. A., Jacobs, D. O., & Rombeau, J. L. (1986). *Nutrition and metabolic support of hospitalized patients.* Philadelphia, PA: W. B. Saunders.

5

Mental Health Assessment

Key Topics and Questions for Health Promotion ——

Key Questions	Rationales/Abnormal Findings
Biographical Data. What is your name? Age? Gender? Race?	Diagnoses early in life may indicate more problems with developmental, cognitive, social, and coping skills. Children are at risk for abuse. Hormonal changes and emotional immaturity may pose risks for teens. Older adults are at increased risk for *depression*. Females are more prone to *depression*, and males are more apt to commit *suicide* or *violence*.
Current Health Status. How are you feeling today?	This generic question opens conversation about mental health concerns.
• Do you have any medical problems: pain, thyroid imbalance, diabetes, hepatitis, renal disease, cerebrovascular accidents, pulmonary diseases, asthma, COPD, irritable bowel syndrome, Crohn's disease, HIV/AIDS, cancer, and surgery that has resulted or may result in disfiguring or incapacitating alteration of function	Physiological changes with or emotional responses to illness can affect mental status. Also consider how the medical condition might affect any psychiatric medications.
• When did you first notice this mental health concern?	Response indicates how long the patient has had a problem.

(text continues on page 74)

Key Questions	Rationales/Abnormal Findings
• Why do you think it started when it did? • How often does it occur? • What changes have you noticed? • Have you ever felt this way before? • What do you think is the cause? • How is this affecting your life?	Identify any possible contributing factors. Response indicates how it might be affecting functioning. Changes include frequency, intensity, or effects on functioning or well-being. This is to assess for any previous episodes, especially if untreated. Assess the patient's understanding and whether it is logical. Assess implications and feelings of self-worth from the patient's responses to the above questions and statements the patient might make about self or illness.
Describe your typical day.	This helps identify the ability to perform activities of daily living.
Have you experienced recent weight loss or gain?	Weight changes may be related to medications, *anxiety*, early *dementia*, *depression*, or *eating disorders*.
Have you noticed any change in your sleeping habits?	Sleep disorders may be associated with *anxiety, mood disorder*, or *substance abuse*.
Medications. What psychiatric medications are you taking? Are you taking them as prescribed?	Consider interactions between medications taken for psychiatric and medical conditions.
Do you use, or have you ever used, any alternative treatments, herbs, or other substances? If yes, list the specific treatments or substances.	
Past Health History. Have you had any surgeries? If so, please list when and why.	Some patients with mental health conditions present with multiple surgeries and psychosomatic symptoms.

Key Questions	Rationales/Abnormal Findings
Have you ever been told that you have a mental health problem? • Have you ever received treatment for a mental health problem before? • Have you ever been hospitalized for a mental problem before?	Assess for patient's history of mental health conditions. Treatment could be outpatient, inpatient, from a general practitioner, or from another health care practitioner. Hospitalization indicates the severity of the condition.
Have you ever been physically, sexually, or emotionally abused? If so, when?	Assess for situational stressors such as bullying at school, family violence, or war violence.
Family History. Has anyone in your family been diagnosed with a mental health condition? • If so, who? • What were the diagnosis and treatment for each relative with a mental health condition? • Is the treatment plan working well for the particular family member?	A family history of mental health conditions is a risk factor for the patient. Answers may help direct line of treatment or medication options for the patient.
Psychosocial Support Network. Do you have a support system? • Whom do you consider as part of your support system? • How well does your support system meet your needs?	Assess the patient's coping skills and resources. Assess members and their effectiveness.
Do you have a significant other in your life: spouse, partner, or close friend? • How do you get along? • How often do you get together with people with whom you don't live?	Assess the stability and effectiveness of the patient's relationships.
Stressors. What are some stresses you have been experiencing? • Have you experienced a loss recently such as death of a family member/friend or loss of job or income?	Assess for current stress. *(text continues on page 76)*

Key Questions	Rationales/Abnormal Findings
• How do you cope with stress?	Coping skills are used to deal with stress.
• How is that working for you?	Evaluate their effectiveness.
Might other factors in your life be contributing to your stress level? • What are your living arrangements? • How many hours a week do you work? • Is this affecting your work? • Is this affecting your level of functioning or thinking?	Factors that contribute to mental health problems include isolation, decreased finances, poor or diminished cognitive abilities, homeless or unsafe environment problems with health care accessibility, language barriers, and literacy problems.
Do you have, or have you had, any legal problems? If so, please specify if you were sent to jail/prison for them and when.	Patients with problems of judgment, substance abuse, or anger management may become involved in the legal system.
Substance Use. Do you drink or use recreational substances? (If you suspect that alcohol use might be a problem, the CAGE is a quick first-step assessment tool. The acronyms are easy to remember and use at any time. See Box 5-1.) • What do you use? • How often? • How is the use of substances affecting your life?	When a patient comes in for treatment of substance use, it is important to be aware of the possibility of an underlying mental health problem.

BOX 5.1 CAGE QUESTIONNAIRE FOR SUBSTANCE USE

- Have you ever felt the need to **C**ut down on drinking?
- Have you ever felt **A**nnoyed by criticism of drinking?
- Have you ever had **G**uilty feelings about drinking?
- Have you ever taken a drink first thing in the morning (**E**ye-opener) to steady your nerves or get rid of a hangover?

Ewing, J. A. (1984). Detecting alcoholism: The CAGE questionnaire. *Journal of the American Medical Association*, 252, 1905–1907.

Key Questions	Rationales/Abnormal Findings
Spirituality. Do you have any religious beliefs regarding your illness? Should I be aware of any religious or cultural beliefs while caring for you?	Asking how the patient views the mental health condition in the context of religion and beliefs allows the nurse to provide culturally sensitive nursing care.
Do you have hope for the future? • What provides you with your emotional support or sense of faith? • What is your religious affiliation? • What are your spiritual beliefs? • What spiritual practices matter to you?	No sense of hope for the future may be an indicator of risk for suicide.

Key Topics and Questions for Common Symptoms

Common Symptoms of Altered Mental Health

- Suicide ideation
- Homicide ideation and aggressive behavior
- Altered mood and affect
- Auditory hallucinations
- Visual hallucinations
- Other hallucinations

Questions to Assess Symptoms	Rationales/Abnormal Findings
Suicide Ideation. Do you have any thoughts of wanting to harm or kill yourself?	Suicide is the 11th leading cause of death for U.S. citizens of all ages. It may accompany any psychiatric illness or occur without a psychiatric diagnosis. A patient is considered to have very "lethal" suicidal ideation if he or she has a history of suicide attempts, a specific plan, and access to the means (eg, owns a gun, has medications).

(text continues on page 78)

Questions to Assess Symptoms	Rationales/Abnormal Findings
Homicide Ideation and Aggressive Behavior. Do you have any thoughts of wanting to harm or kill anyone?	Risk factors for aggressive behavior include male gender, history of violence, and substance abuse. Ethnicity, diagnosis, age, marital status, and education do not reliably identify this behavior. Signs of violence include provocative behavior; angry demeanor; loud, aggressive speech; tense posturing; frequently changing body position, pacing; and aggressive acts.
Altered Mood and Affect. What has your mood been like? *Normal mood is pleasant.*	Assess the intensity, depth, and duration of altered mood. See also Tables 5-1 and 5-2 at the end of this chapter.
On a scale of 0 to 10, with 10 being most intense, how depressed do you feel now?	Mood inappropriate to the situation is abnormal.
Assess the patient's *affect,* an objective observation of how the patient expresses feelings and mood. Assess whether affect matches what the patient says. *Normal affect is congruent with the situation.*	Affect may be temporary and changing compared with mood.
Auditory Hallucinations. Do you hear voices that others do not hear? (Ask this question while closely observing the patient.)	A patient may answer "no" even though he or she is actually experiencing auditory hallucinations. The patient may not realize that others do not hear voices or not want to tell the nurse for fear of ramifications, such as continued hospitalization or starting medications.
Assess the nature of auditory hallucinations. • Does the voice tell you what to do? • Must you listen or do what the voice says or does?	

Questions to Assess Symptoms	Rationales/Abnormal Findings
Visual Hallucinations. Do you see things that others do not?	Causes of visual hallucinations include medications, alcohol withdrawal, and *Parkinson's disease.*
Other Hallucinations. If there is a history of hallucinations or the assessment indicates otherwise, continue to ask questions about other hallucinations (eg, olfactory, tactile).	Some patients with *psychosis* smell smoke or feel someone touching them.

Objective Data Collection

Data for the objective assessment are usually organized by **A** (appearance), **B** (behavior), **C** (cognitive function), and **T** (thought process), plus the Mini-Cog or Mini-Mental Status Examination (MMSE).

Technique and Normal Findings	Abnormal Findings
A: Appearance **Overall Appearance.** Observe overall physical appearance including noticeable physical deformities, weight, and asymmetrical movements. *The patient appears stated age, is of normal weight, and shows symmetrical movements without obvious deformity.*	There may be evidence of cutting or self-harm. Physical problems such as stroke or dementia may exacerbate some mental health conditions. Cradle cap around the face of adults indicates long-term lack of care and is often seen in patients with schizophrenia.
Posture. Assess posture. *Posture is erect but relaxed.*	Abnormal postures are rigid (*anxiety*) or slouching (*withdrawal*). Rigid posture might indicate that the patient is trying to hide, either from a person or thoughts.
Movement. Assess baseline and additional movements. Observe pace, range, and character. *Movements are voluntary, deliberate, coordinated, smooth, and even.*	Immobility (or tremor) might indicate *Parkinson's disease* or *schizophrenia.* The patient may walk a lot or keep physically occupied to distract from "voices" or dealing with emotions. The patient might have a tic or tardive dyskinesia.

(text continues on page 80)

Technique and Normal Findings	Abnormal Findings
Assess gait for steadiness and rhythm. *Gait is steady and even.*	Abnormal gaits include limping, fast or slow speed, pacing, shuffling, and stiff.
Observe activity level. Is it under voluntary control? Do posture and motor activity change with topics under discussion or with activities or people around the patient? *Activity is moderate and relaxed.*	Activity level may be altered from *hypomania* or *ADHD*, medications, or *anxiety*. Activity may be hypoactive, hyperactive, rigid, restless, agitated, gesturing, posturing, with inappropriate mannerisms, hostile/combative, or unusual. See Table 5-3 at the end of this chapter.
Hygiene and Grooming. Note hair, nails, teeth, skin, and, any beard. Observe hygiene and grooming. If the patient is unwashed/unkempt, estimate for how long. Note a change in appearance in a previously well-groomed patient. Compare both sides of the body. *Patient is well-groomed with no unusual body odors.*	Poor hygiene may be from *paranoia*, homelessness, *depression*, or incapacitation. Risk of lice increases with poor grooming. Fastidiousness may accompany *obsessive-compulsive disorder*. One-sided neglect may result from *stroke*, brain trauma, or physical injury. An unkempt state might indicate *depression* or *psychosis*.
Observe for makeup and how it is worn. *Makeup is appropriate to weather, age, gender, culture, and social situation.*	Garish makeup and outside the lines may indicate *mania*. Inappropriate makeup may also indicate a decline in mental status.
Observe the hands for coloration, cleanliness, tremors, pill rolling, or clubbing of the nail bed. Look for signs of itching or scratching.	Hands may provide indicators of health problems, smoking status, drug withdrawal or side effects, or blood glucose level. Clubbing is seen in patients with emphysema or who use recreational drugs with talc; poor oxygenation affects cognition. Itching or scratching may be from hallucination, crystal methamphetamine, or self-harm.

Technique and Normal Findings	Abnormal Findings
Dress. Observe how the patient is dressed. Is clothing clean, pressed, and fastened? How does it compare with clothing worn by people of similar age and social group?	Clothing style and color may indicate an identified social group (eg, gangs, Goth).
Is clothing worn correctly? How many layers is the patient wearing? *Clothing is clean and appropriate.*	Unfastened or incorrectly worn clothes might indicate physical, cognitive, or mental difficulty.
B: Behavior **Level of Consciousness.** Is the patient awake and alert? To assess if the patient is arousable, gently shake the bed or chair that the patient is in; do not directly shake the patient.	Abnormalities include drowsiness, hyperalertness, somnolence, intermittent alertness, and stupor. If the patient is not arousable, assess for breathing, stupor, or psychosis.
• Note if the patient is aware of the surroundings and environment.	This addresses the patient's ability to remain safe.
• Is the patient aware of self? • Does the patient respond appropriately to stimuli? *The patient is awake and alert, responding appropriately.*	Abnormal findings are a lack of awareness of own physical needs and emotional responses.
Eye Contact and Facial Expressions. Assess eye contact. *The patient converses with eyes open and maintains eye contact.*	Abnormal findings are eyes closed, avoiding eye contact, staring, looking vacant, or twitching to side when discussing trauma. A patient who looks away may be responding to voices or easily distracted. Poor eye contact may indicate low self-esteem, shame, embarrassment, *depression,* or a cultural trait.
Observe facial expressions at rest and when the patient is interacting with others. Watch	Facial expressions indicate emotional state. Abnormal expressions are perplexed, stressed,

(text continues on page 82)

Technique and Normal Findings	Abnormal Findings
for variations with topics under discussion. Are they congruent? Is the face relatively immobile throughout? The *patient is calm, alert, and expressive. Facial expressions are congruent with subjects.*	tense, dazed, grimacing, and lacking in expression. Facial expressions may give clues to *depression, anxiety,* hallucinations, physical injury, *mania,* side effects of medications, or possible extrapyramidal symptoms.
Speech. Assess speech for • Rate. *The rate is moderately paced.* • Rhythm. *The rhythm has normal fluctuations.* • Loudness. *Speech is audible with moderate loudness.* • Fluency. *Speech is fluent.*	Slow, fast, latent, pressured, monotone, or disturbed rates are abnormal. Rhyming, slurring, mumbling, or unusual rhythm is abnormal. Note if barely audible or too loud. Note any lengthy pauses, hesitancy, or stuttering (specify frequency).
• Quantity. Does the patient respond only to direct questions? Assess for voluminous speech, poverty of speech, talkativeness, silence, or spontaneity. *There is usually a flow of conversation with pauses.* • Articulation. *Speech is articulate with words clear and distinct.* • Content. *Content is organized and congruent with behavior/ nonverbal communication.*	Too much speech may be covering feelings of discomfort, embarrassment, not knowing answers, or avoiding questions. Too much or too little speech may indicate auditory hallucinations. Too little speech may indicate poverty of thought or developmental delay. Note difficulty. Disorganized, nonsensical, judgmental, religiously preoccupied, or sexually preoccupied speech may indicate impaired judgment and illogical thinking.
• Pattern. *There is a pattern of exchange in conversation.*	See Table 5-4 at the end of this chapter.
C: Cognitive Function *Orientation.* Assess orientation: • Tell me what day of the week, month, and year it is now. • Where are you right now?	Note any inconsistencies regarding orientation. Determine if the patient is new to the area and might not know the place.

BOX 5.2 THE MINI-COG

Administration

The test is administered as follows:
1. Instruct the patient to listen carefully to and remember three unrelated words and then to repeat the words.
2. Instruct the patient to draw the face of a clock, either on a blank sheet of paper or on a sheet with the clock circle already drawn on the page. After the patient puts the numbers on the clock face, ask him or her to draw the hands of the clock to read a specific time.
3. Ask the patient to repeat the three previously stated words.

Scoring

Give 1 point for each recalled word after the clock-drawing test (CDT) distractor.
Patients recalling none of the three words are classified as demented (Score = 0).
Patients recalling all three words are classified as non-demented (Score = 3).
Patients with intermediate word recall of 1-2 words are classified based on the CDT (Abnormal = demented; Normal = non-demented)

Note: The CDT is considered normal if all numbers are present in the correct sequence and position, and the hands readably display the requested time.
Source: Borson, S., Scanlan, J., Brush, M., Vitallano, P., & Dokmak, A. (2000). The Mini-Cog: A cognitive 'vital signs' measure for dementia screening in multi-lingual elderly. *International Journal of Geriatric Psychiatry*, 15(11), 1021–1027. Copyright John Wiley & Sons Limited. Reproduced with permission.

Technique and Normal Findings	Abnormal Findings
• What is your name (first and surname)? • Why are you here right now? *The patient is alert and oriented times 3 (written A&O × 3).*	
Attention Span. Can the patient follow the conversation? Is the patient easily distractible? *The patient can follow conversation and events.*	Attention span indicates current level of cognitive functioning. Note if altered attention span is from restlessness, poor focus, ADHD, or hallucinations.
Memory. Assess short- and long-term memory. Use the Mini-Cog (Box 5-2) or MMSE. *Short- and long-term memory is intact.*	Altered memory may be from *dementia, Alzheimer's disease,* or other processes.

(text continues on page 84)

Technique and Normal Findings	Abnormal Findings
Judgment. Assess judgment by noting the patient's responses to family situations, employment, interpersonal conflict, and use of money. Ask direct questions:	
• How will you get home if you have no money?	Assess the patient's ability to solve problems.
• What will you do if you feel the urge to use alcohol again (in patients with alcoholism)? (They might respond with answers such as seek help, call my AA sponsor, or talk myself out of it.)	Assess the patient's ability to choose among alternatives based on reality.
• What will happen if you hit someone you love, a neighbor, or someone else?	Assess the ability to understand consequences and take responsibility for actions.
• What is your part in this conflict? How might you have contributed?	Note if the patient has poor insight, poor judgment, or poor impulse control and what these findings might indicate.
The patient makes good judgments and takes responsibility for own actions.	

T: Thought Processes and Perceptions

Assess thought processes. *They are easy to follow, logical, coherent, relevant, goal-directed, consistent, and abstract.*

Refer to Table 5-5 at the end of this chapter.

Mental Status Examination

Assess level of cognitive function by using the Mini-Cog (Box 5-2) or the MMSE. The MMSE has 11 questions with a total of 30 points. It is self-explanatory and easy to use. Taking only 5 to 10 minutes to administer makes it easy to use with elderly patients or patients with poor attention span. *A score of 24 to 30 is in the normal range.*

The MMSE and Mini-Cog are both scored tests. A score of 23 or lower on the MMSE indicates cognitive impairment. For more information on this copyrighted tool, contact Psychological Assessment Resources, Inc., 16204 North Florida Avenue, Lutz, Florida 33549. Unsuccessful recall of three items or an abnormal clock drawing test indicates dementia on the Mini-Cog.

Documentation of Normal Findings

Patient denies suicidal or homicidal thoughts. Mood is pleasant; affect is appropriate to situation. Patient denies visual, auditory, olfactory, or tactile hallucinations. Patient appears stated age and is of normal weight with no obvious deformity. Posture is erect and relaxed. Movements are symmetrical, voluntary, deliberate, coordinated, smooth, and even. Gait is steady and even. Activity is moderate and relaxed. Patient is well-groomed with no unusual body odors. Makeup is appropriate to culture and situation. Clothing is clean and appropriate. Patient is awake, alert, calm, and expressive, responding appropriately to voice cues. Converses with eyes open and good eye contact. Facial expressions are congruent with subjects. Speech of moderate pace and volume, fluent, articulate, organized, and congruent with behavior and nonverbal communication. A&O × 3. Patient follows conversation and events; attention span is normal. Short- and long-term memory is intact. MMSE is completed with no deficits. Patient makes good judgments and takes responsibility for actions. Thought processes are easy to follow, logical, coherent, relevant, goal-directed, consistent, and abstract.

▲ Lifespan Considerations

Pregnant Women

Pregnancy is associated with relapse in psychotic disorders, and women with a history of depression are at risk for an episode during pregnancy or postpartum. Pregnant women experience hormonal changes and also may need to stop psychiatric medications because of fetal side effects. Assessment of maternal substance use is critical to protect fetal health.

Children and Adolescents

Older children and teens experience hormonal and physical changes that can affect self-image and self-esteem. Onset of menarche and puberty and social stress can contribute to *depression*, which in turn poses risk for substance abuse, risky behaviors, and *suicide*.

Older Adults

Delirium, dementia, and depression are more common in older adults. Risk factors for mental health issues include female gender; African American or Hispanic background; social isolation; widowed, divorced, or separated marital status; lower socioeconomic status; comorbid medical conditions; uncontrolled pain; insomnia; and functional or cognitive impairment. Older adults may also have physical health changes or end-of-life issues. People who lose interest in work or hobbies, sleep too much, or live alone may be at risk for social isolation. Those experiencing financial pressure may have increased stress.

▲ Cultural Considerations

Patients from different groups tend to selectively express or present symptoms in culturally acceptable ways. Attitudes and beliefs a culture holds influence whether a patient considers an illness "real" or "imagined," and if it is of the body, mind, or both. Cultural meanings of illness have implications for whether people are motivated to seek treatment, how they cope with symptoms, how supportive families and communities are, and where they seek help.

Common Nursing Diagnoses and Interventions Associated with Mental Health

Diagnosis and Related Factors	Nursing Interventions
Risk for suicide	Establish relationship. Assess for suicide risk. Refer for counseling. Remove lethal medications and weapons from the environment.
Risk for self-mutilation	Establish trust. Provide medical treatment for injuries.* Assess for depression, anxiety, impulsivity, and suicide. Secure a contract to notify the staff when experiencing a desire to mutilate.

Diagnosis and Related Factors	Nursing Interventions
Altered thought processes	Reorient as needed. Use concrete, nontechnical words and short phrases. Assess for hallucinations. Convey that you would like to understand what the patient is trying to say, but make sure that the patient does not follow through on harmful processes.
Sensory-perceptual alterations	Validate that the patient is the only person hearing or seeing the hallucination. Provide a safe environment. Encourage expression of responses to hallucinations. Encourage use of alternate coping strategy, such as singing or wearing headphones.
Ineffective individual coping	Assess for causes. Build on the patient's strengths. Set realistic goals.
	Listen and avoid false reassurance.
Self-esteem disturbance	Listen to and respect the patient. Assess strengths and coping abilities. Reframe difficulties as learning opportunities.
Impaired social interaction	Assess social support system. List behaviors associated with being disconnected and alternative responses. Role play social interactions and appropriate responses.

*Collaborative interventions.

Tables of Reference

Table 5.1   Delirium, Dementia, and Depression

Delirium, dementia, and depression can be acute situations. Delirium usually has an acute onset, and the disorganized thoughts can place the patient at risk for injury. Risk of suicide increases with depression. Cues that a patient may have dementia include the following:

• Seems disoriented
• Is a "poor historian"
• Defers to a family member to answer questions directed to the patient
• Repeatedly and apparently unintentionally fails to follow instructions
• Has difficulty finding the right words or uses inappropriate or incomprehensible words
• Has difficulty following conversations

	Delirium	Dementia	Depression
Onset	Acute over a few hours, lasting hours to weeks Occurs in context of medical illness, substance abuse or withdrawal	Slow, lasting months to years	Slow
Description	Impaired recent and remote memory Fluctuating attention Thoughts disorganized Change in cognition	Impaired remote memory Attention preserved Thoughts impoverished	Impaired memory Attention intact Impaired concentration

	Delirium	Dementia	Depression
	Clouding of consciousness		
	Perceptual disturbances— usually disorganized	Global impairment of intellect Alert Aware	If psychosis is present, it is usually systematized and with normal emotional response
	Does not usually present with mood components		Perceptual disturbances Sad affect/ mood

Adapted from Sadock, B. J., Sadock, V. A., & Kaplan, H. I. (2004). *Kaplan & Sadock's comprehensive textbook of psychiatry* (8th ed.). Philadelphia, PA: Lippincott Williams & Wilkins and Edwards, N. (2003). Differentiating the three D's: Delirium, dementia, and depression. *MEDSURG Nursing, 12*, 347–358.

⚠ Table 5.2   Abnormal Findings: Mood Disorders

Euphoria	Excessive Sense of Emotional and Physical Well-being Inappropriate to the Actual Situation or Environmental Stimuli
Flat affect	No emotional tone or reaction
Blunted affect	Severe reduction in emotional expressiveness (often confused with flat affect)
Elation	High degree of confidence, boastfulness, uncritical optimism, and joy accompanied by increased motor activity
Exultation	Reaction extending beyond elation and accompanied by feelings of grandeur

(table continues on page 90)

Table 5.2   Abnormal Findings: Mood Disorders (continued)

Euphoria	Excessive Sense of Emotional and Physical Well-being Inappropriate to the Actual Situation or Environmental Stimuli
Ecstasy	Overpowering feeling of joy and rapture
Anxiety	A feeling of apprehension or worry, especially about the future
Fear	An emotional reaction to an environmental threat
Ambivalence	Having two opposing feelings or emotions at the same time
Depersonalization	Feeling that oneself or one's environment is unreal
Irritability	Feeling of impatience, annoyance, and easy provocation to anger
Rage	Furious, uncontrolled anger
Lability	Quick change of expression of mood or feelings
Depression	Feeling characterized by sadness, dejection, helplessness, hopelessness, worthlessness, and gloom.

Adapted from Department of Health. (2008). *Psychiatry*. Retrieved November 1, 2008, from http://www.doh.gov.ph/zcmc/index.php?option=com_content&task=view&id=101&Itemid=26

Table 5.3   Abnormal Findings: Motor Movements

Akathisia	Motor Restlessness, Inability to Remain Still; Can Also Be a Subjective Feeling
Akinesia	No movement or difficulty with movement
Dystonia	Muscle spasms, spastic movements of the neck and back, can be painful or frightening

Table 5.3	Abnormal Findings: Motor Movements (continued)
Akathisia	Motor Restlessness, Inability to Remain Still; Can Also Be a Subjective Feeling
Parkinsonism	Slow, shuffling gait; masklike facial expression; tremors; pill-rolling movements of the hands; stooping posture; rigidity
Tardive dyskinesia	Involuntary and abnormal movements of the mouth, tongue, face, and jaw, may progress to the limbs, irreversible condition, may occur in months after antipsychotic medication use
Neuroleptic malignant syndrome	Develops as a potentially lethal side effect of antipsychotic medications, with muscle rigidity, tremors, altered consciousness, and incontinence; first warning signs are usually hyperthermia, hypertension, and tachycardia. May be referred to as "lead-pipe" rigidity
Choreiform movements	Irregular, involuntary actions of muscles of the face and extremities
Waxy flexibility	Holding body posture that is imposed by another person for a long time
Hyperkinesias	Excessive movement; destructive or aggressive activity
Compulsive	Unwanted repetitive actions
Automatism	Not consciously controlled, automatic, undirected motor activity
Cataplexy	Temporary loss of muscle tone precipitated by strong emotions.

(table continues on page 92)

Table 5.3 Abnormal Findings: Motor Movements (continued)

Akathisia	Motor Restlessness, Inability to Remain Still; Can Also Be a Subjective Feeling
Catalepsy	Trancelike state with loss of voluntary motion
Stereotypy	Repetitive imitation of another person's movements
Psychomotor retardation	Decreased, slowed activity
Catatonic stupor	Extreme underactivity
Catatonic excitement	Extreme overactivity
Impulsiveness	Outbursts of unpredictable and sudden activity
Tics and spasms	Involuntary twitching and jerking of muscles, usually above the shoulders

Adapted from Department of Health. (2008). *Psychiatry*. Retrieved November 1, 2008, from http://www.doh.gov.ph/zcmc/index.php?option=com_content&task=view&id=101&Itemid=26

Table 5.4 Abnormal Findings: Speech Patterns

Verbigeration	Repetitive, Meaningless Expression of Sentences, Phrases, or Words
Rhyming	Interjecting into conversation regular, recurring, corresponding sounds at the ends of phrases or sentences, as in poetry
Punning	Interjecting clever and humorous uses of a word or words
Mutism	No expression of words or lack of communication over a period of time
Selectively mute	Mostly mute with intermittent periods of verbal expression

Table 5.4	Abnormal Findings: Speech Patterns (*continued*)
Verbigeration	**Repetitive, Meaningless Expression of Sentences, Phrases, or Words**
Aphasia	Partial or total loss of the ability to express self through language or to understand the verbal communication of another person
Neologisms	Words created by the patient that are either not easily understood by others or unintelligible
Spontaneous	Communication initiated by the patient with others
Circumlocutions	Phrases or sentences substituted for a word that the person cannot think of (eg, "what you write with" for a pen).
Paraphasias	Malformed, wrong, or invented words

Adapted from Department of Health. (2008). *Psychiatry*. Retrieved November 1, 2008, from http://www.doh.gov.ph/zcmc/index.php?option=com_content&task=view&id=101&Itemid=26

Table 5.5	Abnormal Findings: Thought Processes
Thought Blocking	**Sudden Cessation of Flow of Thought and Speech Related to Strong Emotions**
Flight of ideas	Rapid conversation with logically unconnected shifting of topics
Word salad	Disconnected and incoherent combination of phrases, words, and sentences
Perseveration phenomena	Repetitive behaviors such as lip licking, finger tapping, pacing, or echolalia

(table continues on page 94)

Table 5.5 Abnormal Findings: Thought Processes (*continued*)

Thought Blocking	Sudden Cessation of Flow of Thought and Speech Related to Strong Emotions
Circumstantiality	Interjection of great detail and incidental material with no primary significance to the central idea of the conversation
Tangential	Deviation from central theme of conversation
Echolalia	Repetitive imitation of another person's speech
Delusion	False belief kept despite nonsupportive evidence
Phobia	Strong, persistent, abnormal fear of an object or situation
Obsession	Persistent, unwanted, recurring thoughts
Compulsions	Repetitive mental act or physical behavior that the patient feels driven to perform to reduce distress, prevent a dreaded event or situation, or respond to an obsession
Hypochondriasis	Morbid concern for one's health and feeling ill without any actual medical basis
Psychosis	Disorderly mental state in which the patient has difficulty distinguishing reality from internal perceptions
Thought broadcasting	Delusion that others can hear one's thoughts
Thought control	Delusion that others can control a person's thoughts against one's will

Thought Blocking	Sudden Cessation of Flow of Thought and Speech Related to Strong Emotions
Thought insertion	Delusion that others have the ability to put thoughts in a person's mind against one's will
Neologisms	Creating and using new words
Loose associations	Changes of conversation in an unrelated, fragmented manner
Incoherent	Not making any sense
Confabulation	Making up answers to cover for not knowing. Demonstrates ability to think and reason with only short-term memory present. Symptom of Korsakoff's syndrome
Ideas of reference	Perception that others or the media are talking to or about the patient
Ruminating	Getting "stuck" on, worrying, or thinking about an idea repetitively

Adapted from Department of Health. (2008). *Psychiatry*. Retrieved November 1, 2008, from http://www.doh.gov.ph/zcmc/index. php?option=com_content&task=view&id=101&Itemid=26

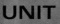

Regional Examinations

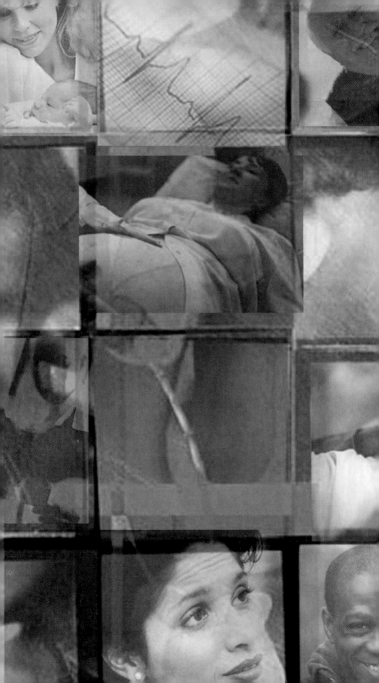

Skin, Hair, and Nails Assessment

Subjective Data Collection

Key Topics and Questions for Health Promotion

Questions to Assess History and Risks

Rationales

Family History. Do you have any first-degree family members (parent, sibling, child) with a history of melanoma?
- Who had the problem?
- Do any first-degree relatives have multiple dark, irregular moles?

Having first-degree relatives with a history of *melanoma* increases the patient's risk for melanoma. Approximately 10% of all patients with melanoma have a family member with melanoma.

Past History. Do you do skin self-examination monthly? When was your last clinical skin examination?

Teach what skin changes warrant further evaluation. A simple method is the **ABCDE**s of melanoma detection:
- **A**symmetry
- **B**order irregularity
- **C**olor
- **D**iameter of more than 6 mm
- **E**volution of lesion over time
See Table 6-1 at the end of this chapter.

Do you have any pigmented skin lesions?
- How many?
- Where are they?
- Have any changed (itching, bleeding, nonhealing, color, size, borders)?

Any **dysplastic nevi** or more than 50 normal moles increases risk for melanoma. Changes in size, color, texture, or shape, onset of itching or bleeding, and nonhealing warrant further evaluation.

(text continues on page 100)

Questions to Assess History and Risks	Rationales
Did you ever have severe sunburn, particularly during your youth? How long can you be in the sun before your skin begins to turn red?	Melanoma on the trunk, arms, or legs is associated with severe (blistering) sunburn during childhood or adolescence.
Have you ever had skin cancer? • When? • Where? • How was it treated?	History of skin cancer significantly increases risk of developing additional cancerous lesions.
Have you had an organ transplant? Do you have HIV/AIDS? Have you had chemotherapy or radiation therapy?	A weakened immune system increases risk for melanoma.
Medications. What medications are you taking? • Do you have allergies to medications, latex, nuts, bees, or other items? • How did you react to the allergy? • Are you allergic to sunscreen?	Medications and substances can cause **photosensitivity**, which usually presents as a rash following sun exposure. Other medications stimulate **phototoxicity**, usually within 24 hours of initial ingestion and resolving readily. **Photoallergy** manifests with blisters and redness on exposed skin after repeated contact with an offending substance.
Lifestyle, Occupational History, and Personal Behaviors. What is your occupation? Hobbies? • Are you exposed to excessive sunlight or other sources of radiation? • How do you protect against excessive sun exposure?	Excessive exposure to sunlight, especially during midday hours, increases risk for melanoma. Determining the protection the patient uses helps establish risk level for melanoma.
Determine the risk for skin breakdown. • Do you have diabetes mellitus, peripheral vascular disease, or any known sensory loss?	Risk is increased in patients with decreased sensory perception.

Health-Promotion Teaching

Self-Skin Examination. Self-examinations of the skin assist patients to identify potentially problematic lesions. The nurse educates that a normal mole is

- A solid tan, brown, black, or skin-toned color
- Smaller than 6 mm in diameter
- With well-defined edges
- Usually round or oval with a flat or dome-like surface
- In existence before age 30.

The nurse teaches the patient the following steps of the self-skin examination:

1. Get fully undressed and stand in front of a full-length mirror.
2. Carefully scan the entire body, using a handheld mirror to look at areas difficult to see (eg, soles of feet).
3. When examining the scalp, use a comb or blow-dryer to part the hair and examine the scalp section by section.
4. Report any suspicious lesion to the health care provider.

Sun Protection. Nurses can simplify patient education about decreasing exposure to harmful ultraviolet light by teaching the phrase "Slip! Slop! Slap!... and Wrap!" Coined by the American Cancer Society, it reminds people to slip on a shirt, slop on sunscreen, slap on a hat, and wrap on sunglasses to protect against UV exposure. Applying sunscreen 15 to 30 minutes before exposure enhances absorption of the sunscreen into the skin and increases protection. Sunscreen application needs to happen every 2 hours for maximum benefit. Another helpful reminder to limit excessive UV exposure is "short shadow, seek shade." Overhead sun casts a shadow shorter than the person and should serve as an alert to seek more shade for protection.

Key Topics and Questions for Common Symptoms

Be sure to review location, characteristics, duration, aggravating factors, alleviating factors, and the patient's viewpoint for each reported symptom.

Common Integumentary Symptoms

- Pruritus
- Rash (multiple lesions)
- Single lesions or wounds

Questions to Assess Symptoms	Rationale/Abnormal Findings
Tell me about your skin problem.	This question encourages the patient to present an unbiased view and perceptions of the problem.
Pruritus (Itching). Do you have a problem with itching? • For how long? • Where? • What do you think is the problem?	Skin lesions or conditions are pruritic, occasionally pruritic, or never pruritic. Pruritus frequently precedes atopic lesions but follows inflammatory lesions.
Rash. Where is/are the lesion(s) located?	Lesions from *contact or allergic dermatitis* are usually on exposed body parts. Lesions over the entire body may be linked to *syphilis. Seborrheic dermatitis* occurs on hair-covered areas. *Herpes zoster* follows a dermatome and is often on the chest, back, abdomen, and face. Genital lesions are commonly sexually transmitted. Single lesions could be *cancer*; multiple lesions could indicate infection.
Has the rash changed since you first noticed it?	*Varicella*, cancer, *pityriasis rosea,* and *contact dermatitis* change over time.
Have you been exposed to anything that would cause itching or rash?	Contacts can be through new occupational or leisure activities, animals, plants, poison ivy, insects, microbials, chemicals, pesticides, medications, vitamin or herbal supplements, new foods, unusual clothes or linens, and communal residences.

Questions to Assess Symptoms	Rationale/Abnormal Findings
Describe your rash.	See Table 6-2 at the end of this chapter.
Do you have any other symptoms?	Fevers and chills may accompany infectious skin disorders. Headache may accompany *mumps* and *meningitis*.
Single Lesion or Wound • Is this wound acute or chronic? • Is it related to medical, surgical, or traumatic causes? • Would any factors delay healing?	Obtain additional information about the wound, its duration, its size, and associated symptoms. Evaluate the nature of events leading to any trauma. Ask about treatments including natural and over-the-counter remedies.

Objective Data Collection

Equipment Needed

- Examination gown
- Tape measure
- Adequate light source
- Magnifying glass

Technique and Normal Findings	Abnormal Findings
Inspection Inspect all body areas. Start at the crown of the head. Part hair to visualize the scalp. Progress caudally to the feet. Make sure to assess the soles and to separate the toes. Note general skin color. *Body pigmentation is consistent. Patients with dark skin may have hypopigmented palms and soles.*	Note pigment changes in any areas, such as with *vitiligo*. Other abnormal color changes include *flushing*, *erythema* (redness), *cyanosis* (bluish discoloration), *pallor* (paleness), *rubor* (dependent redness), *brawny* appearance, and *jaundice* (yellow discoloration). *(text continues on page 104)*

BOX 6.1 LESION CONFIGURATIONS

- Annular: Ring-like, circular
- Arciform: Half-ring
- Linear: Line-shaped
- Polymorphous: Several different shapes
- Punctuate: Small, marked with points or dots
- Serpiginous: Curving, snake-like
- Nummular/Discoid: Coin-shaped
- Umbilicated: Central depression
- Filiform: Papilla-like or finger-like projections (similar to tongue papillae)
- Verruciform: Circumscribed, papular with rough surface

Technique and Normal Findings	Abnormal Findings
Inspect for lesions. If observed, identify morphology, configuration (Box 6-1), distribution pattern (Box 6-2), size, and exact location. *Common benign lesions include freckles, birthmarks, skin tags, moles, and cherry angiomas.*	Lesion morphology is a key determinant in identifying a skin disorder. Primary morphology is the type. Secondary morphology includes shape, size, arrangement, and distribution, which further defines the underlying problem (or normal variant). See Tables 6-2 and 6-3 at the end of this chapter.

BOX 6.2 LESION DISTRIBUTION PATTERNS

- Asymmetric: Distributed solely on one side of body.
- Confluent: With enlargement or multiplication, begin to coalesce to form larger lesion.
- Diffuse: Distributed widely across affected area without any pattern.
- Discrete: Single, separated, well-defined borders.
- Generalized: Distributed over large body area.
- Grouped: Clustered.
- Localized: Located at distinct area.
- Satellite: Single lesion(s) in close proximity to larger lesion, as if "orbiting."
- Symmetric: Distributed equally on both sides of body.
- Zosteriform: Distributed along dermatome.

Technique and Normal Findings	Abnormal Findings
Identify any infections. Be sure to use infection-control principles if infection is suspected.	Infections include *acne, cellulitis, impetigo, German measles (Rubella), herpes simplex* (cold sores), *measles* (Rubeola), *pityriasis rosea, roseola, warts, candida, tinea corporis,* and *tinea versicolor.*
Note any inflammatory lesions.	These include *psoriasis, eczema, urticaria, contact dermatitis,* allergic drug reaction, insect bites, or seborrhea.
Assess for any infestations.	Lice (*pediculosis*), scabies, or ticks are examples.
Observe for growths, tumors, or vascular or other miscellaneous lesions.	See Table 6-4 at the end of this chapter.
Inspect any wounds or incisions. If observed, note the shape and measure the length, width, and depth with a ruler. If a wound is deep or tunneled, insert a cotton applicator to measure depth.	*Partial-thickness wounds* involve the epidermis; *full-thickness wounds* involve the dermis and subcutaneous tissue. Healthy-healing tissue appears pink to red; necrotic tissue may be yellow, white, brown, or black (eschar).
Describe wounds related to trauma. Assess status of the blood supply to the skin; note any bleeding or ecchymosis (bruising).	Traumatic lesions may be *petechiae, purpura, ecchymoses, hematomas, lacerations, abrasions, puncture wounds,* or *avulsions.*
Identify risk for skin breakdown, which is especially important in hospitalized or inactive patients. (See Table 6-5). Visit the Prevention Plus Web page, Home of the Braden Scale, for more information.	The Braden scale scores patients from 1 to 4 in each of six subscales: sensory perception, moisture, activity, mobility, nutrition, and friction.

(text continues on page 106)

Technique and Normal Findings	Abnormal Findings
Classify the wound as partial- or full-thickness; if a pressure ulcer is present identify the stage. Observe and document the size in depth and diameter, margins, condition of surrounding tissues, any varicosities or telangiectasias, status of granulation tissue and epithelial growth, and any drainage, odor, or necrotic tissue. Describe the color and texture of the tissue. Identify the amount, color, consistency, and odor of exudate (drainage). Use appropriate landmarks.	Pressure ulcers may be deep tissue, stage I, stage II, stage III, stage IV, or unstageable. Wound drainage is classified as serous (clear), sanguineous (bloody), serosanguineous (mixed), fibrinous (sticky yellow), or purulent (pus). Note any signs or symptoms of infection.
Assess for nonpressure ulcers; note the characteristics of the wound.	Nonpressure ulcers include neuropathic, venous (vascular), and arterial (vascular) ulcers. See Chapter 13.
Burns are classified based on the depth of tissue destruction and percentage of total body surface area affected. See Table 6-6.	Superficial burns involve the epidermal layers, superficial dermal burns involve the epidermis and part of the dermis, deep dermal burns involve the epidermis and all of the dermis, and total-thickness burns involve all layers of the skin and may extend into the supportive fascia below.
Inspect each fingernail and toenail. Assess for color, thickness, and consistency. *Nails are smooth, translucent, and consistent in color and thickness. Longitudinal ridging is common in aging patients. Longitudinal pigmentation in dark-skinned patients is a normal variant.*	Abnormal findings are splitting of nail tips, thickened nails, and discoloration of the nail bed. See also Table 6-7.

Technique and Normal Findings	Abnormal Findings
Have the patient place the fingernails of both index fingers together to assess the nail angle. *A diamond-shaped opening is visible between the two fingernails, indicating a nail angle of at least 160 degrees.* Inspect the hair, noting color, consistency, distribution, areas of hair loss, and condition of the hair shaft. *Hair is equally and symmetrically distributed across the scalp. Hair shafts are smooth, shiny, of even consistency, and without evidence of breakage.*	*Clubbing* of the nails indicates chronic hypoxia. It exists when the angle of the nail to the finger is more than 160 degrees. In female patients, ovarian dysfunction may be characterized by hair on the beard area, abdomen, upper back, shoulders, sternum, and inner upper thighs.
Note areas of decreased or absent hair. Parting the hair enables visualization of the scalp skin. Note any lesions or color changes there. *Scalp skin is of color consistent with the rest of the body.* Observe hair shafts near the root for lice or nits.	Brittle or broken hair shafts may indicate endocrine or metabolic dysfunction. Lice or nits may be on the hair shaft. The closer to the scalp the nit is located, the more recent the infestation. Excessive dryness and scaling of the scalp are often present in *seborrheic dermatitis*. See Table 6-8.
Palpation Using the dorsal surface of the hands, assess skin temperature. *Skin temperature is consistently warm or cool and appropriate to the environment.*	Further assess any areas of increased temperature for lesions, swelling, and color changes.
Use the palmar surface of the fingers and hands to assess skin moisture and texture. *Moisture is consistent throughout, with evenly smooth skin texture.*	Excessive dryness may be from frequent bathing or *hyperthyroidism*. Excessive moisture may signify a problem with temperature regulation. Cracked or fissured skin may indicate hydration disorders, infections, or chemical injuries.
Assess skin turgor. Gently grasp a fold of the patient's skin between your fingers and pull up. Then,	A persistent pinch, or **tenting**, indicates dehydration.

(text continues on page 108)

Technique and Normal Findings	Abnormal Findings
release (Fig. 6-1). *Skin promptly recoils to its normal position.* 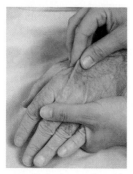 **Figure 6.1** Assessing skin turgor.	
Assess for vascularity by applying direct pressure to the skin surface with the pads of your fingers. *On releasing your finger, color promptly returns to normal.*	Decreased vascular supply is often initially found in the extremities, particularly in the hands and feet. Altered circulation can result in pallor or rubor of an extremity.
Palpate lesions for tenderness, mobility, and consistency.	Tenderness of a lesion or dermatitis may indicate infection. Lesions seemingly fixed in place may be cancerous.
Palpate each fingernail and toenail. *Nails are smooth, nontender, and firmly adherent to the nail bed. Lateral and proximal folds are nontender and nonswollen.*	Swelling, redness, or tenderness in the lateral or proximal folds may indicate *paronychia*. Sponginess of the nail bed may indicate clubbing.
Palpate the hair. Grasp 10 to 12 hairs and gently pull. *Just a few hairs are in your hand.*	Note excessive hair loss (more than 6 hairs) and then assess for presence or absence of the hair bulb. Absent hair bulb may indicate chemical damage to the hair shaft (excessive coloration). Presence of the hair bulb may indicate endocrine dysfunction.

The patient denies pruritus, skin lesions, and excessive dryness of the skin. Denies changes to existing moles. Skin evenly colored, smooth, soft, consistently warm, with intact turgor. No suspicious lesions. Nails smooth and translucent, lateral and proximal folds without swelling or erythema. Hair smooth texture, symmetrically distributed on the scalp, consistent coloration and hydration, without evidence of excessive breakage or loss. Scalp with consistent pigmentation, no lesions noted.

▲ Lifespan Considerations

Pregnant Women

Common benign findings in pregnant women include *melasma; striae gravidarum* (stretch marks); *spider telangiectasias; hyperpigmentation;* enlargement of preexisting keloids; edema of the face, legs, and hands; rapid nail growth; and increased nail brittleness. Pregnant women may report rapid hair growth; postpartum, they may experience excessive hair loss.

Abnormal skin findings in pregnancy include *pyogenic granuloma*, *erythema nodosum*, and *pruritic urticarial papules and plaques of pregnancy* (PUPPP). Pyogenic granuloma usually appears on the oral mucosa or lips as a glistening red papule or nodule that bleeds easily. It commonly develops rapidly in the late second or third trimester. *Erythema nodosum* presents as 2- to 6-cm tender, red, painful nodules on the extensor surfaces of the lower extremities that usually resolve postpartum. *PUPPP* is characterized by intensely pruritic reddish papules and plaques within striae gravidarum.

Newborns and Infants

Evaluation for cyanosis is part of Apgar scoring after birth (see Chapter 22). The more cyanotic the appearance, the lower the score and thus the greater indication of compromised circulation. Persistent cyanosis on the hands and feet can be a normal response to cool environmental temperatures. Bluish mottling of the skin, known as *cutis marmorata*, is from chilling or stress.

Jaundice, always considered pathologic if it appears in the first 24 hours of birth, results from the immature liver's inability to breakdown bilirubin for excretion. Jaundice disappears once the liver can process bilirubin effectively (usually 5 to 10 days after birth).

Pigmented lesions are common in newborns. Café au lait spots larger than 3 cm or more than six café au lait lesions are associated with severe illness. See also Chapter 22.

A newborn's skin is usually thin and almost transparent, especially in premature babies. Vernix or lanugo may appear. *Milia* are tiny white papules on the cheeks, chin, and nose. They result from distended sebaceous glands and generally resolve spontaneously in a few weeks or months. *Erythema toxicum* is a pink papular, vesicular, and occasionally pustular rash on the trunk and extending outward. Lesions are surrounded by an erythematous, blotchy halo and usually resolve spontaneously. Ecchymoses may be from birth trauma. It is common to observe edema of the eyes, scrotum, and labia in neonates.

Children and Adolescents

Children with yellowish palms, soles, and face, but not sclerae, may have carotenemia from excessive ingestion of yellow or orange vegetables or chronic renal disease. Skin findings in children are commonly the result of an infection.

Pubertal adolescents will have maturation of the apocrine glands in the axillae and genitalia areas with production of malodorous sweat. Sebaceous gland secretion increases, as does the predisposition to acne.

Older Adults

Common findings include decreased skin elasticity, thinness, excessive dryness, and age-associated lesions such as seborrheic *keratosis, actinic keratosis,* and *lentigines.* Older adults are at increased risk for skin cancer, abnormal ecchymoses or purpuric lesions, and trauma.

Cultural Considerations

Cultural variations can include a patient's refusal to remove a head covering and a requirement for a chaperone during skin examination, particularly if the health care provider is of a different sex than the patient. Some cultures prohibit directly touching a patient, requiring a nurse to wear gloves.

Integumentary findings in African Americans include ashy dermatitis, keloid formation, traction alopecia, pseudofolliculitis, folliculitis barbae, and perineal follicularis. African American women have increased incidence of melasma in pregnancy; Mongolian spots are common in African American newborns. Pityriasis rosea in African Americans commonly presents with papular, maroon or purple lesions. Skin cancers are more common on the palms, soles, and nail beds in this group than in others.

Southeast Asian men have less body and facial hair than patients of other genetic heritages. Skin adornments (eg, tattoos, body piercings) are common in various Asian cultures. Discolorations from cupping or coining may be found. Pigmentary disorders (eg, vitiligo) in darker-skinned populations may pose psychosocial and emotional distress because of the obvious change in appearance.

Common Associated Nursing Diagnoses and Interventions

Diagnosis	Nursing Interventions
Impaired skin integrity	Classify wound as partial- or full-thickness (stage I or II). Document wound assessment. Assess for risk of skin breakdown. Apply appropriate dressing. Evaluate for use of specialty mattress. Avoid positioning over bony prominences.
Impaired tissue integrity	Determine size and depth of wound (stage III or IV), skin around wound, continence status, and tube/incision placement. Apply appropriate dressing. Collaborate with physician on necessary debridement and surgical intervention.*
Pain related to tissue injury and treatments	Use pain scale to identify current pain intensity and effectiveness of medication. Develop pain goal with patient. Provide pain medications as ordered.* Provide alternatives such as distraction, breathing, and relaxation.
Risk for infection	Practice frequent handwashing and universal precautions. Protect wound with dressing. Monitor for fever, elevated WBCs, wound drainage, or erythema. Discontinue tubes as soon as possible. Encourage adequate nutrition.

*Collaborative interventions.

Tables of Reference

Table 6.1 ABCDEs for Assessment for Melanoma

A: Asymmetry
Does one half look like the other half?

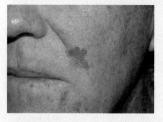

B: Border irregularity
Is the border ragged or notched?

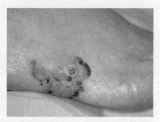

C: Color
Does the mole have a variety of shades or different colors?

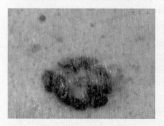

D: Diameter
Is the diameter >6 mm (pencil eraser)?

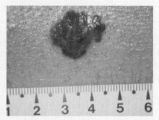

E: Evolution
Has the lesion evolved or changed over time?

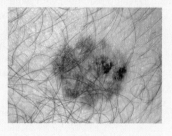

Table 6.2 Primary Skin Lesions

Macule

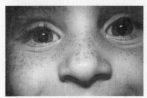

Flat, circumscribed, discolored, <1 cm diameter

Patch

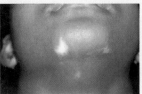

Flat, circumscribed, discolored, >1 cm diameter

Papule

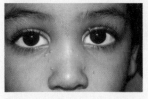

Raised, defined, any color, <1 cm diameter

Plaque

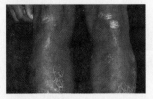

Raised, defined, any color, >1 cm diameter

Wheal

Raised, flesh-colored or red edematous papules or plaques, vary in size and shape

Nodule

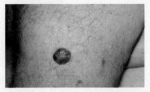

Solid, palpable >1 cm diameter, often with some depth

(table continues on page 114)

Table 6.2 Primary Skin Lesions (*continued*)

Tumor

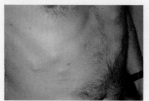

Large nodule

Vesicle

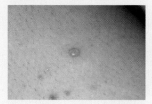

Fluid-filled, <1 cm diameter

Bulla

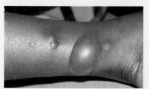

Fluid-filled, >1 cm diameter

Pustule

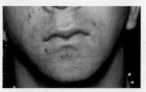

Purulent, fluid-filled, raised to any size

Cyst

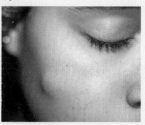

Distinct and walled-off, containing fluid or semisolid material, varied in size

Table 6.3   Secondary Skin Lesions

Atrophy

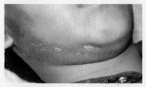

Thinning of skin from loss of skin structures

Scar

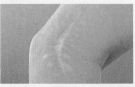

Fibrous replacement of lost skin structure

Keloid

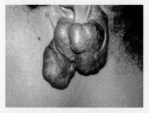

Excessive fibrous tissue replacement resulting in enlarged scar and deformity

Fissure

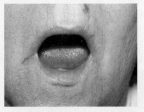

Linear break in skin surface, not related to trauma

Excoriation

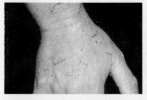

Lesion resulting from scratching or excessive rubbing of skin

Erosion

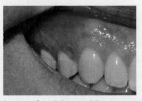

Loss of epidermal layer, usually not extending into dermis or subcutaneous layer

(table continues on page 116)

Table 6.3 Secondary Skin Lesions (*continued*)

Scale

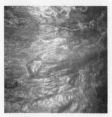

Rapid turnover of epidermal layer resulting in accumulation of and delayed shedding of outermost epidermis

Lichenification

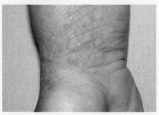

Accentuation of normal skin lines resembling tree bark, commonly caused by excessive scratching

Ulcer

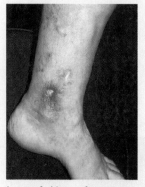

Loss of skin surface, extending into dermis, subcutaneous, fascia, muscle, bone, or all

Crust

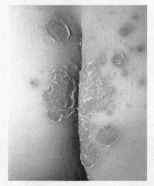

Dried secretions from primary lesion

Table 6.4 Skin Tumors and Growths

Moles or Nevi

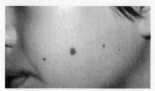

These normal variants can be macular or papular and distributed anywhere. *Congenital nevi* ("birthmarks") exist from birth. *Acquired nevi* usually develop in childhood and adolescence.

Skin Tags

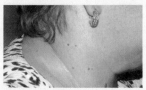

These normal papules are generally <1 cm and found on the neck, axillae, inframammary area, and groin. Skin tags are common in pregnancy and in aging skin.

Lipoma

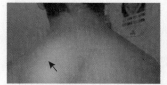

Single or multiple tumors of different sizes and comprising fat cells are commonly found on the back of the neck, torso, arms, and legs. Though benign, some varieties are painful.

Lentigo

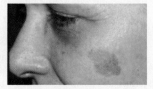

Lentigines are benign, acquired, circumscribed, pigmented macules found generally on sun-exposed skin.

Squamous Cell Carcinoma

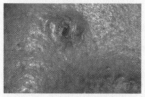

The second most frequent skin cancer is related to actinic keratosis and sun exposure. Lesions are typically papular, nodular, or plaques.

Kaposi Sarcoma

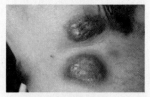

This opportunistic skin infection is a consequence of impaired immune status (eg, AIDS). Lesions occur on the nose, penis, and extremities; with advanced HIV, distribution may be generalized.

(table continues on page 118)

Table 6.4   Skin Tumors and Growths (continued)

Basal Cell Carcinoma

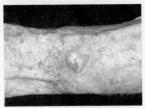

This nodular or papular skin cancer appears shiny with a rolled pearly border and typically has small spider veins on its surface. It grows slowly and rarely metastasizes.

Actinic Keratosis

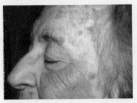

Also called *solar keratoses*, they usually develop on sun-exposed skin, possibly from UV damage. These discrete macules or papules have a rough or scaly surface.

Table 6.5   Pressure Ulcers

Stage	Description
Stage I 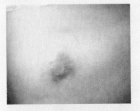	Intact skin with nonblanchable redness of a localized area, usually over a bony prominence. Darkly pigmented skin may not have visible blanching; its color may differ from the surrounding area. The area may be painful, firm, soft, warmer, or cooler as compared to adjacent tissue.
Stage II 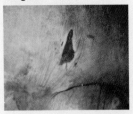	Partial thickness loss of dermis presenting as a shallow open ulcer with a red pink wound bed, without slough. May also present as an intact or open/ruptured serum-filled blister. Presents as a shiny or dry shallow ulcer without slough or bruising (indicates suspected deep tissue injury). This stage should not be used to describe skin tears, tape burns, perineal dermatitis, maceration, or excoriation.

| Table 6.5 | Pressure Ulcers (*continued*) |

Stage	Description
Stage III 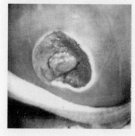	Full-thickness tissue loss. Subcutaneous fat may be visible, but bone, tendon, or muscle is not exposed. Slough may be present but does not obscure the depth of tissue loss. May include undermining and tunneling.
Stage IV	Full-thickness tissue loss with exposed bone, tendon, or muscle. Slough or eschar may be present on some parts of the wound bed. Often include undermining and tunneling.
Unstageable	Full-thickness tissue loss in which the base of the ulcer is covered by slough (yellow, tan, gray, green or brown), eschar (tan, brown or black), or both. Until enough slough or eschar is removed to expose the base of the wound, true depth, and therefore stage, cannot be determined.

Table 6.6 Burns

Depth of Burn	Bleeding	Sensation	Appearance	Blanching
Superficial	Brisk	Pain	Rapid capillary refill	Moist, red
Superficial-Dermal	Brisk	Pain	Slowed capillary refill	Dry, pale pink
Dermal	Delayed	No pain	No capillary refill	Mottled cherry red color
Full thickness	None	No pain	No blanching	Dry, leathery or waxy hard wound surface

Table 6.7 Abnormal Nail Findings

Longitudinal Ridging

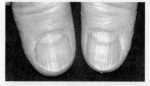

Normal variation, especially in elderly

Koilonychia (Spoon Nails)

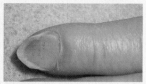

Transverse and longitudinal concavity of the nail, giving the appearance of a spoon. May be normal in infants. Other causes include trauma, iron-deficiency anemia, and hemochromatosis.

Onycholysis

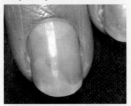

Separation of a portion of the nail plate from the nail bed; results in opaqueness to the affected part, appearing white to yellow to green; causes include trauma, fungal infections, topical irritants, psoriasis, subungual neoplasms, and warts

Pitted Nails

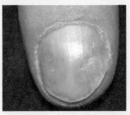

Psoriatic lesions arising from nail matrix that cause pitting on the nail plate as it grows

Beau's Lines

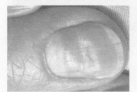

Results from slowed or halted nail growth in response to illness, physical trauma, or poisoning

Clubbing

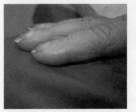

Results from chronic hypoxia to distal fingers, such as with emphysema or congestive heart failure

(table continues on page 122)

Table 6.7 Abnormal Nail Findings (*continued*)

Yellow Nails

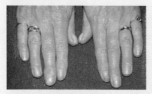

Slowly growing nail, without cuticle, and onycholysis resulting in thickening of nail and yellowish appearance. May be caused by lung disorders or lymphedema

Half-and-half Nails

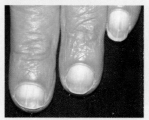

Color changes associated with renal failure; proximal portion of nail is white and distal portion is pink or brown

Dark Longitudinal Streaks

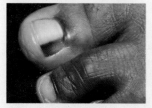

Often normal variant in dark-skinned patients from junctional nevus of nail matrix. Suspicious for malignancy if the streaks blur, spread, or are not solid the full length of the nail.

Splinter Hemorrhages

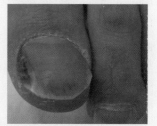

Brownish red longitudinal lines in the direction of nail growth that result from damage to capillaries supplying the nail matrix caused by microemboli, such as with endocarditis, vasculitis, and antiphospholipid syndrome

Alopecia Areata

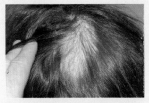

This autoimmune disorder results in noninflammatory loss of hair in a circumscribed distribution.

Trichotillomania

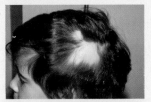

Compulsive hair pulling causes breakage of hair and thinned or balding areas on scalp, although some hair remains present and visible in the affected area.

Traction Alopecia

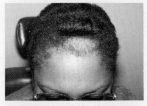

Tight hair braiding practices exert traction force on the hair bulb with subsequent hair loss.

Hirsutism

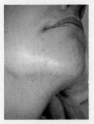

Excessive androgenic hormones in a female patient can cause masculine changes including hair in male distribution patterns.

Head and Neck Assessment

Subjective Data Collection

Key Topics and Questions for Health Promotion

Key Questions	Rationales/Abnormal Findings
Have you ever had an accident that resulted in a loss of consciousness or head injury? Do you wear a seat belt? Bicycle helmet?	Head injuries are a major cause of disability, which can be permanent. They may be preventable with appropriate use of protective gear, such as a helmet.
Were you ever treated with radiation to the neck, chest, or back?	Previously, acne in these areas was sometimes treated with radiation. Patients who received such therapy are at increased risk for thyroid and salivary gland cancers.
Have you had any surgeries involving your head or neck?	Because the head and neck have many structures, surgeries there may result in dysfunction of nerves, muscles, or vascular flow or in endocrine changes.
Do you have a family history of thyroid problems? • Who had the illness? • Was it hypothyroidism or hyperthyroidism? • When did the person have it? • How was it treated? • What were the outcomes?	*Graves' disease*, the most common type of *hyperthyroidism*, is autoimmune and may also be genetic. Some evidence supports that *medullary thyroid cancer* is genetically linked.

Key Questions	Rationales/Abnormal Findings
Do you take any regular medications? How much alcohol do you drink? Do you take any herbal products?	Many medications, including bronchodilators and oral contraceptives, and alcohol can precipitate headaches. Some studies have found feverfew effective in relieving headaches. While patients may use this and other herbal products for relief of symptoms such as headaches, these potentially potent chemicals could actually cause headache and other neurologic side effects.

Health-Promotion Teaching

Reducing Risk of Head and Neck Injury. One method to prevent injury to these areas includes wearing helmets when engaging in sports, bicycling, motorcycling, and other activities that pose risk. The use of seat belts and child safety restraints when driving also help to protect against head and neck injuries. Other causes of injuries to these regions include motor vehicle collisions related to alcohol or drug use or sleepiness. Education for high-risk groups about not driving while under the influence or while sleepy is critical.

Thyroid Screening. Thyroid screening is a particular focus area for pregnant women. Such prenatal care helps to ensure that thyroid levels remain within normal limits, protecting both mother and fetus.

Cancer Screening. Risk factors for neck cancers include male gender, age older than 50 years, tobacco use, and alcohol consumption. For patients with such risk factors, nurses should especially emphasize teaching related to smoking prevention or cessation.

Key Topics and Questions for Common Symptoms

Common Head and Neck Symptoms

- Headache (see Box 7-1)
- Neck pain
- Limited neck movement
- Facial pain
- Lumps or masses
- Hypothyroidism
- Hyperthyroidism

BOX 7.1 LIST OF RED FLAGS FOR HEADACHES

- Onset of new or different headache
- Nausea or vomiting
- Worst headache ever experienced
- Progressive visual or neurological changes
- Paralysis
- Weakness, ataxia, or loss of coordination
- Drowsiness, confusion, memory impairment, or loss of consciousness
- Onset of headache after age of 50 papilledema
- Stiff neck
- Onset of headache with exertion, sexual activity, or coughing
- Systemic illness
- Numbness
- Asymmetry of papillary response
- Sensory loss
- Signs of meningeal irritation

Sobri, M. S., Lamont, A. C., Alias, N. A., & Win, M. N. (2003). Red flags in patients presenting with headache: Clinical indications for neuroimaging. *British Journal of Radiology, 76*(908), 532–535.

Questions to Assess Symptoms	Rationales/Abnormal Findings
Headache. Have you had any unusually frequent or severe headaches? • Where? Does it radiate? Is it on one or both sides? • Describe what the headache feels like? • How bad is it on a 1-to-10 scale, with 10 being worst? • When did it start? How long has it lasted? How often? Do you ever have milder headaches? Is a pattern evident? • What makes it worse or better? What brings it on? Any relationship with food, alcohol, activity, or menstruation? • Do other symptoms accompany the pain (nausea, visual changes, an aura)?	Pay attention to characteristics such as pain worse in the morning on awakening, precipitated or made worse by straining or sneezing (potentially *elevated intracranial pressure*) versus worse as the day progresses (more likely *tension*). A throbbing, severe, unilateral headache that lasts 6 to 24 hours and is associated with photophobia, nausea, and vomiting suggests *migraine*, while a constant, unremitting, general headache described as a feeling of a tight band around the head and lasts for days, weeks, or even months is usually characteristic of a *tension muscle contraction headache*.

Questions to Assess Symptoms	Rationales/Abnormal Findings
• Have you tried any treatments? How often do you take headache relievers or pain pills? Can you function without treatment? • Has there been any recent change in your headaches? **Neck Pain** • Where exactly is the pain? • How long have you had it? • On a scale of 1 to 10, how bad is it? • Describe the pain. • What makes it better? Worse? • What is your pain goal?	Neck pain can be from musculoskeletal injury, tension, or pathologic changes.
Limited Neck Movement. Are you having any difficulty turning or flexing/extending your neck?	Limitation of neck mobility may be from muscle tension/strain or cervical vertebral joint dysfunction.
Facial Pain • Where exactly is the pain? • How long have you had it? • On a scale of 1 to 10 how bad is it? • Describe the pain. • What makes it better? Worse? • What is your pain goal?	Trauma, infection, and neurologic disorders may result in facial pain, which also can be referred from another organ or system. Common causes of facial pain include muscle overuse, oral infections, sinusitis, herpes zoster, trauma, migraine or cluster headaches, jaw pain (if associated with shoulder or arm pain, this could be cardiac and requires immediate evaluation), skull pain, or skin lesions.
Lumps or Masses Have you noted any lumps or masses in your head or neck? • How long have you had this? • How many are there? • How large are any? • Are they changing? • Are they tender or painful?	Differentiate the many structures in the neck by careful questioning of the characteristics of any neck lump, followed by careful physical examination grounded in knowledge of the anatomy of this region.

(text continues on page 128)

Questions to Assess Symptoms	Rationales/Abnormal Findings
Hypothyroidism. Do you have any of these symptoms: fatigue; anorexia; cold intolerance; dry skin; brittle, coarse hair; menstrual irregularities; weight gain or difficulty losing weight; and decreased libido?	Signs and symptoms of thyroid dysfunction are often nonspecific. Nurses should consider that the patient has a thyroid problem when several symptoms are "clustered together." Metabolism is low.
Hyperthyroidism. Do you have any of these symptoms: fatigue; weight loss; anxiety; palpitations; rapid pulse; heat intolerance; fine, limp hair; diaphoresis; and muscle weakness?	Similarly, hyperthyroidism usually presents with several of these signs or symptoms. An overactive thyroid gland increases the metabolic rate.

Objective Data Collection

Equipment

- Ambient lighting
- Penlight or flashlight for tangential lighting
- Gloves, if any lesions of the scalp or skin of head and neck are suspected
- Small cup of water

Preparation

If the patient is wearing a wig or hairpiece, ask him or her to remove it. Wash your hands. The patient is usually seated, facing the examiner. Instruct the patient that the head and neck will be inspected, palpated, and manipulated, but that the procedures should not be painful. Instruct the patient to tell you if any part of the head and neck examination causes discomfort.

Comprehensive Physical Examination

Technique and Normal Findings	Abnormal Findings
Inspection Inspect the head (Fig. 7-1). *The head is centered, proportional to the body (1/7), erect, and without*	Facial asymmetry may indicate damage to CN VII or *stroke.* Enlarged bones or tissues are

tremors, tics, or unusual movements. *The skull is round without obvious deformities. The neck muscles are symmetric.*

associated with *acromegaly.* A puffy "moon" face is associated with *Cushing's syndrome.* Increased facial hair in females may indicate *Cushing's syndrome* or *endocrinopathy.* Periorbital edema occurs with *congestive heart failure* and *hypothyroidism* (*myxedema*). See Tables 7-1 and 7-2 at the end of this chapter.

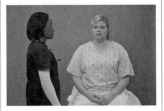

Figure 7.1 Inspecting the head.

Inspect facial features for symmetry and size. *Nasolabial folds are symmetric.*
Inspect the hair (Fig. 7-2) for distribution and quantity, texture, and cleanliness. *Hair is evenly distributed across the scalp, extending from the superior aspect of the forehead to the base of the cranium and to the top of the ears bilaterally.*

If asymmetric, look for signs of trauma. Carefully assess any lesions for infection. Male-pattern baldness occurs when there is both a genetic predisposition and increased testosterone or other male hormones. Adult men may present with baldness in either an "M" pattern on the scalp or, as hair loss continues, a "U" pattern with hair growth around the skull at the level of the temples. Unusual hair distribution and patterns of growth on the face or skull are associated with endocrine abnormalities. Nits attached to hair shafts may indicate *pediculosis* (head lice). See also Chapter 6.

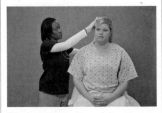

Figure 7.2 Examining the hair and scalp. The nurse wears gloves if there is any possibility of contact with an open sore or lesion.

(text continues on page 130)

Inspect the neck (Fig. 7-3). Look at the neck muscles, sternocleidomastoid, thyroid, and isthmus (may be visualized with tangential light and asking the patient to swallow a sip of water). *Trachea is midline. A slight symmetric elevation may be observed in the midneck.*

Thyroid enlargement or masses can be seen more easily when the patient swallows and while illuminating the neck with a tangential light.

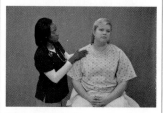

Figure 7.3 Inspecting the neck.

Palpation

Palpate the temporal artery above the cheek bone near the scalp line. *The temporal artery pulse is 2 to 3 on a 4-point scale.*

A biopsy is needed for diagnosis of *temporal arthritis*, painful inflammation of the temporal artery.

Palpate the scalp. Refer to Chapter 13. *Scalp is symmetric without tenderness, masses, lesions, or differences in firmness.*

Bulging or depression of the bony scalp may result from trauma or tumor. Bulging fontanels in infants may be a sign of *hydrocephalus*, or simply from crying (see Table 7-1). Depressed fontanels are most often associated with dehydration.

Palpate the thyroid. *If palpable, the thyroid is smooth, rubbery, nontender, symmetrical, and barely palpable beneath the sternocleidomastoid.*

For the **anterior approach**, have the patient tilt the head slightly back. Locate the thyroid cartilage, which is larger, shield-shaped, in the midneck and sometimes referred to as the "Adam's apple"

Technique and Normal Findings	Abnormal Findings

in males. Below is the ringed cricoid cartilage. Just below the cricoid cartilage the isthmus of the thyroid should be palpable as a smooth rubbery band that rises and falls with swallowing. With the pads of the fingers of one hand gently palpate the thyroid isthmus. Ask the patient to lower the head slightly and turn it slightly to one side. The sterno-cleidomastoid muscle will relax on the side to which the patient turns. Palpate behind the sterno-cleidomastoid muscle (Fig. 7-4).

- Unilateral bulging may be a thyroid *goiter*, cyst, or tumor. Neck masses may also originate from a lymph node or cyst.
- Any new neck mass in a patient older than 35 years should be carefully evaluated to rule out cancer. It could be a lymph node enlarged by metastasis, *primary lymphoma*, or neck tumor.
- Unusual hardness is a dangerous finding, associated with *cancer*.
- A toxic goiter may feel softer than normal thyroid tissue.
- Tenderness is common with *subacute infections*, traumatic injury, and *radiation thyroiditis*.

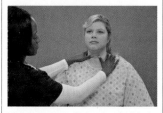

Figure 7.4 Palpating behind the sternocleidomastoid muscle for the anterior thyroid.

For the **posterior approach,** locate the thyroid and cricoid cartilages and the thyroid isthmus by palpation while standing behind the patient. Have the patient bend the head slightly forward and toward one side. Use your index finger to slightly retract the sternocleidomastoid muscle on the side toward which the patient has tilted the head. Use the middle two or three fingers to locate the lobe of the thyroid. The fingers of the other hand should gently displace the trachea and thyroid cartilage on

The parathyroid gland is not independently palpated but may be noted when attempting to

(text continues on page 132)

Technique and Normal Findings	Abnormal Findings

the opposite side, which helps move the thyroid gland slightly forward and prominent and allows for easier palpation. It is, however, not unusual for the thyroid lobes to also be nonpalpable with this approach (Fig. 7-5).

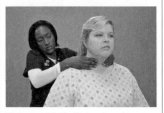

Figure 7.5 Palpating the thyroid from the posterior approach.

Systematically palpate for discernable lymph nodes in the head and neck (Fig. 7-6). Usual order of examination is preauricular, posterior auricular, the pads of the second, third, and fourth fingers to gently palpate with small circles, varying the amount of pressure over each lymphatic region. *No lymph nodes are palpable in the adult.* If a node is palpable, describe the following characteristics:
- Location—which lymphatic chain and where along that chain is the node
- Size—in mm or cm
- Consistency—how hard or soft? It should be smooth, slightly soft, and nontender.
- Mobility—it should be freely movable
- Delimitation—there should not be any matting together of lymph nodes

palpate the thyroid gland. *Parathyroid carcinoma* is a rare form of cancer. The tumors usually secrete parathyroid hormone, producing hyperparathyroidism and increased calcium levels. Parathyroid carcinoma may be suspected, but it usually cannot be confirmed prior to surgery.

Palpable, tender, and warm lymph nodes usually indicate an infection in the area from which the lymph vessels drain to that node:
- Anterior cervical nodes: *pharyngitis*
- Posterior cervical nodes: *mononucleosis*
- Posterior auricular nodes: *otitis media*
- Supraclavicular nodes: must be carefully evaluated as a possible sign of metastatic cancer. Virchow's node, the left supraclavicular, is associated with *lung and abdominal cancers*.
Hard, rubbery, irregular, fixed, and nontender lymph nodes are a possible sign of *lymphoma*.

| Technique and Normal Findings | Abnormal Findings |

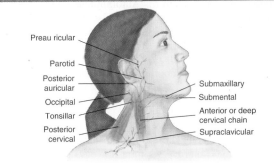

Figure 7.6 Location of lymph nodes.

Labels on figure:
- Preauricular
- Parotid
- Posterior auricular
- Occipital
- Tonsillar
- Posterior cervical
- Submaxillary
- Submental
- Anterior or deep cervical chain
- Supraclavicular

Technique and Normal Findings	Abnormal Findings
Auscultation If the thyroid is enlarged, either unilaterally or bilaterally, auscultate over each lobe for a bruit using the bell of the stethoscope. *No bruit or vascular sounds are audible.*	Bruits are most often found with a *toxic goiter, hyperthyroidism,* or *thyrotoxicosis.*

Documentation of Normal Subjective and Objective Findings

The patient reports no unusual, severe, or frequent headaches. Denies loss of neck mobility or neck pain. Denies any lumps or masses in the neck. Reports no problems with fatigue, weight change, temperature discomfort, skin changes, sweating, or other unusual findings. Thyroid gland is palpable, symmetric, smooth, rubbery, and nontender. No bruit.

▲ **Lifespan Considerations** ─────────────

Pregnant Women

Chloasma may be present on the face of pregnant women. This blotchy and hyperpigmented patch fades in the postpartum period.

Any enlargement of the thyroid gland in pregnant or postpartum women requires further investigation. Detection of thyroid problems is critical to prevent damage to fetal neural development, miscarriage, and preterm birth. Autoimmune thyroid disease is associated with both increased rates of miscarriage and postpartum thyroiditis. Postpartum women may experience slight enlargement of the thyroid. In *silent thyroiditis*, women present with signs and symptoms of hyperthyroidism, followed by hypothyroid symptoms. It may be several months before normal thyroid function returns.

Newborns and Infants

The newborn's head may be slightly asymmetrical, elongated, or both from skull molding during passage through the birth canal. Head shape becomes normal within a few days to weeks. A *caput succedaneum* is a swollen and ecchymotic area caused from squeezing of the head during birth. It usually resolves in the first few days. A *cephalohematoma* is a defined hemorrhage over one cranial bone. It appears shortly after birth, increases in size, and then resolves on its own; however, this infant is at risk for jaundice because of the breakdown of red blood cells.

Two *fontanels* (skull areas with a soft, nonossified matrix) enable the head and underlying structures to grow as the child develops. Assessing the size of the fontanels at each evaluation of the infant is important to determine timely ossification. The posterior fontanel closes by 3 months of age; the anterior fontanel closes by 18 months. Fontanels should be flat—neither bulging nor retracted. A bulging fontanel may be normal when an infant cries but otherwise needs further evaluation for increased intracranial pressure. A depressed fontanel may indicate dehydration. An unusual head shape may be noted if fontanels close prematurely but may also be from prolonged positioning of the infant in one way. Parents should change their infants' position regularly while babies are awake to enhance normal physical development. Infants should be able to hold up the head by 4 months of age.

Children and Adolescents

In children 1 to 5 years of age, small (<10 mm), nontender, movable nodes in the head and neck may be normally palpable. The thyroid gland and lymph nodes are usually nonpalpable in school-age children. Note any limitations in neck range of motion. If the child holds the head to one side with the chin pointing toward the opposite, the sternocleidomastoid muscle may be injured.

Older Adults

With aging, facial subcutaneous fat decreases, making the skeleton more pronounced. Skin may sag and wrinkle across the forehead, surrounding the eyes, at the tip of the nose, and on the cheeks. Thinning of the hair is also a normal aging process. The neck may have reduced range of motion with chronic conditions (eg, arthritis). Concave curve of the spine is exaggerated.

Cultural Considerations

The most noticeable difference among racial groups is skin color. Shape of the eyes, nose, and lips also varies based on background and genetics. Variations in skull or neck shape or size relate more to height and weight than to specific racial or cultural background.

Common Nursing Diagnoses and Interventions Associated with the Head and Neck

Diagnosis and Related Factors	Nursing Interventions
Activity intolerance related to hypothyroidism	Determine cause.* If appropriate gradually increase activity. Monitor response to activity. Refer patient to physical therapy.
Fatigue related to low T3 and high TSH	Assess severity. Evaluate sleep and nutritional status. Gather data to help determine if the cause is physiological or psychological.
Chronic pain related to cervical spine injury	Assess characteristics. Work with pain team to determine appropriate medical treatment. Use nonpharmacologic interventions.

*Collaborative interventions.

> ⚠️ **Table 7.1 Head and Neck Problems More Common in Childhood**

Hydrocephalus

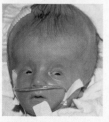

Collection of cerebrospinal fluid in the brain ventricles causes enlargement of the cranium. Affected infants may have separation of the cranial sutures, bulging fontanels, and dilated veins across the scalp.

Fetal Alcohol Syndrome (FAS)

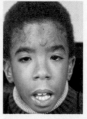

Maternal alcohol intake during pregnancy may result in developmental delays and congenital abnormalities in the child. Manifestations include microcephaly, flat cheekbones and upper lip, small eyes, and multiple developmental and learning disabilities.

Down's Syndrome (Trisomy 21)

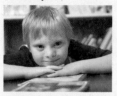

This congenital condition results from an extra chromosome 21 or translocation of chromosome 14 or 15 with 21 or 22. Manifestations include microcephaly, flattened occipital bone, slanted small eyes, depressed nasal bridge, low-set ears, and protruding tongue.

Cretinism (Congenital Hypothyroidism)

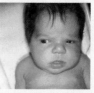

Affected infants have puffy facial features and often a larger than normal tongue. This syndrome is more common in parts of the world where diets are deficient in iodine.

Table 7.1   Head and Neck Problems More Common in Childhood (*continued*)

Torticollis

Congenital or acquired contraction of the sternocleidomastoid muscle causes the patient to incline the head to one side. Range of motion of the head and neck is decreased.

Craniocytosis

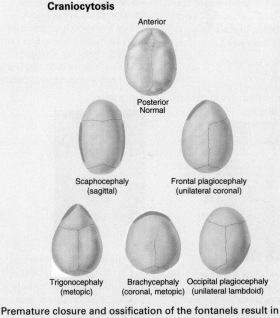

Anterior

Posterior
Normal

Scaphocephaly
(sagittal)

Frontal plagiocephaly
(unilateral coronal)

Trigonocephaly
(metopic)

Brachycephaly
(coronal, metopic)

Occipital plagiocephaly
(unilateral lambdoid)

Premature closure and ossification of the fontanels result in skull deformities and microcephaly. Early diagnosis and surgical correction minimize malformations.

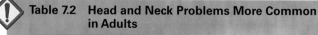

⚠️ **Table 7.2 Head and Neck Problems More Common in Adults**

Cushing's Syndrome

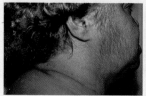

Excessive production of exogenous ACTH results in a round "moon" facies, fat deposits at the nape of the neck, "buffalo hump," and sometimes discoloration around the neck (*acanthosis nigra*).

Scleroderma

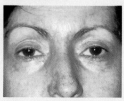

Hardening of the skin usually occurs first in the hands and face. Skin becomes firm and loses mobility, seemingly fixed to underlying tissues. Facial scleroderma presents with shiny taut immobile skin, making speaking, chewing, and swallowing difficult. It can affect other organs and tissues

Cerebral Vascular Accident (CVA/Stroke)

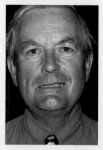

Also know as a "brain attack." Embolism, hemorrhage, or vasospasm in the brain results in ischemia of surrounding tissue and neuro logic damage. Symptoms depend on the part of the brain affected.

Bell's Palsy

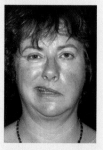

Paralysis, usually unilateral, of CN VII can be transient or permanent. Causes include trauma, compression, and infection.

Acromegaly

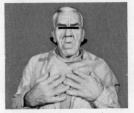

Overproduction of growth hormone in adults results in thickening of the skin, subcutaneous tissue, and facial bones and coarsening of facial features.

Parkinson's Disease

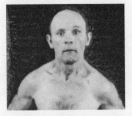

With this degenerative neurologic disease, patients present with a masklike facial appearance, rigid muscles, diminished reflexes, and a shuffling gait.

Myxedema

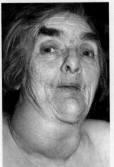

With severe hypothyroidism, patients present with periorbital swelling and edema of the face, hands, and feet. These patients must be identified and treated quickly and chronically with exogenous thyroid hormone.

Goiter

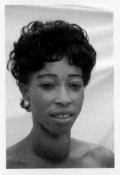

Enlarged thyroid gland can be associated with hyperthyroidism, hypothyroidism, or normal thyroid function. Enlargement can compress other structures in the neck, making surgical removal necessary. After thyroidectomy patients must be treated with exogenous thyroid hormone for the rest of their lives.

Eyes Assessment

Key Topics and Questions for Health Promotion

Key Questions	Rationales
Current Problems. Are you having any eye problems now?	This general question opens discussion.
Family History. Do any family members have myopia, hyperopia, strabismus, color blindness, cataracts, glaucoma, retinitis pigmatosa, or retinoblastoma?	Some conditions and diseases that affect vision have a genetic or familial link (eg, *glaucoma*).
Personal History **Eye Conditions** • Do you have a history of cataracts, glaucoma, high blood pressure, diabetes, or thyroid disease? • Do you have any history of eye injury? • Have you had injuries or accidents, foreign bodies, or trauma to your eyes?	The focus is conditions that could affect vision and eye function.
Eye Surgery • Have you ever had surgery on your eye(s)? • Have you ever had any facial surgery? • Have you ever had cataract removal, lens implant, or LASIK?	The focus is eye or facial surgeries, which can change the landscape of eye structures.

Key Questions	Rationales

Medications. Do you use artificial tears, decongestants, corticosteroids, antibiotics, antihistamines, or any prescribed eye drops?

These medications can affect the eye and its functioning.

Risk Factors
Allergies
- Do you have any allergies?
- Are they seasonal?
- Are your eyes sensitive to pollen or animal dander?
- How do you react to insect stings/bites: any swelling around the eyes?

Response to allergens can affect the eyes through excessive tearing, allergic conjunctivitis, and itching. Insect stings/bites may lead to periorbital edema and erythema. Previous occurrences increase risk with repeat exposure.

Exposure to Viruses. Has anyone ever told you that you were exposed to rubella in the womb? Were you diagnosed with congenital syphilis?

Fetal exposure to rubella and congenital syphilis can lead to eye problems, including cataracts and blindness.

Environmental Exposure
- Are you exposed to toxins, chemicals, infections, or allergens at work?
- How would you relate your current stress level: low, moderate, or high?

Many activities can increase risk for eye injury, infections, or trauma. Stress has been linked with decreased vision.

Eye Health
- When was your last eye examination?
- Were you screened for glaucoma?

The nurse needs to determine how the patient cares for the health of the eyes.

Corrective Prescriptions
- Do you wear glasses and/or contacts?
- Do you wear contacts for the recommended time frame only?
- How do care for your contacts?
- How often do you change your contacts?

These questions address risks based on *Healthy People* goals to reduce the number of people with uncorrected refractive errors.

(text continues on page 142)

Key Questions	Rationales
Eye Protection • Are you exposed to any hazards that could affect your eyes? • Do you wear goggles or a face shield when you play sports or do home projects? • Do you wear your protective eyewear 100% of the time?	Questions address *Healthy People* goals to reduce injuries to the eyes of people whose occupation or leisure activities put them at risk.
Nutritional Status. Do you generally eat a well-balanced diet?	Assess for any vitamin deficiencies that could affect the eyes.

Health-Promotion Teaching

Diabetes mellitus increases risks for diabetic retinopathy, cataracts, and glaucoma. Sunlight exposure also increases risks, so use of sunglasses is important, especially if the patient lives in a sunny climate. Poor diet has been linked to eye problems. Foods that promote eye health include deep-water fish, fruits, and vegetables (eg, carrots, spinach). Because the lens has no blood supply, staying well-hydrated keeps the lens supple and moist.

Key Topics and Questions for Common Symptoms

In assessing the patient's health history, it is important to immediately determine if an eye problem results from trauma, is related to changes in vision, or involves visual symptoms. Failure to obtain an accurate and complete history can lead to loss of sight.

Common Eye Symptoms

• Pain	• Discharge
• Trauma	• Change in activities of daily
• Visual change	living (ADLs)
• Blind spots, floaters, or halos	

Questions for Common Symptoms	Rationale/Abnormal Findings
Pain. Do you have any eye pain or discomfort? (Ask about location, intensity, duration, description, aggravating factors, alleviating factors, functional impairment, and pain goal.)	Pain in the eye is never normal and should always be further explored.
Trauma or Surgery. Is your problem related to trauma or an injury? • How was the injury/trauma sustained? • Was this a high-velocity injury? • Was this a blunt force trauma?	High-velocity injuries are typically penetrating. Blunt force trauma often results in fracture of the orbit.
Visual Change. Have you noticed any recent changes to your vision? • What is the nature of it? • When did the change begin? • Was onset sudden or gradual? • Have you noticed any double vision or halos/rainbows around objects?	If the patient describes loss of vision, it is critical to ascertain a timeline. Sudden vision loss requires an emergent referral.
Blind Spots, Floaters, or Halos. Have you noticed any blind spots? • Any difficulty seeing at night? • Do you see any spots (floaters)? • Do you have associated symptoms (eg, flashing lights, floaters, halos around lights)?	Loss of night vision is associated with *optic atrophy, glaucoma*, and *vitamin A deficiency*. Floaters (translucent specks that drift across the visual field) are common in people older than 40 years and nearsighted patients. No additional follow-up is needed.
Discharge. Are you having any eye discharge? • Is there any pain or grittiness, redness, or discharge associated? • Are one or both eyes affected? • Have you noticed any excessive tearing, dryness, or itching?	Discharge is associated with inflammation or infection.
Change in ADLs. How has your eye problem (eg, diplopia, dry eyes) affected your ability to perform ADLs?	Assess functional limitations.

Objective Data Collection

Equipment

- Penlight
- Cotton wisps and cotton-tipped applicators
- Ophthalmoscope
- Snellen chart for far-vision testing
- Jaeger chart for near-vision testing
- Occlusive covers for individual eye testing
- Ishihara plates (optional for testing color vision)

Technique and Normal Findings	Abnormal Findings
Visual Acuity Visual acuity tests include testing for distance, near, peripheral, and color vision. Perform these before using any solution to dilate the pupil.	
Distance Vision. Has the patient read the Snellen or Allen chart (based on age or reading ability). Give the patient an opaque card or eye occluder so that he or she can cover one eye at a time during assessment. Stand by the chart and request that the patient reads through it to the smallest letters (or pictures) possible, occluding one eye at a time. Request that the patient reads the next smallest line. If the patient wears lenses, they should remain on; only reading glasses should be removed for the assessment. Acuity for distance vision is documented in two numbers, with reference to what a person with normal vision sees 20 ft from the test.	Abnormal findings include leaning forward, squinting, hesitation, misidentification of more than three of seven objects, or more than a two-line difference between eyes. Refer to Table 8-1, Refractive Errors, at the end of this chapter.

Technique and Normal Findings	Abnormal Findings

Someone with "20/20" (normal) vision can read at 20 ft what the normal eye can read at 20 ft. On top, mark the distance in feet the patient was from the test (eg, 20). On bottom, mark the number under the smallest line the patient correctly identified (eg, 40, 200). Also document the number of letters missed and if patient wore corrective lenses. The larger the bottom number, the worse the visual acuity. *Refractive index is 20/20 bilaterally.*

Near Vision. Near vision is usually assessed in patients older than 40 years or younger patients who report difficulty reading. If no Jaeger test (pocket screener) is available, ask the patient to read newsprint (eg, newspaper, magazine).

Patients older than 40 years often have a decreased ability to accommodate; therefore, they move the card further away to read it.

Instruct the patient to hold the Jaeger chart 14 inches (35 cm) from the eye. The person should read through to the smallest letters possible, occluding one eye at a time (with corrective lenses on) (Fig. 8-1). *Near vision is 14/14 bilaterally.*

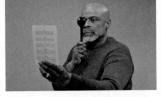

Figure 8.1 Assessing near vision.

Color Vision. Color vision is assessed with Ishihara cards (Fig. 8-2) or by having the patient identify color bars on the Snellen chart. *The patient correctly identifies embedded figures or colors bars.*

A patient who incorrectly identifies the embedded figures or color bars may have color blindness.

(text continues on page 146)

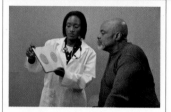

Figure 8.2 Testing color vision.

Visual Fields

Visual field refers to what is visible in the environment when the eye fixates on a stationary object. When evaluating for visual field defects, the visual field is divided into four quadrants—inferior, superior, left, and right.

Visual injury or disease usually causes defects in the normal full visual field.

Static Confrontation. The static test can detect gross differences in all four quadrants and effectively screens for differences from side-to-side (hemianopias) and inferior and superior (attitudinal). The examiner does not move the fingers but presents one to four fingers in each quadrant.

Stand 2 to 3 ft (an arm's length) directly in front of the patient. Your eyes and the patient's eyes should be on the same level. Ask the patient to cover the left eye with the palm of the left hand (without applying pressure). Close your right eye and instruct the patient to look only at your open eye at all times. Present one to four fingers midway between yourself and the patient in each of the four field quadrants (Fig. 8-3).

This screening test assumes that the nurse's visual field is normal and serves as the comparison for the patient's test.

Technique and Normal Findings	Abnormal Findings

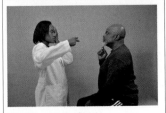

Figure 8.3 Static confrontation test.

Ask the patient to report the number of fingers, without looking directly at them. Repeat the test with the other eye. The *patient accurately reports the number of fingers presented in all four quadrants.*

Reports of an incorrect number of fingers indicate a visual field defect.

Kinetic Confrontation. The kinetic test assesses the gross peripheral boundaries of the visual field. It is performed when the nurse moves an object or fingers from the periphery toward fixation at the point that the patient first becomes aware of the target. As with static confrontation, your eyes and the patient's eyes must be on the same level. Instruct the patient to say "now" when the fingers first come into view. Wiggle your fingers from a far distal point and move them toward the center of each quadrant (Fig. 8-4). Your fingers should not be immediately visible (except in the inferotemporal quadrant). The *patient sees the fingers at about the same time as the nurse if the peripheral visual field is normal in that quadrant.*

A patient who sees fingers presented on either side only on one side may have a hemianopic defect. If the patient sees only from an inferior or superior position, an attitudinal defect is suspected.

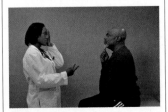

Figure 8.4 Kinetic confrontation test.

(text continues on page 148)

Technique and Normal Findings	Abnormal Findings
Extraocular Muscle Movements Three basic tests assess movements of the eye in several planes: up and down, side-to-side, diagonally from right superior to left inferior, and diagonally from left superior to right inferior (Fig. 8-5).	

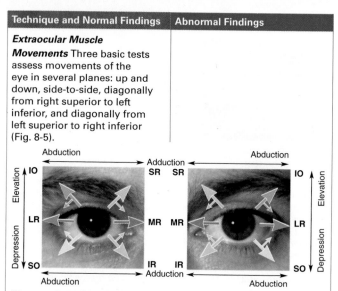

Figure 8.5 Extraocular movements.

Corneal Light Reflex. To test for strabismus, instruct the patient to stare straight ahead at the bridge of your nose. Stand in front of the patient and shine a penlight at the bridge of the patient's nose. Note where the light reflects on each cornea (Fig. 8-6). *Light reflection is in exactly the same spot in both eyes.*	Abnormal findings indicate improper alignment and appear as asymmetric reflections. Document abnormal findings using the face of the clock as a guide.

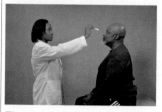

Figure 8.6 Testing corneal light reflex.

Technique and Normal Findings	Abnormal Findings
Cover Test. To assess ocular alignment, stand in front of the patient and ask him or her to focus on a near object movement of the uncovered eye that may indicate refixation of the gaze. Remove the cover and observe the previously covered eye for refixation. Repeat the procedure for the other eye. *Gaze is steady and fixed.*	Any refixation is from muscle weakness in the covered eye (ie, while covered the eye drifted into a relaxed position).
Cardinal Fields of Gaze. Further testing of the extraocular muscles assesses for symmetrical movements of the eyes in all nine cardinal fields of gaze. Tell the patient to hold the head steady and to follow the movement of your finger or pen with the eyes. Hold your finger or pen approximately 12 to 14 inches from the patient's face. Move slowly through position 2–9, stopping momentarily in each, then back to center. Proceed clockwise. The *patient's eyes move smoothly and symmetrically in all fields of gaze.*	Document a deficit by noting in which field there is an abnormality. Mild nystagmus at the extreme lateral angles is normal; in any other position it is not.

External Eyes

Stand directly in front of and facing the patient. Inspect eyebrows, lashes, and eyelids; note eye shape and symmetry.

Eyebrows show no unexplained hair loss. Lashes curve outward away from the eyes and are distributed evenly along the lid margins. Eyelids open and close completely, with spontaneous blinking every few seconds. Eye shape varies from round to almond but is symmetrical. | **Eyebrows:** Unexplained hair loss; with normal aging, the outer third of the eyebrow thins

Eyelashes: Curved inward away toward the eye, distributed unevenly along lid margin, or both

Eyelids: Incomplete opening or closing; no spontaneous blinking; improper positioning with respect to iris and limbus

Eye shape: Asymmetry |

(text continues on page 150)

Technique and Normal Findings	Abnormal Findings
Note general appearance of the eyes. *Eyes are in parallel alignment.*	Eyes not in parallel alignment require further assessment. **Ptosis**, drooping of the eyelids, is a common finding with **stroke** (Fig. 8-7).

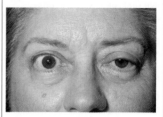

Figure 8.7 Ptosis.

Lacrimal Apparatus. Inspect and palpate the lacrimal apparatus (if the patient reports eye fatigue or dry eyes). Identify the punctual opening at the inner canthus. Use your thumb to gently stretch the bottom eyelids downward. Gently press your index finger against the nasolacrimal sac (Fig. 8-8). *Lacrimal apparatus is not enlarged or tender.*	An enlarged lacrimal apparatus is rare. If you palpate an enlarged lacrimal apparatus, evert the eyelid and inspect the gland. Suspect conditions such as *sarcoid disease* and *Sjögren's syndrome* (Fig. 8-9).

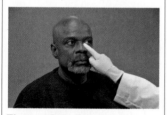

Figure 8.8 Palpating the lacrimal apparatus.

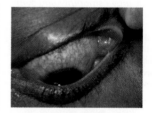

Figure 8.9 Sjögren's syndrome.

Bulbar Conjunctiva. Gently lift the upper eyelid. Instruct the patient to look down and then to the right and left. Note the surface for color, injection (redness), swelling, exudates,	Erythema, cobblestone appearance, or both may indicate allergy or infection. Sharply defined bright red blood indicates a *subconjunctival hemorrhage* (Fig. 8-10).

Technique and Normal Findings	Abnormal Findings

or foreign bodies. Gently stretch down the lower lid. Instruct the patient to look up and to the right and left. Again note the surface for color, redness, swelling, exudates, or foreign bodies. *Bulbar conjunctiva is normally transparent with small blood vessels visible*.

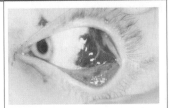

Figure 8.10 Subconjunctival hemorrhage.

Abnormal thickening of the conjunctiva from the limbus over the cornea is known as a *pterygium* (Fig. 8-11). Risk for development is heavy exposure to ultraviolet light, most commonly in equatorial areas.

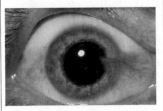

Figure 8.11 Pterygium.

Sclera. During inspection of the bulbar conjunctiva you can also inspect the sclera for color, exudates, lesions, and foreign bodies. *Sclera is clear, smooth, and white*.

Scleral abnormalities include jaundice, bluing, and drainage. Refer to Table 8-2 at the end of this chapter.

Exterior Ocular Structures

Cornea and Lens. Stand in front of the patient. Use a penlight or ophthalmoscope split light to inspect the cornea. Shine the light directly on the cornea.

A narrow angle indicates *glaucoma*.

(text continues on page 152)

Technique and Normal Findings	Abnormal Findings
Move the light laterally toward the bridge of the nose. Repeat on the other eye. Observe the angle of the anterior space and the clarity and translucence of the lens. *A normal angle allows full illumination of the iris. Lens is transparent.*	Cloudiness of the lens can indicate a *cataract,* which is associated with increased age, smoking, alcohol intake, and sunlight exposure. Risk factors for cataracts are primarily environmental. See also Table 8-2.
Iris. Inspect for color, nodules, and vascularity. *Color is even, smooth, and without apparent vascularity. A normal variation is mosaic.*	See Table 8-2.
Pupils. Stand in front of the patient. Use your light to observe the pupil shape and size (mm). *Pupil is black, round, and equal with a diameter of 2 to 6 mm.* Gently place your open hand along the patient's nose. Shine the light into the right eyes, as you observe pupillary constriction (direct) (CNIII) (Fig. 8-12). Repeat, except observing the left eye for pupillary constriction (consensual) (CN III). Repeat these two procedures in the left eye. *Pupils constrict directly and consensually.*	See Table 8-3 at the end of this chapter for abnormal pupils. 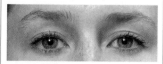 **Figure 8.12** Pupillary constriction.
To test for accommodation (CN III), instruct the patient to stare at a distant object for 30 seconds. Hold an index finger or penlight about 14 inches (10 cm) in front of the nose. Ask the patient to focus on your finger, as you move it toward the patient's nose (Fig. 8-13). *Pupils constrict (accommodation) and eyes cross (converge).*	Accommodation is necessary for far-to-near focus. Documentation of this sequence of assessments is easily accomplished with the acronym PERRLA: Pupils Equal, Round, Reactive to Light, and Accommodation. Several abnormalities can be seen in the pupil during assessment. See Table 8-3. 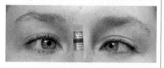 **Figure 8.13** Accommodation.

Internal Ocular Structures

Examination of internal ocular structures is in the domain of the advanced practice nurse (APRN). The ophthalmoscope has some basic features that make inspecting the interior ocular structures easier. See Box 8-1.

First set the ophthalmoscope on the 0 lens and aperture on small round light. When examining the right eye, grasp the ophthalmoscope in your right hand and then turn on the light source. When examining the left eye, grasp the ophthalmoscope in the left hand. This helps you to avoid bumping noses with the patient.

Ask the patient to focus on a distant object across the room. Place your hand on the patient's head, which puts you about 2 ft from the

---

BOX 8.1 USING THE OPHTHALMOSCOPE

*T*he ophthalmoscope contains (1) a light source, (2) viewing aperture, and (3) a lens refraction adjustment. These features allow nurses to direct the light source toward the pupil by looking through the viewing aperture.

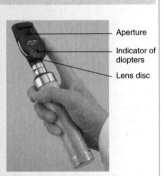

Aperture

Indicator of diopters

Lens disc

The *aperture*, which has a lens selector wheel, allows for adjustment of refraction to bring the internal ocular structures into sharp focus, compensating for refractive errors of the patient or nurse. The aperture is set on large for the dilated pupil or small for the constricted pupil. The slit aperture is used to examine the anterior portion of the eye and evaluate lesions at the fundal level. The grid feature is used to locate and describe fundal-level lesions. The green beam (red-free filter) is often used to evaluate retinal hemorrhaging (which appears black with this filter) or melanin spots (which appear gray).

Proper inspection of the posterior ocular structures with an ophthalmoscope requires slight dilation of the pupils. The optometrist or ophthalmologist will often use mydriatic eye drops, which are short-acting ciliary muscle paralytics that dilate the pupil. However, accommodation reflexes may be lost with the use of eye drops. Mydriatic drops are not used if a neurological assessment is necessary, because they may obscure pupil size and reactivity parameters used to determine neurological status.

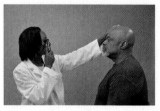

Figure 8.14 Ophthalmoscopic positioning.

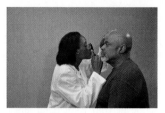

Figure 8.15 Inspecting anterior ocular structures.

patient. From an angle of 15 degrees lateral to the patient's line of vision, shine the ophthalmoscope toward the pupil of the right eye (Fig. 8-14).

Look through the ophthalmoscope's viewing hole. Note and focus on the red reflex. Now, move toward the patient until you are about 10 inches (25 cm) away from the patient's forehead. Move the lens selector from 0 to the + or black numbers to focus on the anterior ocular structures. Inspect for transparency (Fig. 8-15). Now move the lens selector from the + black numbers to the – or red numbers to focus on structures progressively more posterior.

Adjust the focus with an index finger on the lens focus until the retina comes into focus. Look toward the nasal side of the retina. If you are having difficulty, ask the patient to look toward the right. Inspect the prominent optic disc.

The direct ophthalmoscope technique is difficult to master and takes months of practice. The easiest way to find the optic disc is to find a blood vessel and then follow it back to its origin at the optic disc. Inspect the shape (round or oval), color (creamy yellow-orange to pink), disc margins (distinct and sharply demarcated), and size of the disc cupping (brighter yellow-white than rest of disc) (Fig. 8-16).

The blood vessels can be directly observed in the retina. Systemic diseases of the body are often reflected in the blood vessels and can be directly observed in the eye. When examining the vascularity of the eye, make note of the number, color, artery-to-vein ratio, tortuousity, and arteriovenous (AV) crossing. Also make note of the ratio of arteries to veins width, which is normally 2:3 or 4:5.

The final retinal structure to be assessed is the macula. Move the ophthalmoscope approximately two disc diameters (2DD) temporally to view the macula. You can also ask the patient to look at the light. It can be difficult to find because the macula is light sensitive. You may find that turning the aperture to green light (red-light filter) may

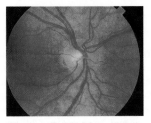

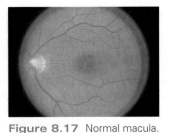

Figure 8.16 Normal optic disc.

Figure 8.17 Normal macula.

make it easier to assess. The macula is a darker, avascular area with an ophthalmoscope light reflective center known as the fovea centralis. The color of the macula varies with ethnicity and age (Fig. 8-17).

Review the structures and what you are looking for:

- **Disc**: What is the cup-to-disc ratio? Do the rims look pink and healthy?
- **Vessels**: Any signs of AV nicking?
- **Macula**: Does it look flat? Is there a good light reflex off the surface?
- **Periphery**: Any lattice or tears?

See Table 8-4 at the end of this chapter.

Documentation of Normal Subjective and Objective Eye Findings

The patient denies pain, trauma, visual changes, blind spots, floaters, halos, and discharge. No changes in the ability to perform ADLs. Visual acuity 20/20. The patient accurately reads newsprint. The patient identifies color bars on Snellen chart correctly. The patient sees the finger at about 50 degrees superior, 90 degrees temporal, 90 degrees inferior, and 60 degrees nasal. Alignment symmetrical/corneal light reflex. Gaze fixed and steady. EOMs intact. Eyebrows full and appropriate to age. Eyelashes evenly distributed. Blinking every 2 to 3 seconds. Eyes round, symmetrical, and in parallel alignment. Lacrimal apparatus not enlarged or tender. Conjunctiva with small vessels visible. Sclera clear and white. Lens is transparent. Iris is brown, smooth, and without vascularity. PERRLA.

▲ Lifespan Considerations ————————————

Pregnant Women

The most common eye problem during pregnancy is dry eyes from decreased conjuctival capillaries. Corneal thickening can make use of contact lenses uncomfortable. Corneal curvature also may increase. Visual field changes may be related to the pituitary gland affecting the optic nerve. Decreased intraocular pressure is significant if the woman has glaucoma; adjustment of medications may be necessary. Chloasma around the eyes may result from increased progesterone levels.

Newborns, Infants, Children, and Adolescents

At birth, the visual system is the least mature sensory system. Development progresses rapidly over the first 6 months and reaches adult level by 4 to 5 years. Newborns are sensitive to light and often keep their eyes closed for long periods. Ability to focus is limited, but by age 3 months they can follow objects. The pupils are reactive to light, the blink reflex is intact, and the corneal reflex is easily stimulated.

Assess vision in infants through testing for pupillary light reflex and observing behavior. Assess a toddler's visual acuity through the Allen test, which uses picture cards of common objects. Normal findings in toddlers are 20/200 bilaterally. In preschool children (3 to 5 years old), assess visual acuity with the Snellen E chart, with normal findings being 20/40 and improving to 20/30 or better by 4 years. The Snellen E chart is used to assess visual acuity in school-age children until the children acquire reading skills. By 5 to 6 years of age, normal visual acuity should approximate that of adults or 20/20 in both eyes. Children should be screened for color blindness between 4 and 8 years of age. Depth perception develops throughout childhood. Vision changes, such as nearsightedness, are common in adolescents.

Older Adults

Older adults have changes both in eye structures and vision. Eyelids may droop and become wrinkled from loss of skin elasticity. The eyes sit deeper in the orbits from loss of subcutaneous fat. Eyebrows become thinner, and the outer thirds of the brows may be absent. Conjunctivae are thinner and may appear yellowish from decreased perfusion. The iris may have an irregular pigmentation. Tearing decreases as a result of loss of fatty tissue in the lacrimal apparatus. Vision may decline. Because the pupil is smaller, there is loss of accommodation, decreased night vision, and decreased depth perception. The lens enlarges and transparency decreases.

Visual impairments can begin to affect the older adult's functional capacity, decreasing the ability to drive and perform usual activities. Cataracts and age-related macular degeneration (AMD) are the two leading causes of loss of vision and blindness in the United States and are diseases primarily seen in the elderly. Glaucoma is also more common with increased age.

Cultural Considerations

Eye color differs among people of various genetic backgrounds, with lighter eyes more prevalent in more Northern countries. Genetic background also influences the diameters of eyelids and eyebrows. Variations are found in the sclera: in light-skinned people, the sclera appears white with some superficial vessels. In dark-skinned people, the sclera often has tiny brown patches or is grayish-blue. African Americans are at a significantly higher risk for glaucoma compared to other races.

Common Nursing Diagnoses and Interventions Associated with the Eyes

Diagnosis and Related Factors	Nursing Interventions
Disturbed sensory perception related to vision disturbance	Converse with and touch the patient frequently. Use lighting for reading. Use a magnifying glass for shaving or to apply makeup.
Risk for injury related to impaired vision	Refer to the optometrist for corrective lenses. Ensure that the patient wears lenses and that eyeglasses are clean. Make sure that objects are out of the path. Remove hazards from room, such as razors and matches.

*Collaborative interventions.

Tables of Reference

Table 8.1   Refractive Errors

Asthenopia (Eye Strain)

Eye strain develops after reading, computer work, or other visually tedious tasks from tightening of the eye muscles after maintaining a constant focal distance. Symptoms include fatigue, red eyes, eyestrain, pain in or around the eyes, blurred vision, headaches, and, rarely, double vision.

Astigmatism

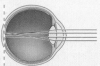

Focal point of light rays: multiple areas of the retina

Abnormal (football-shaped) curvature of the cornea prevents light from focusing on the retina. Images appear blurred because not all optical planes are focused. This condition is corrected with a cylindrical lens that has more focusing power in one access than the other.

Myopia (Nearsightedness)

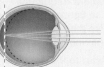

Focal point of light rays: in front of the retina

Images of distant objects focus in front of, instead of on, the retina from an imperfection in the shape of the eye or lens. People with myopia can see clearly objects up close but have difficulty seeing distant objects. Myopia is corrected with a concave lens that moves the focus back to the retina.

Hyperopia (Farsightedness)

Focal point
of light rays:
behind the
retina

Images of near objects focus behind, instead of on, the retina from an imperfection in the shape of the eye or lens. People with it can see distant objects clearly but have difficulty seeing objects up close. A convex lens is used to treat hyperopia, moving the focus forward onto the retina.

Presbyopia

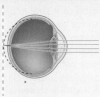

Focal point
of light rays:
behind
the retina

This symptom, considered a natural part of aging, is believed to result from loss of elasticity of the crystalline lens. As this happens, the ciliary muscles that bend and straighten the lens lose their power to accommodate. This condition affects near vision and therefore is corrected with a convex lens in front of the eye in the form half-glass or as bottom of a bifocal or multifocal lens if other correction is needed for distance viewing.

Color Blindness

Color blindness (inability to distinguish colors) has a genetic component. The cones of the eye, located in the macula, contain blue, green, a nd red pigments that allow color sight. Color blindness results with damage to the cones or a cone that has missing pigment. The most common form is the red/green. No effective treatment for color blindness exists.

(table continues on page 160)

Table 8.1 Refractive Errors (*continued*)

Blindness

Blindness means loss of vision or visual acuity that cannot be corrected with glasses or contact lenses. Partial blindness refers to those with very limited vision; complete blindness means an inability to see anything, including light. People with vision worse than 20/200 are classified as legally blind in most U.S. states.

Table 8.2 External Eye Abnormalities

Chalazion

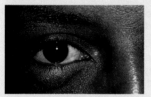

A cyst (meibomian gland lipogranuloma) in the eyelid resulting from inflammation of the meibomian gland. Sometimes confused with a hordeolum (stye), it can be differentiated because it is usually painless and tends to be larger.

Iris Nevus

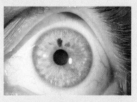

Rare condition affecting one eye, with abnormalities in appearance of the iris, pain, and decreased vision; patients may also have glaucoma on the same side

Blepharitis

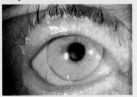

Inflammation of the margin of the eyelid. Most common type is seborrheic, followed by staphylococcal, and then rosacea-associated

Jaundice

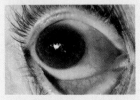

Yellowing of the sclera, which indicates liver disease

Exophthalmos

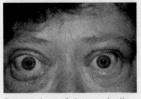

Protrusion of the eyeball anteriorly out of the socket. The most common cause is a thyroid disorder known as Graves' disease.

Bacterial Conjunctivitis

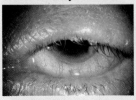

Should be suspected if there is purulent discharge (yellow or green), injected (red), and numerous follicles. Occasional blurring is common

Hyphema

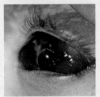

Blood in the anterior chamber of the eye, usually caused by blunt trauma

Hordelum (Stye)

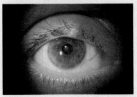

Caused by a blockage and infection of the sebaceous gland at the base of the eyelashes. While painful and unsightly, generally has no lasting damage

(table continues on page 162)

Allergic Conjunctivitis

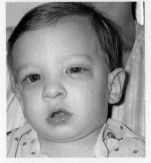

Usually bilateral and common in people with ectopic (allergic) conditions; associated with slight watery discharge and itching of the eyes

Viral Conjunctivitis

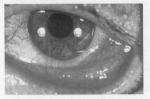

Most often associated with a watery discharge from the eye that may be accompanied by sinus congestion and rhinorrhea (runny nose), slightly injected (diffusely pink), and numerous follicles on the inferior conjunctiva

Osteogenesis Imperfecta

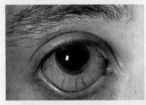

A blue sclera is due to a thinning of the sclera and is indicative of osteogenesis imperfecta.

Cataracts

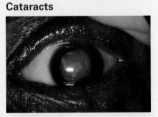

Opacity of the crystalline lens of the eye, which obstructs the passage of light. The most common causes are long-term exposure to ultraviolet light, radiation, diabetes, hypertension, and advanced age

Glaucoma

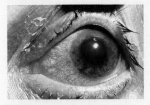

The leading cause of irreversible blindness and most common chronic optic neuropathy. Disease of the optic nerve that involves loss of retinal ganglion cells. A significant risk factor is increased intraocular pressure. Impaired flow of aqueous humor leads to increased intraocular pressure.

Amblyopia (Lazy Eye)

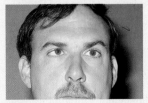

Condition in which the vision in one eye is reduced because the eye and brain are not working together. It is the most common cause of visual impairment in children. The eye upon examination looks normal, but vision is not normal because the brain is favoring the other eye.

⚠ **Table 8.3   Abnormal Findings in the Pupil**

Key Hole Pupil (Coloboma)

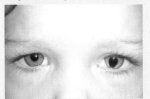

A gap appears in the iris. It can be congenital or caused during cataract or glaucoma surgery.

Miosis (Small Fixed Pupil)

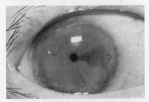

Pupils are constricted and fixed. Miosis occurs with eye drops for glaucoma, iritis, brain damage to pons, and narcotic drug use.

(table continues on page 164)

Anisocoria (Unequal Pupils)

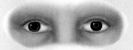

These usually result from a defect in the efferent nervous pathways controlling the oculomotor nerve.

Argyle Robertson

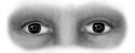

Bilateral pupils accommodate but do not dilate when exposed to bright light. Direct and consensual pupil reflexes are absent.

Mydriasis (Dilated Fixed Pupil)

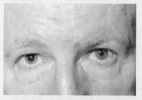

Pupils are dilated and fixed, usually from eye drops or stimulation of sympathetic nerves as a consequence of CNS injury, circulatory arrest, deep anesthesia, acute glaucoma, or recent trauma.

Horner's Syndrome

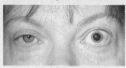

Pupillary miosis (constricted pupil) and dilation lag on the affected side. Also often present is ptosis.

Adie's Pupil

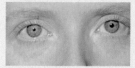

Pupils are fixed, dilated, and tonic. Direct and consensual pupil reactions are weak or absent.

Oculomotor (CN III) Nerve Damage

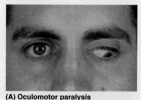

(A) Oculomotor paralysis

(B) Abducent paralysis

A unilateral dilated pupil has no reaction to light or accommodation.

Age-related Macular Degeneration (AMD)

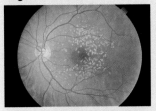

AMD gradually causes loss of sharp central vision, needed for common daily tasks (eg, driving, reading). The macula degenerates (dry) or abnormal blood vessels behind the retina grow under the macula (wet). The more common dry AMD occurs slowly in stages: early, intermediate, and advanced. Wet AMD develops quickly without stages.

Retinopathy

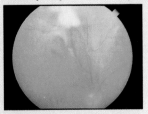

Retinopathy occurs from damage to retinal blood vessels. The two most common causes are diabetes and hypertension. *Diabetic retinopathy* is the most common cause of blindness in the United States. *Hypertensive retinopathy* presents with a dry retina, while diabetic retinopathy presents with a wet retina.

Retinitis Pigmentosa

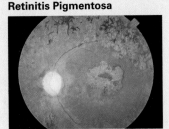

In this genetically transmitted disease, the retinas in both eyes progressively degenerate. It starts with loss of night vision, then loss of peripheral vision, progressing to tunnel vision, and finally no vision.

(table continues on page 166)

Table 8.4   Retinal Abnormalities (*continued*)

Copper Wiring

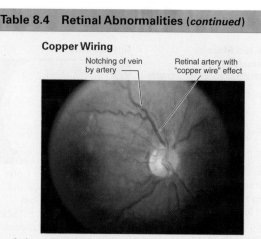

Notching of vein by artery —

Retinal artery with "copper wire" effect

Chronic hypertension causes the retinal arterioles to thicken. The name *copper wiring* comes from the initial bronze appearance of the retina light reflection. As uncontrolled hypertension continues, the retina takes on a silvery or whitish appearance.

Ears Assessment

Key Topics and Questions for Health Promotion

Questions on History and Risk	Rationales
Family History. What is your family's history of ear or hearing problems, if any? • Who had the illness? • What was the illness? • When did the person have it? • How was the illness treated? • What were the outcomes?	Identifying a family history of possible inherited and chronic disorders (eg, *Meniere's disease, otosclerosis*) is important in determining the patient's risk and providing anticipatory guidance.
Personal History. How do you protect your skin from the sun? • How often do you wear a hat? • How often do you apply sunscreen? • What SPF is the sunscreen you use? • When are you usually in the sun? • How long are you in the sun?	The ear is commonly forgotten when it comes to sun protection. Melanomas are commonly found in the head and neck region, including the external ear.
Have you been diagnosed with ear infections, hearing loss, tinnitus, or vertigo? (Explore the specific illness, when it occurred, how it was treated, and its outcomes.)	In children, ear infections are extremely prevalent. Children are at risk for tympanic membrane rupture, scarring, and hearing loss.

(text continues on page 168)

167

Questions on History and Risk	Rationales
Provide details on any ear-related surgeries you have had, including any complications or lasting effects (sequela).	Surgeries may be performed for artificial eustachian tube placement, tympanic membrane repair, and cochlear implants. Ear surgery increases the risk of exposure to ototoxic drugs (eg, aminoglycosides).
Medications. What prescription and over-the-counter medications are you taking? • How often do you take them? • What dosage? • What route?	Several drugs have possible adverse effects on the ears. Examples of ototoxic agents include all aminoglycosides, anti-inflammatory agents, antimalarials, diuretics, nonnarcotic analgesics with salicylates, antipyretics with salicylates, quinidine sulfate, erythromycin, and antineoplastic drugs.
What immunizations have you received? • What were your last vaccinations? • Have you received all required doses?	*Mumps* can cause sensorineural deafness in those who have not been vaccinated, did not develop immunity with vaccination, or had decreased immunity over time. Maternal exposure to *rubella* can cause congenital deafness in the newborn.
Risk Factors. What type of loud noises have you been exposed to over your lifetime? • When were you exposed to them? • How long was the exposure? • What protective ear equipment did you use? • How did you monitor the exposure?	Hearing loss from loud noises is a major worldwide health issue. Workers at high risk for harmful noise exposure are farmers, fire fighters, police, emergency medical technicians, heavy machinery operators (eg, construction workers), military personnel, and members of the music industry.
What exposure to cigarette, pipe, or cigar smoke have you had over your lifetime? • When were you exposed to it? • How long were you exposed?	Those exposed to smoke are at increased risk for early-onset hearing loss.
What allergies have you had? • To what are you allergic? • When did you have this problem? • What were the symptoms? • How were these treated? • What were the outcomes?	Allergy symptoms such as runny nose and stuffy sinuses may lead to eustachian tube dysfunction in some patients.

Questions on History and Risk	Rationales
How often do you travel by airplane? What related ear problems have you experienced, if any?	Air pressure changes with altitude. Air travelers commonly experience middle ear discomfort during the aircraft's descent. The eustachian tubes help equalize pressure on both sides of the tympanic membrane. Eustachian tubes may malfunction with upper respiratory infections and ear conditions. When eustachian tubes cannot equalize pressure, intense middle ear and sinus pain can occur.
What experience with diving do you have? • How often do you dive? • What ear problems have you experienced, if any?	Air pressure changes with altitude; those who dive are at risk for middle ear trauma. Those at highest risk suffer from eustachian tube malfunction (as discussed under air travel).
How do you clean your ears?	Inserting cotton-tipped applicators into the external ear canal may lead to impaction of cerumen, which can contribute to hearing loss.

Health-Promotion Teaching

Preventing Hearing Loss. The most significant topic for patient teaching based on thorough risk assessment of the ears is general hearing loss. Although ability to hear decreases somewhat with age, much hearing loss is preventable. Ask patients about exposure to noise and protective equipment used. Educating patients on the types, effectiveness, and instructions for use of protective ear equipment allows them to make decisions based on their needs.

Preventing Skin Cancer. Many melanomas are found near or on the helix of the ear. Teaching patients how to protect themselves from unnecessary sun exposure increases the likelihood of preventative behaviors. See Chapter 6.

Performing Safe Hygiene. Address how the patient cleans the ears. Many people associate cerumen in the ear with lack of hygiene and therefore clean their ears routinely with cotton-tipped applicators. This unsafe self-care behavior increases risk for cerumen impaction. Reinforce proper cleaning techniques.

Key Topics and Questions for Common Symptoms

Common Eye Symptoms

•Hearing loss	•Tinnitus
•Vertigo	•Otalgia

Questions to Assess Symptoms	Rationales/Abnormal Findings
Hearing Loss. Describe your hearing. What changes, if any, have you noticed? • When did this start? • Did it start suddenly or gradually? • In what situations is it hardest to hear? • What have you done for it? • What were the outcomes? • Is there a family history of hearing loss? • Have you been exposed to loud noises such as machinery or gunshots?	Determining onset of hearing loss may help uncover cause and if it can be reversed, such as with a cerumen or foreign-body obstruction. Sudden hearing loss indicates trauma or obstruction. Family history of hearing loss indicates **presbycusis**. Environmental damage to hearing may involve consistent or onetime exposure to loud noise.
Vertigo. Have you ever felt dizzy or had problems with balance? • Describe what has happened. • How long does this continue? • Does it feel like you are, or the room is, spinning? • How have you treated the problem? • What were the outcomes?	Transient vertigo and persistent vertigo have different etiologies and thus necessitate different treatments. *Vertigo,* the sensation of the room spinning, indicates dysfunction of the bony labyrinth in the inner ear.
Tinnitus. Do you ever have a sensation of a buzzing or ringing that no one else can hear? • Is there any time that this seems louder? • Are you taking any medications, vitamins, or herbal supplements?	Tinnitus is thought to be an inability to filter internal noise from external sound input. Ototoxic agents can cause tinnitus. Stopping their use may resolve it, although some ototoxic agents cause lasting damage.

Questions to Assess Symptoms	Rationales/Abnormal Findings
Otalgia. Do you experience pain in either ear? • Is it in both ears or just one? • Have you ever had this pain before? • If so what was the cause? • Is the pain inside or outside? • Does it hurt to touch your ear? • Is the pain persistent or intermittent? • What makes the pain better or worse? • Is there any drainage from your ears? • What color was the drainage? • Did it have an odor? • Were there any recent surgeries or illnesses? • How do you clean your ears?	Otalgia usually indicates ear dysfunction, most commonly *otitis media or otitis externa.* Pain in the ear can be referred from the pharynx. It is not uncommon for a patient recovering from tonsil surgery to complain of ear pain. Severe pain followed by relief and drainage indicates a *ruptured tympanic membrane.* External ear sensitivity indicates *otitis externa,* which may result from self-induced trauma, such as inserting bobby pins, keys, or fingernails into the external ear canal.

Objective Data Collection

Equipment

- Otoscope
- High-pitched tuning fork

Technique and Normal Findings	Abnormal Findings
Inspection Inspect the ears. *Ears are symmetrical, equal size, and fully formed.*	*Microtia, macrotia, edematous ears,* cartilage pseudomonas infection, carcinoma on auricle, cyst, and frostbite are abnormal findings. See Table 9-1 at the end of this chapter.
Inspect the face. *Facial tone is uniform with ears. Skin is intact.*	

(text continues on page 172)

Palpation

Palpate the auricle. *Ears are firm without lumps, lymph tissue is not palpable, ears are nontender, and no pain is elicited with palpation of the auricle or mastoid process.*

Enlarged lymph nodes indicate pathology or inflammation. Pain with palpation indicates *otitis externa* or furuncle.

Whisper Test

The **whisper test** evaluates for loss of high-frequency sounds. Instruct the patient to plug (or plug for the patient) the ear opposite to the one you are testing. With your head 18 inches from the patient's ear and your mouth not visible, whisper a simple sentence (Fig. 9-1). Have the patient repeat what you have said. Repeat on the opposite side. The *patient repeats the entire sentence to you without errors.*

Not being able to repeat the sentence clearly or missing components may indicate hearing loss of higher frequencies and requires follow-up with formal testing.

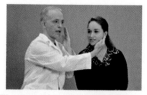

Figure 9.1 The whisper test.

Rinne's Test

The use of a tuning fork in the Rinne's test helps establish if hearing is equal in both ears and if there is either a conductive or sensorineural hearing loss by allowing comparison of the difference in bone conduction (BC) versus air conduction (AC). AC has less resistance than BC.

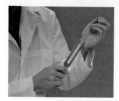

Figure 9.2 Striking the tuning fork against the back of the hand.

1. Grasp and tap the handle of the tuning fork against the back (heel) of your hand (Fig. 9-2).
2. Place the base of the handle on the patient's mastoid process (Fig. 9-3). Note the time on the second hand of your watch.
3. Instruct the patient to say when he or she no longer hears the sound of the fork. Note the number of seconds.

BC that is longer or the same as AC is evidence of conductive hearing loss. Conductive hearing loss on one side may indicate external or middle ear disease. Patients with conductive hearing loss should have

Technique and Normal Findings	Abnormal Findings

4. Once the patient no longer hears the sound, move the tip of the tuning fork to the front of the external auditory meatus. Again note the time on the second hand of your watch.
5. Instruct the patient to report when he or she no longer hears the sound. *AC is twice as long as BC.*

an assessment of the auricle and external auditory canal to look for blockage. The tympanic membrane should be assessed to ensure that there is no middle ear abnormality, such as fluid or a tympanic membrane perforation.

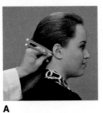 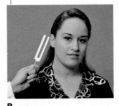

A **B**

Figure 9.3 Rinne's test. **(A)** Placing the tuning fork on the mastoid process. **(B)** Moving the tip to the front of the external auditory meatus.

Weber's Test

The Weber's test helps differentiate the cause of unilateral hearing loss. After activating the fork, place its handle on the midline of the parietal bone in line with both ears (Fig. 9-4). The *patient hears the sound in both ears and at equal intensity*.

Unilateral identification of the sound indicates sensorineural loss in the ear that the patient did not hear or had reduced sound perception. Sensorineural hearing loss on one side may be related to *Meniere's disease* or a *vestibular schwannoma* (*acoustic neuroma*).

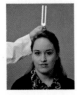

Figure 9.4 Weber's test.

Otoscopic Evaluation

In this advanced practice examination, inspect the external meatus and canal. Choose a

Redness, swelling of the external auditory canal, and discharge are signs of
(text continues on page 174)

Technique and Normal Findings	Abnormal Findings

speculum size that fits into the external canal without discomfort. *The canal has fine hairs; some cerumen lining the wall skin is intact, with no discharge.*

Hold the otoscope so that your thumb is by the window and you are bracing the shaft with your fingers along the patient's cheek. This allows you to stabilize the otoscope and it decreases risk of scraping the external auditory canal with the speculum.

Hold the patient's ear at the helix and lift up and back to align the canal for best visualization of the tympanic membrane (Fig. 9-5A).

external otitis. Either a foreign body or cerumen can obstruct the canal.

Swelling or bulging of the tympanic membrane indicates acute otitis media (Table 9-2). A diffuse cone of light indicates *otitis media with effusion.* Air bubbles caused by a functioning eustachian tube allow drainage of effusion and aeration of the middle ear. A perforated tympanic membrane may allow for direct visualization into the middle ear.

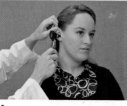

A

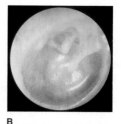

B

Figure 9.5 (A) Correct position of the patient's ear to optimize visualization of the tympanic membrane. **(B)** Normal tympanic membrane.

After visualization of the canal, rotate the otoscope slightly to visualize the entire tympanic membrane. Look at portions of the malleus, umbo, manubrium, and short process through the translucent membrane (Fig. 9-5B). A well-aerated middle ear allows visualization of part of the incus as well. *Tympanic membrane is intact and translucent and allows*

Technique and Normal Findings	Abnormal Findings
visualization of the short process of the malleus. The cone of light is visible in the anterior inferior quadrant. Once the tympanic membrane is visualized you may use the bulb insufflator attached to the head of the otoscope (Fig. 9-6) to observe tympanic membrane movement. First apply positive pressure that forces air into the external auditory canal and pushes down the tympanic membrane. Then release pressure and note the negative pressure pulling the tympanic membrane outward. *The tympanic membrane moves inward when inflated and outward with release.*	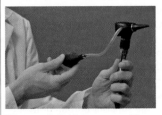 **Figure 9.6** Otoscope with bulb insufflator attached.

Documentation of Normal Subjective and Objective Findings

Patient alert and follows conversation with no evidence of hearing loss. Denies hearing difficulty, vertigo, tinnitus, and otalgia. Right and left pinnas normal, canals well aerated, and tympanic membranes translucent with visible bony prominences of the malleus and sharp cones of light. Hearing intact bilateral with whisper test. Rinne's and Weber tests normal.

🔺 Lifespan Considerations

Pregnant Women

Estrogen levels in pregnancy stimulate blood flow throughout the body. Subsequent vessel changes in the middle ear may cause a sensation of fullness in the ear or intermittent otalgia. Vertigo in pregnant women can result from increased vascularity and edema.

Newborns, Infants, and Children

Shorter, wider, and more horizontal eustachian tubes, frequent upper respiratory infections, and immature anatomy increase risk for otitis media in young children. While ear infections can cause severe discomfort and difficulty, they rarely lead to permanent hearing loss. Following an episode, fluid can remain in the middle ear for 3 months. Repeated infections or persistent effusion does cause temporary conductive hearing loss, which may delay speech. Hearing will become normal once the effusion is gone. Placement of small tubes through the tympanic membrane to treat otitis media is the most common U.S. surgery. Otitis media also can be treated with topical instead of oral antibiotics.

When assessing the ears, approach and involve young children playfully and as developmentally appropriate. Note the placement of the external ear. The superior portion of the pinna should be congruent with the outer canthus of the eye. There should be no more than a 10-degree deviation from the medial fold of the lobe to attachment of the superior portion of the helix.

Parents may need to hold young children during the otoscopic examination to reduce risk of injury. Toddlers are best examined sitting on their parents' lap facing forward while the parents "hug" them with one arm and hold their heads steady with the opposite arm. Preschoolers usually need to be held down on an examination table. Older children can sit on the examination table, but it may be easier for them to be supine with their heads turned toward the parents.

To insert the otoscope tip into a child's ear canal, the pinna must be manipulated differently than with an adult. Gently grasp the child's lobe and pull downward.

Screening for hearing acuity includes evaluation of developmental milestones. If there is a developmental lag or concern by caregivers, a pediatric audiologist should perform a formal evaluation. See also Chapter 22.

Older Adults

Cartilage formation continues over the lifespan, which may make ears seem more prominent in older adults. Extra cartilage can lead to loss of rigidity and potential collapse of the external auditory canal. In addition, fine hairs lining the ear canal become coarser and stiffer, which can interfere with sound waves as they move toward the tympanic membrane, decreasing hearing.

With decreased hair mobility, cerumen accumulates more readily and is compounded by cerumen itself becoming drier. Removing mechanical blockage can restore hearing and enhance socialization. It also helps to prevent injury by preserving the sense of hearing.

Over time some people experience a natural sensorineural loss called *presbycusis*. Difficulty distinguishing sounds increases, especially in noisy environments. Garbled or mumbled speech is a symptom. Amplification of sound, such as with simple hearing aids, does little to alleviate presbycusis.

▲ Cultural Considerations

Socioeconomic status and environmental exposure are indicators of risk for otitis media. Lower socioeconomic status corresponds to higher rates of otitis media. Exposure to cigarette smoke, propping bottles for babies to feed, and bottle-feeding in a supine position are all environmental factors that increase risk for otitis media.

Color and consistency of cerumen differ with cultural background. Yellow to dark brown cerumen, varying from liquid to firm paste (known as *wet cerumen*), is most common in Caucasians and African Americans. Flakey gray to white cerumen (*dry cerumen*), often misdiagnosed as eczema, is most prevalent in Asians and Native Americans.

Common Nursing Diagnoses and Interventions

Diagnosis and Related Factors	Nursing Interventions
Disturbed auditory sensory perception related to hearing loss	Minimize background noise. Sit directly in front of the patient. Allow the patient to see your face. Do not overenunciate or shout at the patient.
Pain related to inflammation of ear canal	Use pain scale to identify current pain intensity and effectiveness of medication. Develop pain goal collaboratively with the patient. Provide pain medications as ordered.* Provide alternatives such as distraction, breathing, and relaxation.
Risk for infection	Follow frequent handwashing and universal precautions. Protect wound with dressing. Monitor for fever, WBC, wound drainage, or erythema. Discontinue tubes as soon as possible. Encourage adequate nutrition.

*Collaborative interventions.

Table 9.1 Abnormalities of the External Ear

Microtia

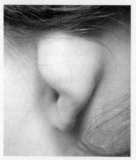

Small or deformed auricle that may be associated with a blind or absent auditory canal

Macrotia

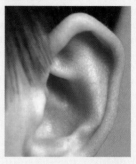

Excessive enlargement of the auricle; usually congenital

Edematous Ears

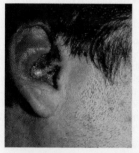

An external ear canal that is swollen with inflammation or infection

Cartilage *Staphylococcus* or *Pseudomonas* Infection

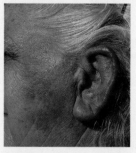

Painful, reddened ear usually surrounding incisions, ear piercing, or an area of traumatic injury

Table 9.1 Abnormalities of the External Ear (*continued*)

Carcinoma on Auricle

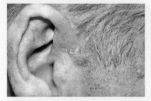

Common site of carcinoma related to sun exposure; either basal cell or squamous cell tumors may be present

Cyst

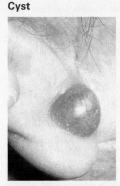

A sac or pouch with a membranous lining filled with fluid or solid material

Tophi

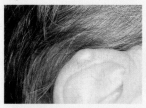

Uric acid crystals associated with gout; may appear as hard nodules on the ear surface

External Otitis

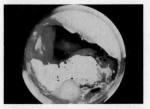

Inflammatory and infectious discharge in the external canal; associated with pain, itching, fullness, and reduced hearing

Tympanic Membrane Rupture

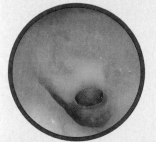

A nonintact tympanic membrane; associated symptoms include clear, purulent, or bloody discharge; hearing loss in the affected ear; buzzing in the ear; and ear pain

Acute Otitis Media

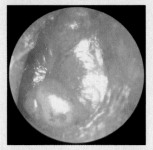

Acute infection in the middle ear. Onset is usually sudden and may be with fever and pain. Fluid may be in the middle ear. Causes may be viral or bacterial.

Otitis Media with Effusion

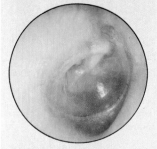

Purulent discharge associated with a bacterial infection. Redness and bulging on the eardrum

Scarred Tympanic Membrane

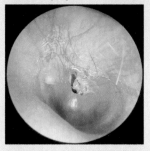

Caused by frequent ear infections with perforation of the tympanic membrane. Scars are dense white patches on the tympanic membrane.

Table 9.2 Abnormal Findings in the Internal Ear (*continued*)

Foreign Body

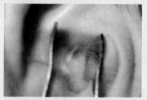

Tympanostomy Tubes

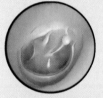

Most commonly these are found in the canal of a child who puts a bean or bead in the ear. If the object has been in the ear for several days, the patient may present with purulent discharge, pain, or hearing loss.

Tympanostomy tubes are indicated for chronic otitis media and its complications, recurrent acute otitis media, and antibiotic failure in children.

Nose, Sinuses, Mouth, and Throat Assessment

Subjective Data Collection

Key Topics and Questions for Health Promotion ———

Key Questions	Rationales
Family History. Do you have a family history of mouth or upper respiratory illness? • Who had the illness? • What was the specific illness? • What management was implemented? • What was the outcome?	Hereditary prevalence for *atopy* (allergy) is strong. Family history of *cancer*, genetic disorders (eg, *cystic fibrosis*), autoimmune disease (eg, *Wegener's granulomatosis*), *Churg-Strauss syndrome*, and *Sjögren's syndrome* increases the patient's risk for the same problem.
Personal History. Have you ever been diagnosed with a mouth or upper respiratory condition? • What was the specific condition? • When did it occur? • How was the condition treated? • What were the outcomes?	Positive history of frequent *upper respiratory infections* suggests underlying allergy, chronic hypertrophy of the adenoids and tonsils, or *chronic sinusitis*.
Did you have a history of chronic upper respiratory infections as a child?	A positive response raises suspicion of *allergy*. Chronic respiratory inflammation may lead to mucosal damage.
Current Health Status. Do you have known sensitivities to inhalant allergens (dust mites, mold, pollen, animal dander)? Have you had allergy testing?	Allergy can affect any target organ in the body. The nose and respiratory mucosa are the entry port for inhalants and thus common inflammatory targets.

Key Questions	Rationales
Medications/Supplements. What medications do you currently take? (Find out names, doses, and frequency of administration.)	Some medications have side effects that affect the mouth, nose, and sinuses. Blood-pressure drugs may produce cough. Anticoagulants may lead to bleeding problems. Medication that dries the mouth may affect oral health.
Do you take over-the-counter, natural, or herbal supplements? (Note what they are and how frequently.)	Used for a short time, topical decongestant sprays provide relief, facilitate vasoconstriction, and treat nosebleeds. With persistent use, they produce rebound congestion and are addictive. Ginkgo biloba and garlic cause increased clotting times and are contraindicated in those with frequent nosebleeds. Other herbs may stimulate *allergic rhinitis*.
Dental Health. How often do you brush and floss? When were your teeth last cleaned? Any tooth or gum problems?	Regular dental cleanings keep teeth and gums healthy and identify problems early.
Psychosocial History. Do you currently smoke cigarettes, pipes, or cigars? • How many packs per day? • How many years have you smoked? • Have you ever tried to stop? • Are you interested in stopping? • Do you currently or have you ever chewed tobacco?	Smoking increases respiratory inflammation, exacerbating *allergic rhinitis* and *chronic sinusitis*. It also increases risks for *head and neck carcinoma*. Chewing tobacco increases risk for *oral cancer*.
Are you frequently around smokers? What measures do you take against exposure?	Secondhand smoke increases risks for *head and neck cancer*, *allergic rhinitis*, *pharyngitis*, and *sinusitis*.
Have you ever inhaled marijuana, cocaine, methamphetamine,	These substances can irritate the upper airway. Regular *(text continues on page 184)*

Key Questions	Rationales
heroin, glue, or spray paint? Are you interested in information to reduce associated risks or to help you quit?	marijuana use may lead to injury, infection, and *head and neck cancer*. Cocaine may permanently damage the nasal mucosa, resulting in perforation. Methamphetamines may damage the teeth.
What is your history of exposure to chemical substances or irritants at work? • Do you take precautions to protect the respiratory tract? • Do you monitor your exposures?	Chemical exposures may damage the cilia, affecting the natural self-cleaning ability of the mucosal lining. Repeat exposures may produce allergic reactions in atopic patients. Chemicals may also be toxic.
Do you have hobbies that increase risk for upper respiratory problems: farming; frequent exposure to animals; exposure to paint, chemical fumes, and wood dust; airplane flying; scuba diving; and swimming?	Farming may expose patients to allergens. Fumes from paints and solvents may irritate or damage the respiratory mucosa. Scuba diving and flying may lead to barotrauma. Chronic chlorine exposure may produce or aggravate *sinusitis* or *allergy*.

Health-Promotion Teaching

Smoking and Tobacco Use. Smoking is a major risk to the respiratory tract and the leading cause of preventable death. At every encounter, question patients about smoking and their interest in stopping. Offer multiple choices for discontinuing smoking and provide information on resources, such as support groups or individual counseling.

Oral Health. Visits to dental care providers are an excellent opportunity to improve oral health. Reduction of dental caries through oral hygiene, good nutrition, community water fluoridation, and application of dental sealants after the eruption of permanent teeth are all examples of opportunities for improvements. Daily brushing and flossing are essential in decreasing dental caries as well as reducing gingivitis and periodontal disease.

Key Topics and Questions for Common Symptoms —

Common Mouth and Upper Respiratory Symptoms

- Facial pressure/pain/headache
- Snoring/sleep apnea
- Obstructive breathing
- Nasal congestion
- Epistaxis (nosebleeds)
- Halitosis (bad breath)
- Anosmia (decreased smell)
- Cough
- Pharyngitis/sore throat
- Dysphagia (difficulty swallowing)
- Dental aching/pain
- Hoarseness/voice changes
- Oral lesions

Questions to Assess Symptoms	Rationale/Abnormal Findings
Describe your upper respiratory (nasal) breathing.	Patients can offer unbiased descriptions of how they feel their upper airway performs.
Facial Pressure/Pain/Headache. Do you have any pain, pressure, or a headache?	Sinus pain or pressure is common with *colds, influenza*, and *sinusitis*.
Snoring/Sleep Apnea. Do you have sleep problems: snoring, restless sleep, breathing that stops while asleep, daytime drowsiness, or drooling at night?	All patients with *sleep apnea* snore, but not all who snore have sleep apnea. Patients with sleep apnea are at risk for stroke, hypertension, heart attack, and accidents.
Obstructive Breathing. Is nasal breathing decreased? • Is this unilateral or bilateral? • Is it related to any facial trauma? • Does the congestion alternate? • Does anything aggravate or improve your nasal breathing?	Inflammation from allergy or irritant exposure may decrease breathing. *Deviated nasal septum, nasal polyp,* or tumor may cause nasal obstruction. Trauma may lead to *deviated septum* or *hematoma.*
Nasal Congestion. Do you experience excessive nasal discharge? • Is it clear or cloudy? • What color is it? • Is it bilateral or unilateral?	Clear rhinorrhea may be *allergic* or *nonallergic rhinitis.* Unilateral clear discharge unresponsive to treatment may be a rare *cerebrospinal fluid leak.* Discolored or cloudy discharge indicates inflammation.

(text continues on page 186)

Questions to Assess Symptoms	Rationale/Abnormal Findings
Epistaxis. Do you have difficulty with nosebleeds? Do you habitually pick or remove nasal crusts?	Nasal inflammation causes dilatation of its blood vessels. Digital manipulation or nose picking may aggravate nasal bleeding.
Halitosis. Have you ever been told that your breath smells bad?	Foul breath suggests infection.
Anosmia. Do you have a decreased sense of smell? Is this a long-term or sudden problem?	*Anosmia* (decreased smell) may accompany chronic nasal inflammation or obstruction of one or more paranasal sinuses.
Cough. Do you have a cough? • Does it feel like the cough comes from your chest or upper airway? • Is your cough wet or dry? • Productive or nonproductive? • What makes the cough worse? Better?	Sinus drainage, allergen or irritant exposure, or *chronic sinusitis* may produce cough. Reactive airway in *asthma* may produce cough. Cough may be secondary to *gastroesophageal reflux disease* (*GERD*).
Pharyngitis. Do you experience sore throats?	Causes include chronic tonsillar hypertrophy or enlargement and recurrent strep infections.
Dysphagia. Do you have difficulty swallowing?	*Dysphagia* may accompany a growth or lesion or result from inflammation secondary to *GERD*.
Dental Pain. Do you experience toothaches? Are your teeth sensitive to cold or heat?	*Sinusitis* may produce dental aching, particularly of the upper teeth. *Dental caries* or *abscess* may produce tooth pain.
Voice Changes. Have you experienced hoarseness or voice changes?	Common causes include postnasal drainage; inflammation secondary to *GERD*, *allergy*, or *irritant exposure*; or lesions.
Oral Lesions. Do you have any mouth sores? If so, has there been any change in size or appearance of the sore?	Smoking or chewing tobacco increases risk for *oral cancer*. Persistent or changing lesions may indicate *oral cancer*.

Much of the physical examination of these areas is performed by inspection. Palpation for masses or tenderness is performed if abnormal findings are suspected. It is common to perform assessments in this region as focused examinations.

Equipment Needed

- Handheld otoscope
- Nasal speculum
- Tongue blades
- Cotton gauze 4 × 4
- Gloves
- Penlight
- Scratch or sniff test card
- Nasopharyngeal-laryngeal mirror

Technique and Normal Findings	Abnormal Findings
External Nose *Inspection.* Inspect the nose. It is symmetrical, midline, and proportional to face. Skin surface is smooth without lesions; color is consistent with facial complexion.	Asymmetry, swelling, or bruising may result from *trauma* or accompany lesions or growths. See Table 10-1.
Palpation. Generally, the RN does not palpate unless there is a specific problem. For the APRN, gently palpate with thumb and forefinger. *There is no pain, tenderness, or break in contour.*	Tenderness on palpation and crepitus suggest *fracture.*
Internal Nose The APRN generally inspects the internal nose with an otoscope, nasal speculum, or both (Fig. 10-1).	See Table 10-1.

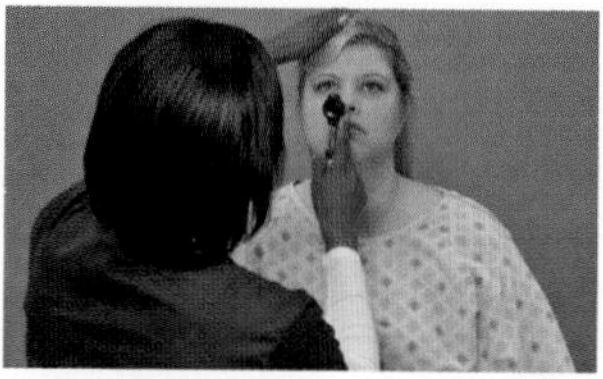

Figure 10.1 Using the otoscope.

(text continues on page 188)

Technique and Normal Findings	Abnormal Findings
Gently insert a wide-tipped speculum into the nasal vestibule or naris. Open vertically while lifting up the tip of the nose. Never open the nasal speculum horizontally—this puts uncomfortable pressure on the septum. Observe the color of the mucous membranes. Inspect any mucus. Note the color and character of the nose. The inferior turbinate is the first structure visualized. The middle turbinate can be noted superior and lateral (Fig. 10-2). Assess airflow by asking the patient to breathe out while holding the mouth closed. Gently manipulate the external nose to assess how changes affect airflow. *Septum is midline; mucosa is pink and moist; and no prominent blood vessels or crusts. Drainage is clear. Airflow is adequate.*	Infection and inflammation of nasal mucosa may be present with *viral, bacterial,* or *allergic rhinitis.* Excessive clear watery drainage suggests *allergic rhinitis.* Thick discolored mucus or gross pus may accompany *infection.* Absence of normal structures (eg, turbinates), suggests previous surgery. Deviation of the nasal septum may be congenital or acquired. Note any crusting or prominence of nasal vessels with special attention to the anterior septum. A *septal perforation* is a hole in the midline septum. It may be secondary to trauma, surgery, or illicit drug use. **Polyps,** grapelike swollen nasal membranes, may appear white and glistening.

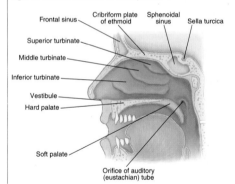

Figure 10.2 Inspecting the nasal mucosa.

If the patient notices a loss of smell, ask to identify common scents with the use of sniff test cards. The *patient correctly identifies scents.*	Anosmia may occur with *trauma,* congestion, *polyps,* or *sinus infection.* Sudden loss of smell may be from *intracranial mass.*

Technique and Normal Findings	Abnormal Findings

Sinuses

Inspection. Inspect the sinus areas for redness or swelling. *Findings are symmetrical with no redness or swelling.*

Redness and swelling may represent acute *infection*, *abscess*, or *mucocele*. See Table 10-1.

Palpation and Percussion. Palpate and percuss the maxillary, ethmoid, and frontal sinus areas (Fig. 10-3).

Tenderness or fullness suggests infection.

No tenderness or fullness is present.

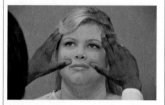

Figure 10.3 Palpating the sinus area.

Mouth

External Inspection. Inspect lips, noting color, moisture, lesions, and oral competence. *Lips are pink and moist with no lesions.*

Dryness or cracking may be from inadequate hydration. Lesions or aphthous ulcers may be with *viral infection*. Lip swelling or edema suggests *allergy*. Oral incompetence may occur in cleft lip.

Internal Inspection. Buccal Mucosa. Hold a light in the nondominant hand and a tongue blade in the dominant one. Gently separate areas to fully inspect the buccal mucosa (Fig. 10-4).

Poor oral hygiene has been linked to *pneumonia*. Inflamed buccal mucosa suggests *infection*. White patches (leukoplakia) may suggest a growth or lesion. Ulceration may represent viral infection or tumor. Petechiae or small red spots resulting from blood, which escapes the capillaries, may occur with trauma, infection, or decreased platelet counts. Redness or swelling of Stensen's duct may represent infection or blockage of the parotid gland. See also Table 10-2.

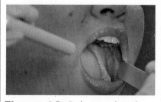

Figure 10.4 Inspecting the U-shaped area under the tongue.

(text continues on page 190)

Technique and Normal Findings	Abnormal Findings
Inspect the entire U-shaped area in the floor of mouth. Note the parotid (Stensen's) duct appearing as a small dimple opposite the second upper molar. Small isolated and insignificant white or yellow papules (**Fordyce's granules**) may be noted on the cheeks, tongue, and lips.	
Teeth and Gums. Note numbers and position of teeth, appearance, signs of decay, and alignment. Note breath odor.	Teeth may be stained or have *decay*. Swollen or red gums with bleeding may indicate *gingivitis*. Foul breath may suggest infection. See Table 10-3.
Uvula. Note uvula position (Fig. 10-5). Have the patient say "ah" and watch the rise of the uvula.	Uvula may be swollen with allergic reactions. It may be bifid or have a notch or cleft.

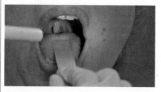

Figure 10.5 Observing the uvula.

Technique and Normal Findings	Abnormal Findings
Hard and Soft Palate. Inspect the color and surface of the hard and soft palate.	With *cleft palate*, nasopharyngeal incompetence may be present along with resultant nasal air leak during speech.
Tongue. Inspect the tongue, including dorsum, sides, and underneath. Note papillae. Ask the patient to stick out the tongue. To test the gag reflex, gently place a tongue blade on the posterior dorsum.	Tongue may have lesions or ulcers. A white coating may be oral candidiasis. This condition is very common in patients taking antibiotics. See Table 10-4 at the end of this chapter.
Wharton's Ducts and Salivary Flow. Inspect Wharton's ducts in the floor of the mouth. Evaluate salivary flow from the submandibular salivary gland.	Swelling or redness of Wharton's duct suggests inflammation of the submandibular gland.

Technique and Normal Findings	Abnormal Findings

Palpation. Palpate the parotid, submandibular, and sublingual glands for swelling or tenderness (see Chapter 7). *There is no swelling or tenderness.*

Swelling may occur with mumps, blockage of a duct, abscess, or tumor. Duct obstruction can occur as a result of aging, dehydration, or use of anticholinergics.

Palpation of the mouth is usually part of a specialty assessment. Place a gloved hand inside the cheek to assess Stensen's duct. Assess for a stone or growth. Palpate for any lesions. *Ducts are soft and nontender without lesions.*

Firmness of either Stensen's or Wharton's duct or lesions may represent a stone or growth. Hard fixed lesions have a higher incidence of cancer. Soft, mobile lesions are more often cysts or benign disease.

Throat

Inspection. Press down slightly with the tongue blade on the midpoint of the tongue. Visualize the pharynx, tonsils, soft palate, and anterior and posterior tonsillar pillars. Note color, symmetry, enlargement, and any lesions (Fig. 10-6).

Mucosal inflammation may indicate *infection* or allergy. Tonsillar hypertrophy occurs with persistent recurrent infection. Frequent infections may leave superficial scars or crypts that collect food and oral debris, appearing as embedded white curdlike material. With chronic tonsillitis and hypertrophy, findings are symmetrical. Asymmetrical tonsillar enlargement raises suspicion of *neoplasia.* Peritonsillar abscess (*quinsy*) may occur with collection of fluid in the anterior tonsillar pillar. Sleep apnea should be suspected with a squeezed appearance of the general proportion of the throat. Strep throat presents with red and white patches in the throat, difficulty swallowing, tender or swollen lymph nodes, or red and enlarged tonsils.

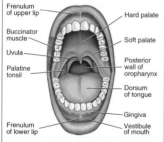

Frenulum of upper lip

Buccinator muscle

Uvula

Palatine tonsil

Frenulum of lower lip

Hard palate

Soft palate

Posterior wall of oropharynx

Dorsum of tongue

Gingiva

Vestibule of mouth

Figure 10.6 Inspecting the internal mouth and throat structures.

Tissue is pink and moist with symmetrical margins. No enlargement or lesions are noted. Grade the tonsils using the scale in Box 10-1. *Tonsils are absent or 1+.*

(text continues on page 192)

BOX 10.1 TONSILLAR GRADING SCALE

- 1+ tonsil obstructs 0%–25% to midline
- 2+ tonsil obstructs 25%–50% to midline
- 3+ tonsil obstructs 50%–75% to midline
- 4+ tonsil obstructs 75%–100% to midline

Source: Newland, D. (2003). Pediatric otolaryngology. In M. Layland & T. Lin (Eds.), *The Washington manual survival guide series. Otolaryngology survival guide* (pp. 153–166). Philadelphia, PA: Lippincott Williams & Wilkins.

Palpation. An APRN will find palpation of the neck helpful to assess inflammatory and other throat changes. Anterior and posterior cervical chain lymph nodes and submental areas are palpated as part of a normal neck examination (see Chapter 7). *Nodes are symmetrical, soft, and nontender.*

Lymph nodes are quick to respond to inflammation and slow to resolve.

Swallowing Evaluation

Evaluation of swallowing is a technique typically performed by a speech therapist, APRN, or physician. Position the thumbs and index finger on the laryngeal protuberance. Ask the patient to swallow; feel the larynx elevate. Ask the patient to cough. Observe for signs associated with swallowing problems: coughing; choking; spitting of food; drooling; difficulty handling oral secretions; double or major delay in swallowing; watering eyes; nasal discharge; wet or gurgly voice; decreased ability to move tongue and lips, chew food, or move food to the back of mouth; pocketing of food; and slow or scanning speech. *Swallowing takes less than 1 second with no sign of aspiration.*

Patients with *stroke*, *head injury*, or other neuromuscular disorders are at risk for dysphagia. Swallowing problems are common in hospitalized patients and may prolong length of stay because of an inability to obtain adequate nutrition for healing. Dysphagia may be from a growth in the airway or enlargement of surrounding glands or tissue. Dysphagia may be secondary to *GERD*, which should be suspected when inflammation of the larynx is visualized on indirect or direct view. Aspiration into the larynx may be observed with incomplete closure of vocal cords or impeded movement of the epiglottis.

Documentation of Normal Subjective and Objective Findings

Patient states breathing is comfortable and quiet. Denies facial pressure, pain, headache, snoring, sleep apnea, obstructive breathing, or nasal congestion. Reports no epistaxis, halitosis, anosmia, or cough. States no pharyngitis, dysphagia, dental pain, hoarseness, or oral lesions. Nose is symmetrical, midline, and proportional to facial features. Skin surface is smooth without lesions; coloration is consistent with facial complexion. Sinus areas are symmetrical with no redness or swelling. Lips are pink and moist with no lesions. Buccal mucosa and soft and hard palates are pink with no lesions. Gingiva is pink and moist without inflammation. Breath has no foul odor. Tongue is smooth and midline. Teeth are well aligned with no evidence of decay. Uvula rises symmetrically with "ah." Ducts are smooth without inflammation. Tonsils are absent.

▲ Lifespan Considerations

Pregnant Women

Rhinitis during pregnancy results from the increased vascularity of the respiratory tract as well as hormonal effects on the mucosal lining. Increased nasal congestion or obstruction is common in pregnant women. Sinus infections, epistaxis (nosebleeds), or both may occur. Gums may become hyperemic and softened, leading to bleeding with toothbrushing. Localized gingival enlargement may lead to a tumor-like mass known as *epulis* forming on the gums.

Infants and Children

The nasal and oral examination can be difficult with children. An APRN commonly performs it in the clinic setting. With the child sitting on the parent's lap facing the examiner, the parent uses one hand to hold the child's head, the other arm to restrain the child's arms, and one leg to secure the child's legs. If the child refuses to open the mouth, gently closing the nostrils results in an open mouth for air within seconds. Flavored tongue blades may encourage small children to cooperate. Examiners can encourage children to growl "like a lion" to afford a thorough view of the oral cavity and throat.

Special considerations include checking for competency of the palate. Infants may have small white bumps (*milia*) across the nasal bridge. Older children with allergies may develop a traverse ridge across the nasal bridge from habitually performing the "*allergic salute.*"

Examining the child's nose is best accomplished by gently pressing upward on the tip and visualizing the interior with the bright light from an otoscope. Assessing nasal breathing should include feeling for symmetrical airflow from each nostril. Holding a laryngeal mirror beneath the nose should demonstrate bilateral fogging. Nasal flaring or narrowing with inspiration is an indicator of respiratory distress. Foul odor or unilateral thick mucus suggests a foreign body. A normal finding in infants is a small pad of tissue in the middle of the upper lip (*sucking tubercle*).

Note age-appropriate tooth eruption. For children younger than 2 years, the age in months minus 6 should equal the number of deciduous teeth. After 2½ years, all 20 deciduous teeth should be present. Discoloration of the tooth enamel with plaque is a sign of poor dental hygiene. Brown spots in the crevices of the tooth may be caries (cavities).

Tongue mobility should extend to the alveolar ridge. *Ankyloglossia* (short lingual frenulum) may be congenital, restricting tongue movement and speech. An extremely narrow, flat roof or a high-arched palate can cause speech and feeding problems.

Tonsils are not visible in newborns but gradually enlarge. They remain proportionally large in small children and decrease in size as they mature.

Older Adults

Loss of subcutaneous fat may cause the nose to appear more prominent. *Gustatory rhinitis* (clear rhinorrhea stimulated by the smell and taste of food) is common. Olfactory sensory fibers start to decrease after age 60.

In the oral cavity, the soft tissue of the cheeks and tongue thins and increases risks for ulcerations, infections, and oral cancers. Saliva production and the number of taste buds decrease. Resorption occurs in gum tissue, surrounding teeth, and the mandible. Natural tooth loss accompanies the breakdown of the tooth surface and receding gums. These problems may lead to malocclusion and temporomandibular joint pain.

Edentulous (without any teeth) older adults may develop a pursed-lip appearance. Malocclusion may lead to skin maceration at the corners of the mouth (*angular cheilitis*). Teeth may appear yellow from worn enamel and larger as gums recede.

The tongue and buccal mucosa may appear smoother and shiny from papillary atrophy and thinning of the buccal mucosa, a condition called *smooth, glossy tongue. Fissures* (*scrotal tongue*) can become inflamed with accumulation of food or debris.

● Cultural Considerations

Incidence of dental caries varies with sociodemographic group. While spending trends for dental care have increased, many people still do not have dental insurance. *Gingivitis* (gum inflammation and bleeding) is high among Hispanics, American Indians, Alaskan Natives, and adults of low socioeconomic status. Cleft lip and palate have increased incidence in Native Americans and Asian Americans.

Oral and pharyngeal cancers vary by race and ethnicity, most likely related to tobacco use, and the 5-year survival rate from them is lower among African Americans than Caucasians. Asians are at increased risk for nasopharyngeal cancer.

The nasal bridge may be flat in African Americans and Asians. Dark-skinned patients have more deeply colored gums and sometimes a brownish ridge along the gum line.

Common Nursing Diagnoses and Interventions

Diagnoses	Nursing Interventions
Impaired dentition	Teach toothbrushing and flossing. Provide assistance as needed. Perform mouth care if the patient cannot do so independently.
Altered oral mucous membrane	Provide fluids and mouth care. Moisturize mucous membranes. Treat infections.*
Impaired swallowing	Evaluate swallowing ability. Provide sips of fluids before giving dry foods. Elevate head of bed. Thicken liquids if needed.
Altered breathing pattern	Use tissues to clear upper airway. Elevate head of bed. Give frequent fluids to liquefy secretions.

*Collaborative interventions.

⚠️ **Table 10.1   Common Assessment Findings: Nose and Sinuses**

Epistaxis (Nosebleed)

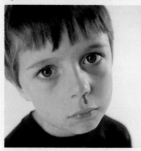

Bleeding; dry sensations or crusting in nose; prominent vessels, scabs, or crusts on anterior septum; blood in nasal vestibule.

Foreign Body

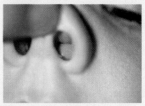

Any object not commonly found in the upper aerodigestive tract. May result from nasal piercing, deliberate placement of objects, and postsurgical remnant of cotton or gauze.

Rhinitis

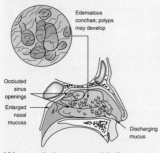

Edematous conchae; polyps may develop

Occluded sinus openings

Enlarged nasal mucosa

Discharging mucus

Watery, itchy nose with frequent sneezing, congestion, clear nasal drainage, pale blue, boggy mucosa, or redness and inflammation.

Nasal Polyps

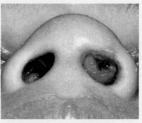

Grapelike swelling of the nasal and sinus mucosa leading to nasal obstruction; associated with inflammation, congestion, and facial pain and pressure.

Deviated Septum

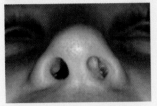

Congenital or traumatic deflection of the center wall of the nose (septum). The patient may experience a unilateral decreased ability to breathe through the nose, pressure or headache, and narrowing of the nasal chamber.

Perforated Septum

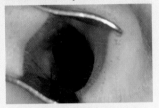

A hole in the nasal septum, which may be accompanied by crusting, purulent drainage, foul odor, whistling sound, and recurrent nosebleed.

Sinusitis

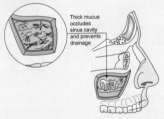

Thick mucus occludes sinus cavity and prevents drainage

Acute or chronic infection of one or more paranasal sinuses resulting from allergy, irritants, chemicals, or inflammation secondary to GERD. The patient has facial pain or pressure, thick nasal discharge, fever, cough, halitosis, and redness and inflammation of nasal mucosa.

Cleft Lip/Palate

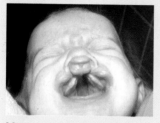

Most common congenital malformation of oral cavity; an opening or fissure of the lip/alveolus and palate; represents a fusion abnormality of the midfacial skeleton and soft tissues.

Bifid Uvula

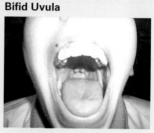

Congenital complete or partial split of uvula; adenoidectomy may be contraindicated. Usually asymptomatic.

Kaposi's Sarcoma

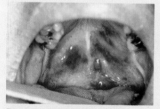

Rapidly proliferating malignancy of the skin or mucous membranes; oral involvement includes the tongue, gingiva, and palate. The biggest risk factor is infection with HIV.

Acute Tonsillitis or Pharyngitis

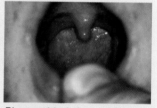

Pharyngitis: inflammation of the pharyngeal walls—may include tonsils, palate, and uvula.
Tonsillitis: inflammation in lymphoid tissue of oropharynx including Waldeyer's ring, palatine or lingual tonsils, pharyngeal bands, nasopharynx, and adenoids.

Strep Throat

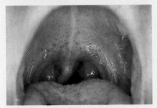

Infection of the tonsils involving *Streptococcus* bacterium.

Torus Palatinus

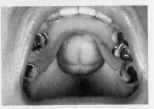

A bony prominence in the middle of the hard palate. Congenital; no clinical significance.

Herpes Simplex Virus (HSV)

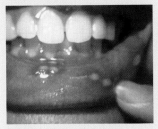

Painful, clear, vesicular oral lesions with indurated base that frequently appear at the lip–skin juncture. Lesions evolve into pustules that rupture, weep, and crust; typical course is 4–10 days.

Candidiasis

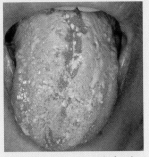

Opportunistic yeast infection of the buccal mucosa and tongue that results in white sticky mucus on the affected areas.

(table continues on page 200)

Aphthous Ulcers (Canker Sores)

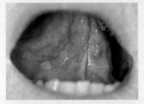

Vesicular oral lesion that evolves into a white ulceration with a red margin. Pain at and around site.

Leukoplakia

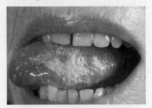

White patchy lesions with well-defined borders and firmly attached to the mucosal surface.

Black Hairy Tongue

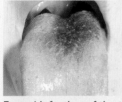

Fungal infection of the tongue involving elongation of the papillae and a brown/black hairy coating on tongue.

Carcinoma

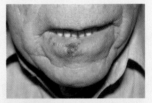

An initially indurated lesion with rolled irregular edges; later may crust or scab but does not heal. The lesion may be painful or limit tongue mobility; adjacent lymph nodes may be swollen.

⚠ **Table 10.4 Findings of the Gums and Teeth**

Dental Caries

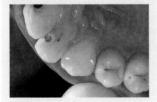

Progressive tooth destruction resulting from poor oral hygiene. Findings include pain with hot and cold substances and a tooth area that early appears chalky white and later becomes brown or black and forms a cavity.

Table 10.4   Findings of the Gums and Teeth
(*continued*)

Gingival Hyperplasia

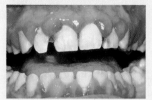

Painless gum enlargement that may accompany hormonal fluctuations leukemia; side effect of drugs (eg, phenytoin [Dilantin])

Gingivitis

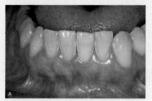

Painful, red, swollen, and bleeding gums resulting from poor oral hygiene, hormonal fluctuations, and vitamin B deficiency

Baby Bottle Tooth Decay

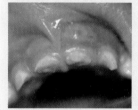

Decay of deciduous teeth from pooling of liquid carbohydrate around front teeth, which ultimately destroys tooth enamel. Results from children taking bottles to bed and bottle-feeding past age 1 year.

Ankyloglossia (Tongue-tie)

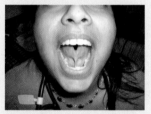

A congenitally shortened lingual frenulum. Findings include limited tongue movement and speech disruption, particularly with a, d, and n sounds.

11

Thorax and Lung Assessment

Subjective Data Collection

Key Topics and Questions for Health Promotion

Key Questions	Rationales/Abnormal Findings
Family History. Do you have any family history of respiratory problems? Provide details.	Note genetic problems (eg, *cystic fibrosis*), contagious diseases with possible familial transmission, and *lung cancer*.
Past Medical History. Have you ever been diagnosed with asthma, bronchitis, emphysema, or pneumonia?	History of chronic respiratory diseases increases risk for recurrence.
Did you have frequent respiratory infections as a child?	Frequent childhood infections may lead to problems later in life.
Do you now or have you ever had allergies? Provide specific details.	Common respiratory allergens include pollens, dust mites, grasses, molds, animal dander, and latex; exercise also may induce allergies.
When was your last tuberculosis (TB) skin test or chest x-ray? When did you receive your last influenza or pneumococcal vaccine?	Influenza vaccine is recommended annually for people at high risk. Pneumococcal vaccine is recommended every 5 years for at-risk populations.
Medications. Are you taking any medications for respiratory problems? Provide details.	Trends of increased use of respiratory medications may indicate a worsening condition.

Key Questions	Rationales/Abnormal Findings
Are you taking any natural supplements or over-the-counter medications? Provide details.	Beta 2 receptor blockers may exacerbate bronchoconstriction. Sensitivity to nonsteroidal anti-inflammatory agents may cause wheezing in patients with asthma.
Lifestyle and Personal Habits. Do you smoke or have you ever smoked cigarettes, pipes, or cigars? • How many packs per day do you smoke? • How many years have you smoked? • Have you ever tried to stop smoking? • Are you interested in quitting?	Smoking is described by number of **pack years** (number of years × number of packs per day). A patient who has smoked ½ pack per day for 30 years has a 15 pack year history. Increased pack years increase the risk for respiratory problems.
Are you frequently around smokers? What measures do you take to control this?	Secondhand smoke increases respiratory disease risks.
Do you use or have you ever inhaled marijuana, cocaine, methamphetamine, glue, or spray paint? Are you interested in information about how to quit or reduce your risk?	These inhaled substances can irritate the linings of the upper or lower airway.
Do you have any hobbies that might increase risk for respiratory problems: exposure to paint fumes or wood dust, bird breeding, mushroom growing, scuba diving, swimming, and high-altitude activities?	Such hobbies may cause lung injury. See also Chapter 10.
Occupational History. Have you ever been or are you now exposed to substances or irritants at work? What protective steps do you take?	See Chapter 10 for more on respiratory risks.
Environmental Exposures. Have you ever been or are you now exposed to substances or irritants at home?	Common household irritants can contribute to *asthma* and allergens.

(text continues on page 204)

Key Questions	Rationales/Abnormal Findings
Have you recently traveled to any high-risk areas for respiratory conditions?	Potential high-risk locations include the Midwestern and Southwestern United States, Central and South America, southern Africa, parts of Asia, and Turkey.

Health-Promotion Teaching

Smoking Cessation. Smoking is the leading cause of preventable death. At every appointment ask all patients who smoke about their readiness to stop—when health care providers ask patients to do this, smoking cessation is more likely. Patients can be given several choices to assist with quitting (eg, individual or group counseling, medical treatment, or nicotine replacement).

Prevention of Occupational Exposure. Review how to modify the work environment to limit exposure to irritants. In some cases, consultation with employees at work sites is recommended. Occupational health and safety guidelines should be followed.

Prevention of Asthma. Asthma triggers include tobacco smoke, dust, dust mites, molds, furred and feathered animals, and cockroaches and other pests. For patients with allergies, modification of the home may be recommended. Examples include covering the bed and pillows and ensuring that pets sleep separately from owners.

Immunizations. Counsel all adults to obtain the influenza vaccine annually. This consideration is especially important for health care providers.

Key Topics and Questions for Common Symptoms

Common Respiratory Symptoms

- Chest pain or discomfort
- Dyspnea
- Orthopnea or paroxysmal noctural dyspnea
- Cough
- Mucus or phlegm
- Wheezing or tightness in chest
- Change in functional ability

For each symptom, be sure to review location, characteristics, duration, aggravating factors, alleviating factors, accompanying symptoms, treatment, and the patient's view of the problem.

Questions to Assess Symptoms	Rationales/Abnormal Findings
Chest Pain. Do you have chest pain or discomfort?	Pleuritic chest pain is sharp or stabbing, worsening with deep breathing or coughing, and often lateral or posterior in the lung. Pain from **tracheobronchitis** is burning in the upper sternum and associated with a cough. Chest wall pain may be secondary to frequent coughing and achy; muscles may be tender.
Dyspnea. Have you had any difficulty breathing? Note cause, onset, association with anxiety, or history of chronic obstructive pulmonary disease (*COPD*) or congestive heart failure (*CHF*).	**Dyspnea** may be normal with exercise or heavy activity. Patients with *lung disease* may experience dyspnea with normal activities or at rest.
Paroxysmal Nocturnal Dyspnea. Do you have difficulty breathing when you sleep? • How many pillows do you use? • Do you have difficulty breathing when lying flat? • Do you wake up suddenly at night short of breath? • Do you snore or stop breathing when you sleep? • Do you have night sweats?	Patients with **orthopnea** (difficulty breathing when supine) may use two or more pillows or sleep in recliners. Night wakening with shortness of breath is **paroxysmal nocturnal dyspnea**, caused by fluid overload from elevation of the legs. The heart cannot pump the excess fluid, which suddenly accumulates in the lungs and causes dyspnea.
Cough. Do you have a cough?	Causes include *sinus congestion*; throat, laryngeal, or lung irritation; *pneumonia*; *common cold*; smoking; *bronchitis*; *sinus drainage*; *heart failure*; *asthma*; gastroesophageal reflux disease (*GERD*); or *hernia*.
Sputum. Do you cough up mucus or phlegm? • How much? • Has the amount increased or decreased?	Quantifying amount provides clues about severity; color may differentiate cause. **Mucoid** sputum of *bronchitis* is clear, *(text continues on page 206)*

Questions to Assess Symptoms	Rationales/Abnormal Findings
• What color is it? • Is it thick or thin? • Do you notice an odor? • Has the amount, consistency, or color changed?	white, or gray. **Purulent** yellow or green sputum indicates *bacterial infection*. Rust-colored sputum is found with *TB* and *pneumococcal pneumonia*. **Tenacious thick sputum** may be from *dehydration* or *cystic fibrosis*; sputum from *heart failure* is thin, frothy, and slightly pink. Sputum may be bloody (hemoptysis) with *lung cancer, TB,* or an irritated throat or sinus.
Wheezing. Do you have any wheezing or chest tightness? • Do you use a peak flow meter? • What are the usual values? • Is wheezing associated with allergies? What are they? • What makes the problem worse? • How often do you use your inhalers?	Wheezing, associated with *asthma, CHF,* and *bronchitis,* is a response to narrowed bronchioles. Patients with asthma use a peak flow meter to provide objective data about how much they can inhale with each breath. If airways are greatly constricted, breaths will be small and patients may need to use their inhalers.
Functional Ability. Have breathing difficulties changed any normal activities? How do you plan the day and pace activities? (In addition to eating, grooming, and dressing, also consider the patient's ability to perform home maintenance, such as vacuuming, bed making, cooking, cleaning, and buying groceries.)	Patients with respiratory problems commonly have more energy in the morning and need frequent rest. Some are short of breath even at rest. Others are breathless with activity. Patients with declining health may need plans for assistance. Ask what they like to do and if they can do them.

Objective Data Collection

Equipment

- Examination gown
- Stethoscope and alcohol swab
- Marking pen and small ruler for diaphragmatic excursion (optional)

Technique and Normal Findings	Abnormal Findings
Initial Survey	
Closely assess position for breathing. *Posture is relaxed and upright.*	Patients in respiratory distress may lean forward (tripod position).
Observe for **pursed lips** and **nasal flaring**. *Facial expression is relaxed.*	Patients in *respiratory distress* may look anxious or show nasal flaring. Patients with *COPD* may have pursed lips.
Evaluate the level of consciousness. The *patient is alert, cooperative, and normally oriented.*	Patients with *hypoxemia* may be irritable, somnolent, restless, confused, or combative.
Observe skin color. Document absence of cyanosis or pallor. *Skin color is appropriate tone for race.*	Signs of respiratory problems include cyanosis, pallor, grayness, rubor, or erythema.
Observe respiratory movements. Note if the patient uses the upper or lower chest to breathe. *Expiration is twice as long as inspiration* (*inspiration:expiration* = 1:2).	Patients with disease that impedes outflow may have forced expiration. Guarding may accompany respiratory pain.
As you observe respiratory movements, count rate. *Respiratory rate is 12 to 20 breaths/ min for adults, with regular rhythm.*	Wheezing may be audible in severe *asthma* or *bronchitis*. Tachypnea is greater than 24 breaths/min; bradypnea is less than 10 breaths/min. See Table 11-1 at the end of this chapter.
Assess oxygen saturation level. *Normal is 95% to 100%.*	*Pulmonary embolism* produces hypoxemia.
Assess muscles used for breathing. *Diaphragm and external intercostals do most of the work.*	Patients with *respiratory distress* may use accessory muscles.
Note any retractions. *Retractions are absent.*	Retractions accompany resistance to airflow (eg, in *severe asthma*).
Observe fingers for clubbing. *Normally no clubbing is present.*	Clubbing is noted with chronic lung disease.

(text continues on page 208)

Technique and Normal Findings	Abnormal Findings

Posterior Chest

Inspection. Note thoracic shape and configuration. Observe spontaneous chest expansion. *Spinous processes of vertebrae are midline; scapulae are symmetric. Chest wall is cone-shaped, symmetric, and oval. Transverse* (side to side)*:anterior-posterior ratio is 1:2 to 5:7. Any visible ribs slope at 45 degrees. Chest expansion is symmetric.*

See Table 11-2 at the end of this chapter for abnormal thoracic configurations.

Palpation. Start with fingertips above the scapula over the lung apex. Move from one side to another; compare bilateral findings. End at lung base; move laterally to midaxillary line (Fig. 11-1). Palpate for crepitus if the patient has had rib fractures, recent chest surgery, or chest tubes. *Nontender thorax has no lesions, lumps, masses, or crepitus.*

Tender areas may indicate *muscle strain, rib fracture, or soft tissue damage.* With trauma, air can enter lungs and escape, creating a crackling sensation (crepitus). *Subcutaneous emphysema* migrates and may be found in the head and neck. If the amount is large, mark borders with a pen to note changes.

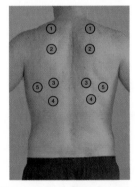

Figure 11.1 Sites for and sequence of palpation of the posterior thorax.

Technique and Normal Findings	Abnormal Findings

Technique and Normal Findings

Test for symmetric chest expansion when there are concerns about reduced lung volumes. With thumbs at T9-10, wrap the palms laterally and parallel to the rib cage (Fig. 11-2). Slide thumbs and hands medially to pinch a small skinfold between thumb and vertebra. Ask the patient to inhale deeply; observe the thumbs. *Thumbs move apart symmetrically, 5 to 10 cm.*

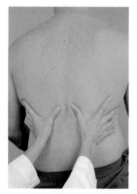

Figure 11.2 Testing for chest expansion.

Test tactile fremitus if concern exists about lung obstruction or consolidation. Follow the palpation sequence, avoiding the scapulae. Place the palmar or ulnar hand surface on the chest above the scapula. Ask the patient to say "ninety-nine." Vibrations of air in the bronchial tree are transmitted to the chest wall when the patient speaks.

Abnormal Findings

Asymmetrical movements indicate collapse or blockage of lung. Patients with muscle weakness, respiratory disease, recent surgery, chest wall abnormalities, or obesity may have reduced chest expansion.

Conditions that may lead to decreased or absent fremitus include obstructed bronchus, *COPD, pleural effusion, fibrosis, tumor, pneumothorax*, obesity, or an extremely large chest. Increased fremitus may accompany severe localized *pneumonia* or *lung tumor*.

(text continues on page 210)

Technique and Normal Findings	Abnormal Findings

Assess for intensity and symmetry of fremitus. If fremitus is difficult to palpate, ask the patient to speak louder. *Normal variations are wide-ranging.*

Percussion. Percussion is used when lung obstruction or consolidation is suspected. Begin at the apex of the lungs. Percuss from one side to another (Fig. 11-3). Work toward the bases in the intercostal spaces (ICSs). Move fingers approximately 5 cm apart. When fingers are below the level of lung tissue, sound changes from resonant to dull; from around T10 move laterally to percuss near the anterior axillary line and 7th and 8th ICSs. Avoid the area over the ribs and scapulae, because normal bone is flat. *Healthy lung tissue sounds resonant.*

Percussion may be dull with *lobar pneumonia, hemothorax, tumor, empyema,* or *pleural effusion.* Generalized hyperresonance may be heard with *COPD* or *emphysema.* Unilateral hyperresonance may be with *pneumothorax.*

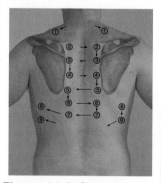

Figure 11.3 Sites and sequence for posterior chest percussion.

Technique and Normal Findings	Abnormal Findings

Technique and Normal Findings

Test **diaphragmatic excursion** in cases of concern about chest expansion. Ask the patient to deeply exhale and hold it; then percuss in the ICSs down the scapular line (Fig. 11-4A). Hold the breath at the same time as the patient to remember to let the patient breathe after a short time. When the sound changes from resonant to dull, go back to the previous resonant rib space. This marks the location of lung tissue on deep expiration (it also may be marked with a pen) (Fig 11-4B). Allow the patient to breathe if needed or ask the patient to take in and hold a deep breath. Percuss in the previously resonant spot; *it should remain resonant*. Move down into the previously dull ICS;

Abnormal Findings

Diaphragmatic excursion may be reduced in *emphysema*, *atelectasis*, extreme *ascites*, advanced pregnancy, and extreme obesity. S*pinal cord injury, stroke, Guillian-Barré syndrome*, or *muscular dystrophy* can also inhibit respiratory excursion. Lag in expansion may occur with *atelectasis, pneumonia*, or postoperative pain.

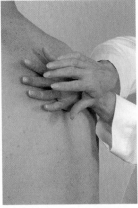
A

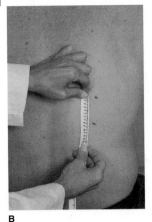
B

Figure 11.4 Assessing diaphragmatic excursion. **(A)** Percussing in the intercostal spaces. **(B)** Marking the location of lung tissue.

(text continues on page 212)

Technique and Normal Findings	Abnormal Findings

it should now be resonant at deep inspiration. Move down one or two more rib spaces until the sound is dull again; *the difference should be one or two rib spaces, or 3 to 5 cm and 7 to 8 cm in well-conditioned adults.*

Auscultation. Listen from top to down alternating left and right. **Ensure that the stethoscope is in direct contact with the skin.** Listen for extra, abnormal sounds of breathing. Ask the patient to breathe through the mouth. Place the flat side of the diaphragm on the chest wall firmly to block extraneous noise. Listen to one full breath in each location. Move from one side to another.

Stand behind and beside the patient. Listen from lung apices to bases and then laterally in the same sequence as percussion. If sounds are too soft, ask the patient to breathe deeper.

The bases often are the first area to collapse with atelectasis and to collect fluid in CHF or fluid overload.

Identify vesicular, bronchovesicular, and bronchial breath sounds. Listen for intensity, quality, pitch, and duration of inspiration versus expiration. *Normal breath sounds are vesicular. Expiration is longer than inspiration, similar to normal breathing. See Table 11-3.*

Breath sounds are abnormal when heard outside normal location. See Table 11-4.

Note the absence of adventitious sounds when documenting.

Adventitious (added) sounds are layered on underlying breath sounds. If heard, listen for loudness, pitch, duration, number, timing, location, variation, and any change after a cough or deep breath.

Technique and Normal Findings	Abnormal Findings
Auscultate voice sounds when an area of consolidation or compression is suspected. They may be assessed if other findings suggest these conditions.	Bronchophony, egophony, and whispered pectoriloquy are all found with increased consolidation or compression, as with *lobar pneumonia*, *atelectasis*, or *tumor*.
Ask the patient to say "ninety-nine" as you auscultate the chest wall, comparing sides. *Sounds are muffled and difficult to distinguish.*	The word "ninety-nine" sounds as if the patient is directly talking into the stethoscope (**bronchophony**).
Ask the patient to say "ee." *This sound is also muffled and difficult to hear.*	In **egophony**, the "ee" sounds like a loud "A."
Ask the patient to whisper "one-two-three." *Sounds are faint, muffled, and difficult to hear.*	Sounds are loud and clear, as if the patient is directly whispering into the stethoscope (**whispered pectoriloquy**).

Anterior Chest

Inspection. Use the same techniques as for the posterior chest (Fig. 11-5). *Normal findings are similar as for the posterior chest.*

Abnormal findings are similar to those for the posterior chest.

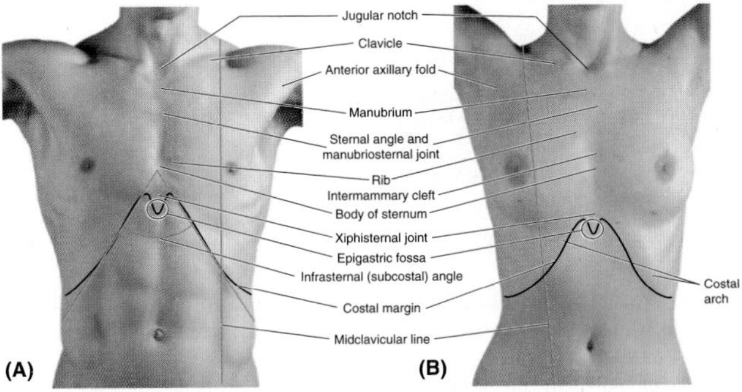

Figure 11.5 Landmarks of the thoracic cage.
(A) Male. **(B)** Female.

(text continues on page 214)

Technique and Normal Findings	Abnormal Findings
Palpation. Palpate bilaterally for tenderness, masses, or lesions. Begin at the lung apices; end below the costal angle and laterally to the midaxillary line.	Abnormal findings are similar to those for the posterior chest.
Palpate with the thumbs along each costal margin (Fig. 11-6). Slide the thumbs medially so that they raise a small skin fold between them. Ask the patient to inhale deeply; observe thumb movement. Feel for extent of symmetric chest expansion. *Anterior chest expansion is greater because the rib cage has more anterior mobility.*	Abnormal findings are similar to those for the posterior chest.

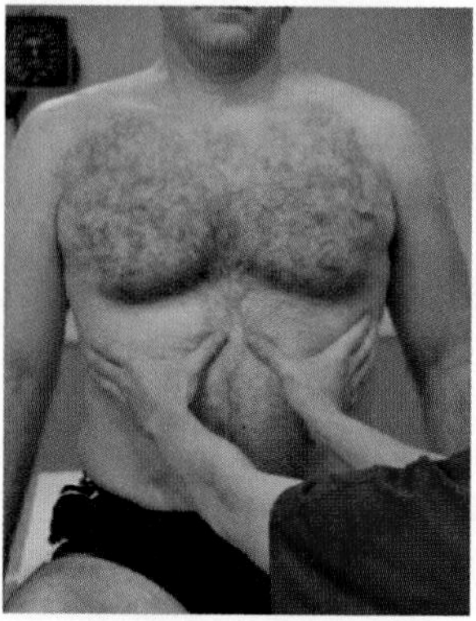

Figure 11.6 Assessing anterior chest expansion.

Technique and Normal Findings	Abnormal Findings
Assess for tactile fremitus. Begin at the lung apices and continue to the bases and laterally. Compare sides. Ask female patients to lift or to displace their breast to the side, because fremitus is decreased over this soft tissue.	Abnormal findings are similar to those for the posterior chest.

Technique and Normal Findings	Abnormal Findings
Fremitus is decreased or absent over the precordium. Fremitus is greatest over large airways in the second and third ICS.	
Percussion. Percuss the anterior and lateral chest in the ICSs and laterally, comparing findings. Women may need to displace the breast. Avoid percussing over bone, which produces a flat tone. *The heart produces dullness from the third to fifth ICS to the left of the sternum. The upper border of liver dullness is percussed in the fifth ICS in the right midclavicular line (MCL). Tympany is percussed over the stomach in the fifth ICS in the left MCL.*	Abnormal findings are similar to those for the posterior chest.
Auscultation. Begin at the trachea. Listen to the apices. Move the stethoscope from one side to another. Place the stethoscope around the breasts in women. Listen to the sixth ICS bilaterally or when breath sounds become absent, signaling the end of the lung fields. *Breath sounds are louder in the upper chest. Bronchial breath sounds are audible over the trachea; bronchovesicular sounds are heard over the second to third ICSs to the right and left of the sternum over the bronchi. Vesicular sounds are heard in other areas.*	Abnormal findings are similar to those for the posterior chest.
Auscultate for transmitted voice sounds.	Abnormal findings are similar to those for the posterior chest.

Documentation of Normal Subjective and
Objective Findings

The patient denies chest pain or discomfort, dyspnea, orthopnea, paroxysmal noctural dyspnea, cough, mucus, wheezing or
tightness in chest, and decrease in functional ability. Breathing,
posture, and facial expression are relaxed. Respirations are 16
breaths/min without accessory muscle use or retractions. Skin is
pink without cyanosis or pallor. Symmetrical chest shape without
kyphosis or scoliosis. Vesicular breath sounds over lung fields. The
patient denies chest pain or tenderness. No crackles or wheezes.

▲ Lifespan Considerations

Pregnant Women

The woman's chest may appear wider and the costal angle larger in
late pregnancy as the uterus pushes up on the diaphragm. Pregnant
women may have strained or fractured ribs because of expansion of
the thoracic cage.

Newborns, Infants, and Children

Respiratory function develops throughout childhood, with increases
in airway size and alveolar size and number. The newborn chest is
round and consistent with head size until approximately age 2 years.
The thin chest wall makes the ribs more prominent. Increased cartilage makes the chest wall more compliant and flexible than in adults.
Newborns noticeably use the diaphragm and abdominal muscles for
respiratory effort. Crepitus around the clavicle may indicate a pneumothorax, especially following forceps delivery. Percussion is not
useful in newborns because an adult's hands are too large for the
small chest. When auscultating the lungs, make sure to use the pediatric diaphragm on the stethoscope appropriate for the newborn's size.
If the baby is crying, wait for a quiet moment to auscultate. Also, take
advantage of sleep in newborns to listen to breath sounds; listen for
fine differences in quality. Expect to auscultate crackles or gurgles
because of small amount of fluid that remains in the lungs. If adventitious lung sounds are asymmetrical, meconium aspiration may have
occurred in one section of the lung. If gastrointestinal gurgling sounds
are heard in the chest, communicate these findings to a primary health
practitioner, because the newborn may have a diaphragmatic hernia.

In newborns, Apgar scores taken at 1 and 5 minutes after birth help determine health status and need for interventions. Apgar scoring includes respirations and skin color, which the nurse evaluates using a sliding scale. See Chapter 22.

Respiratory patterns in infants vary based on feeding, sleep state, and body temperature. Because of this irregularity, respirations in infants should be counted for 1 minute. Respiratory rates are fastest in newborns; they decrease with age.

Parents may hold a hesitant child or a child may want to sit on the parent's lap. Children are curious about stethoscopes; gain trust by having them listen to their own breath sounds first. Detecting expiratory sounds in children with rapid respirations is difficult. Asking them to blow out the penlight will prolong expiratory sounds and wheezing may be detected. A child may also like to breathe like a hot or tired dog during auscultation. A child's breath sounds are louder and harsher; therefore, bronchovesicular breath sounds may normally be heard through the chest.

Children begin using their intercostals muscles to breathe by 6 to 7 years of age. A round chest shape that persists past 5 to 6 years may indicate pulmonary disease. If the child is crying, auscultate the chest during the deep breath that follows a sob.

Older Adults

With aging, respiratory strength declines. Lungs lose elasticity, cartilage in the ribs loses flexibility, and bones lose density. These changes result in smaller breaths (decreased inspiratory volumes) and more air remaining in the lungs after exhalation (increased residual volume). The anterior to posterior depth of the chest widens, causing the thorax to become more rounded or barrel shaped. When the thorax is rounded, it is harder to inhale deeply. Costal cartilages are calcified, creating a less flexible thorax and more use of the upper lung fields, which are less efficient than the bases. As breathing becomes shallower, older adults inhale less air and may need to increase rate of breathing to maintain oxygenation.

The alveoli are less elastic and more rigid, and the lungs may become "stiff." It takes more work to ventilate stiff lungs. Loss of alveoli renders less surface area available for gas exchange. Their decreased reserves make it difficult to maintain ventilation during stress, such as exercise or illness. Additionally, decreased function of the cilia leads to the pooling of secretions in the lungs. Weaker chest muscles also decrease the older person's ability to cough up secretions. Thick, pooled secretions increase risks for pneumonia.

Immobility creates a risk for airway collapse (atelectasis), reduced air exchange, hypoxia, hypercapnia, and acidosis. Reduced gag and cough reflexes can place older people at risk for aspiration of secretions and, potentially, aspiration pneumonia. Postoperative pulmonary complications are another possibility because of impaired cough reflex, weaker muscles, and decreased inspiratory capacity.

Respiratory assessment may be tiring for people of this age group, so allow frequent rest periods. Postpone those activities that can wait until strength has returned so that these patients can use energy for breathing.

◗ Cultural Considerations

Chest size influences how much a person can inhale and exhale. There is no significant difference in the chest volumes of Caucasians, African Americans, or Hispanics. Variability is more closely linked to body size versus ethnicity. Genetic patterns of inheritance increase risks for respiratory problems such as cystic fibrosis and alpha-1 antitrypsin deficiency (associated with COPD).

Common Associated Nursing Diagnoses, Outcomes, and Interventions

Diagnosis and Related Factors	Nursing Interventions
Impaired gas exchange related to alveolar-capillary membrane changes	Administer oxygen,* deep breathing, incentive spirometer, inhalers*
Ineffective airway clearance related to thick tracheobronchial secretions	Cough and deep breathe, increase fluids, expectorants,* postural drainage*
Ineffective breathing pattern related to fatigue	Position to decrease workload of breathing, pace activity, provide rest, reduce fever
Excess fluid volume related to congestive heart failure	Elevate head of bed, administer diuretics,* intake and output, daily weights

*Collaborative interventions.

Tables of Reference

Table 11.1 Respiratory Patterns

Normal

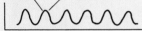

Rate of 10–20 breaths/min; ratio of respiration:pulse is approximately 4:1; 500–800 mL/breath; regular rhythm

Hyperventilation

Rate >24 breaths/min; >800 mL/breath, deep; regular rhythm

Hypoventilation

Rate <10 breaths/min; <500 mL/breath, shallow; irregular rhythm

Biot's respiration

Rate variable; depth variable; irregular irregular rhythm

Tachypnea

Rate >24 breaths/min; <500 mL/breath, shallow; regular rhythm

Bradypnea

Rate <10 breaths/min; 500–800 mL/breath, shallow; regular rhythm

Cheyne-Stokes respiration

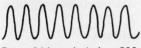

Hyperpnea   Apnea

Rate variable; depth variable; regular irregular rhythm that cycles from deep and fast to shallow and slow, with some periods of apnea

Apnea
No breaths

Table 11.2 Thoracic Configurations

Normal Adult

Anterior-posterior:lateral ratio is 1:2, wider than it is deep, oval shaped. Cone shaped from head to toe.

Pectus Excavatum (Funnel Chest)

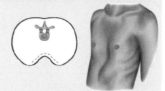

Depression in lower part of and adjacent to sternum. Congenital condition may compress heart or great vessels and cause murmurs.

Kyphoscoliosis

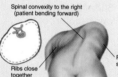

Spinal convexity to the right (patient bending forward)

Ribs close together

Ribs widely separated

With kyphosis, the thoracic spine curves forward, compressing the anterior chest and reducing inspiratory lung volumes. With scoliosis, a lateral S-shaped curvature of the spine causes unequal shoulders, scapulae, and hips. In severe cases, asymmetry may impede breathing.

Barrel Chest

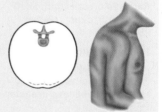

Anterior-posterior:lateral ratio near 1:1, round shaped. Ribs are more horizontal and costal margin is widened. Associated with COPD, chronic asthma, and normal aging.

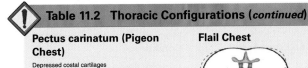

Table 11.2 Thoracic Configurations (*continued*)

Pectus carinatum (Pigeon Chest)

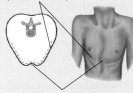

Depressed costal cartilages

Anteriorly displaced sternum

Sternum is displaced anteriorly, depressing the adjacent costal cartilages. Congenital condition with increased anteroposterior diameter.

Flail Chest

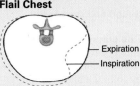

— Expiration
— Inspiration

When multiple ribs are fractured, paradoxical movements of the chest may occur. As the diaphragm pulls down during inspiration, negative pressure causes the injured area to cave inward; during expiration it moves out.

Table 11.3 Normal Breath Sounds

Sound	Characteristics Intensity and Pitch
Bronchial	**Intensity and pitch:** Loud and high **Quality:** Coarse or tubular **Duration:** Inspiration < expiration **Locations:** Larynx and trachea
Bronchovesicular	**Intensity and pitch:** Intermediate and intermediate **Quality:** Intermediate **Duration:** Inspiration = expiration **Locations:** Anteriorly between first and second interspaces; between scapula
Vesicular	**Intensity and pitch:** Soft and low **Quality:** Whispering undertones **Duration:** Inspiration > expiration **Locations:** Over most of the lung fields

Table 11.4 Adventitious Breath Sounds

Sound and Description	Mechanism and Associated Conditions
Fine crackles (rales): High-pitched, soft, brief crackling sounds that can be simulated by rolling a strand of hair near the ear or stethoscope	Deflated small airways and alveoli will pop open during inspiration. In early CHF, small amounts of fluid in the alveoli may cause fine crackles. Late inspiratory crackles are associated with restrictive disease. Early inspiratory crackles occur with obstructive diseases.
Coarse crackles (rales): Low-pitched, moist, longer sounds that are similar to Velcro slowly separating	Small air bubbles flow through secretions or narrowed airways. Associated conditions include pulmonary fibrosis, pulmonary edema, COPD.
Wheeze: High-pitched or sibilant musical sounds heard primarily during inspiration	Air passes through narrowed airways and creates sound, similar to that of a vibrating reed. Note if inspiratory or expiratory. Found with asthma, bronchitis, emphysema.
Rhonchi: Gurgle, low-pitched wheeze, or sonorous wheeze sound that may clear with coughing	Airflow passes around or through secretions or narrowed passages in cases of pneumonia.
Pleural friction rub: Loud, coarse, and low-pitched grating or creaking sound similar to that of a squeaky door during inspiration and expiration; more common in the lower anterolateral thorax	With pleuritis, inflamed pleural surfaces lose their normal lubrication and rub together during breathing.
Stridor: Loud high-pitched crowing or honking sound louder in upper airway	Laryngeal or tracheal inflammation or spasm from epiglottitis, croup, or aspiration of a foreign object can cause stridor.

12

Heart and Neck Vessels Assessment

Subjective Data Collection

Key Topics and Questions for Health Promotion

Key Questions	Rationales
Obtain from the chart age; heredity; gender; and dates and results of last blood pressure measurement, cholesterol level, C-reactive protein level, B-type natriuretic peptides, and thyroid levels.	Risk factors for cardiovascular disease include increased age; male gender; African American, Mexican American, American Indian, native Hawaiian, and Asian American heritages; elevated cholesterol, and C-reactive protein, and thyroid levels.
Family History. Do you have any family history of cardiovascular problems? Provide details.	*Premature* (onset before 55 years of age in men and 65 years in women) *coronary artery disease* in a first- or second-degree relative increases the patient's risk for the same. Other family history risk factors are high blood pressure, high cholesterol, diabetes, heart disease, and obesity.
Past Medical History. Have you been diagnosed with chest pain, heart attack, heart failure, or irregular rhythm?	Past problems provide information that can assist with anticipating future needs.
Do you have high blood pressure, high blood cholesterol, or diabetes mellitus? Do you take anything for these?	Untreated hypertension, elevated cholesterol, and diabetes mellitus are risk factors for cardiac disease.

(text continues on page 224)

Key Questions	Rationales
Medications. Are you taking any medications for cardiac problems? • What are they? • How often? • How well are you following your prescribed regimen?	Note drug, dose, and frequency. Obtain the reason for the medication—some drugs have several purposes. Compliance with medications is essential; many cardiac medications have side effects that cause patients to stop taking them.
Do you use any natural supplements or over-the-counter (OTC) medications? What are they? How often?	Some supplements have cardiac side effects. Note any potential drug interactions between prescribed and OTC medications.
Lifestyle/Behavior. Do you smoke or use tobacco products? • How long? • How many packs per day?	Smokers are at significantly increased risk for *coronary heart disease* and sudden cardiac arrest.
What is your usual physical activity and exercise? How long and how often?	Low activity level is associated with increased risk for cardiovascular disease.
What is your typical diet?	A diet low in fruits and vegetables and high in fat and cholesterol increases risk.
How much alcohol do you usually drink per day? Week? Month? Do you use any recreational drugs such as cocaine?	More than two drinks per day for men or one drink per day for women can raise blood pressure, contribute to *heart failure*, elevate triglyceride levels, contribute to obesity, and produce irregular heartbeats. Cocaine increases risk of *myocardial infarction (MI)* and *coronary vasospasm*.

Health-Promotion Teaching

Smoking Cessation. Ask patients who smoke about their willingness to quit at every visit. Patients who quit reduce their risk of cardiac events. Give patients choices about tools to help them quit (eg, referrals to behavioral therapy, information about support groups, medication).

Control of Blood Pressure and Cholesterol Level. High blood pressure should be controlled with medication if diet, exercise, and weight reduction are unsuccessful. High cholesterol can be modified by eating a low-cholesterol diet, with reduced animal fat. Lean cuts of grilled or roasted meat are better than deep-fried, fatty cuts. If diet alone is unsuccessful, the physician may prescribe a statin medication.

Key Topics and Questions for Common Symptoms

For each of the symptoms, be sure to assess features such as onset, location, duration, character, aggravating factors, associated factors, and treatments.

Common Cardiovascular Symptoms

- Chest pain
- Dyspnea, orthopnea, and cough
- Diaphoresis
- Fatigue
- Edema
- Nocturia
- Palpitations

△ *SAFETY ALERT 12-1*

Always assume that a patient's chest pain is heart pain until another cause can be found. If chest pain is ischemic, rapid treatment is necessary to prevent the death of cardiac cells. If medication or angioplasty can open the artery, the size of the MI can be reduced.

Questions to Assess Symptoms	Rationales/Abnormal Findings
Chest Pain. Do you have chest pain or discomfort?	Pain of *MI* typically is on the left side of the chest, radiates down the left arm or into the jaw, and is diffuse. Onset can be sudden or gradual. Patients may describe the pain as crushing, viselike, pressure, or discomfort. Some patients have nausea or vomiting; others describe indigestion. Associated symptoms include diaphoresis, pallor, anxiety, and fatigue.

(text continues on page 226)

Questions to Assess Symptoms	Rationales/Abnormal Findings
Dyspnea. Have you had any shortness of breath? Describe features.	Patients with *heart failure* may be short of breath from fluid accumulation in the pulmonary bed. Onset may be sudden with *acute or chronic pulmonary edema.* **Dyspnea on exertion** is common with physical activity. Note the amount of activity that elicits dyspnea.
Orthopnea. Have you had difficulty sleeping? How many pillows do you use? Do you awaken short of breath?	Patients with *heart failure* may have fluid in their lungs, making it difficult to breathe when flat. They may wake up suddenly as the fluid is redistributed from edematous legs into the lungs (**paroxysmal nocturnal dyspnea or PND**), typically after a few hours of sleep. They may waken feeling tired, anxious, or restless.
Cough. Have you noticed a cough? Describe features.	Coughing occurs for the same reason as dyspnea.
Diaphoresis. Have you noticed any excessive sweating? Describe features.	Nighttime diaphoresis is associated with *tuberculosis.* Diaphoresis in response to exercise or activity may be related to cardiac stress.
Fatigue. Have you been especially fatigued or tired?	Fatigue occurs when the heart cannot pump enough blood to meet the needs of tissues. It is the most common symptom of MI in women.
Edema. Have you noticed any swelling in your feet, legs, or hands?	Fluid may accumulate in organs and dependent areas as a result of problems with blood flow.

Questions to Assess Symptoms	Rationales/Abnormal Findings
Nocturia. Do you need to get up at night to use the bathroom?	**Nocturia** is a common symptom associated with redistribution of fluid from legs to core when flat.
Palpitations. Do you notice that your heart is beating faster? Are you having skipped or extra beats?	Tachycardia may be from decreased contractile strength of the heart muscle. With reduced stroke volume, pulse increases to maintain cardiac output. **Palpitations** (rapid throbbing or fluttering of the heart) are associated with *arrhythmias*.

Objective Data Collection

Equipment

- Stethoscope with bell and diaphragm
- Watch with second hand
- Penlight or examination light for visualizing neck veins

Technique and Normal Findings	Abnormal Findings
Jugular Venous Pulses Inspection of the subtle pulses requires practice with several patients. Rather than identify all the waves, nurses more commonly observe pattern and rhythm.	If severe *heart failure* is suspected, invasive hemodynamic monitoring may be used.
Position the patient with the head of the bed 30 to 45 degrees (Fig. 12-1). Remove the pillow to improve vein exposure. Move any long hair away. The right side is easiest to see.	If the patient is unusually dehydrated, it may be necessary to lower the head of the bed to visualize the vein, while the patient with fluid overload may need to have the head of the bed elevated.

(text continues on page 228)

Technique and Normal Findings	Abnormal Findings

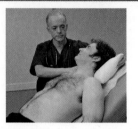

Figure 12.1 Lower the head of the bed to a 45-degree angle to better visualize the soft jugular venous pulses.

Technique and Normal Findings	Abnormal Findings
Light the area. Indirect lighting is best from 45 degrees. *There are usually two pulsations with a prominent descent. The carotid pulse has one pulsation and a prominent ascent with systole.*	**Distended** veins can extend all the way to the ear. Patients with *dehydration* or *volume depletion* have barely visible neck veins, described as **flat neck veins**.
Jugular Venous Pressure After locating the internal jugular vein, identify the top height of the pulsation. Locate the sternal angle in the 2nd intercostal space (ICS). Using a line parallel to the horizon, from the sternal angle estimate the difference between the parallel line and the top of the pulsation in the external jugular vein (Fig. 12-2). *Findings are up to 3 cm above the sternal angle.*	Jugular venous distention (JVD) is associated with *heart failure* and *fluid volume overload.* The neck veins appear full, and the level of pulsation may be >3 cm above the sternal angle.

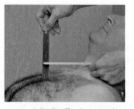

Figure 12.2 Estimate the jugular venous pressure.

Technique and Normal Findings	Abnormal Findings

Hepatojugular Reflux

Apply gentle pressure over the right upper quadrant or middle abdomen for at least 10 seconds to increase venous return (Fig. 12-3). *Pulsation increases for a few beats and returns to normal <3 cm above the sternal angle.*

The highest level of pulsation stays above 3 cm for more than 15 seconds.

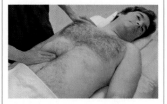

Figure 12.3 To assess hepatojugular reflux, press gently on the liver.

Carotid Arteries

Inspection. Inspect for a double stroke seen with S1 and S2. *Contour is smooth with a rapid upstroke and slower downstroke.*

Pulse is bounding and prominent (*hypertension, hypermetabolism*). It is low in amplitude and volume with a delayed peak (*aortic stenosis*). If diminished unilaterally or bilaterally, the cause may be *carotid stenosis from atherosclerosis.*

Palpation. Palpate carotid arteries one at a time (Fig. 12-4). Palpate strength of the pulse; grade it as with peripheral pulses (see Chapter 13). *Strength is 2+ or moderate. Pulses are equal bilaterally.*

A diminished or thready pulse may accompany decreased stroke volume. Pulse strength may be reduced with *heart failure, atherosclerosis,* exercise, or stress.

(text continues on page 230)

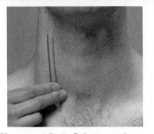

Figure 12.4 Palpate each carotid artery medial to the sternomastoid muscle in the neck.

Auscultation. Lightly apply the bell over the artery medial to the sternomastoid muscle, in the middle of the neck, and near the clavicle. Do not compress the artery. *No sounds or bruits are heard.*

Bruits (swooshing sounds similar to the sound of blood pressure) result from turbulent blood flow related to *atherosclerosis.*

Precordium
Inspection. Assess for lesions, masses, or tenderness. Observe for the point of maximum impulse (PMI) in the apex at the 4th to 5th ICS at the left midclavicular line (MCL). *Impulses are absent or in the 4th to 5th left ICS at the MCL with no lifts or heaves.*

The enlarged heart of *cardiomegaly* displaces the PMI laterally and inferiorly.

Palpation. Palpate for lesions, masses, or tender areas. Use the palmar surface. Begin at the apex of the heart; feel for the pulse in the location observed during inspection. Use the finger pads; depress in the 5th left ICS at the MCL (Fig. 12-5). The PMI, which may or may not be palpable in adults, is usually a light tap from S1 to halfway through systole and <1 to 2 cm. *PMI is in the 5th left ICS at the MCL.*

An abnormal PMI is displaced left or downward, raises a larger than normal area, or is sustained throughout systole. It may result from *heart failure, MI, left ventricular hypertrophy,* or *valvular heart disease.*

Technique and Normal Findings	Abnormal Findings

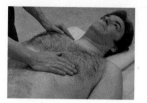

Figure 12.5 Location of the apical impulse.

Palpate in the sternoclavicular area, right and left upper sternal borders, right and left lower sternal borders, apical area, and epigastric area. *No pulsations are palpated in other areas.*

Abnormal sensations include lifts and heaves. **Thrills** are vibrations detected on palpation from *incompetent valves, pulmonary hypertension, or septal defects.*

Percussion. Chest x-ray has largely replaced chest percussion.

Auscultation. Auscultation is the most important technique of cardiovascular examination.

Rate and Rhythm. Using the diaphragm, listen to Erb's point to identify S1, S2, rhythm, and rate (Fig. 12-6). *Heart rate is 60 to 100 bpm and regular in adults.*

No detectable pattern is characteristic of *atrial fibrillation*. Refer to Chapter 3 for rate variations.

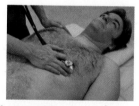

Figure 12.6 Auscultating at Erb's point.

S1 and S2. Identify S1 as lub and S2 as dub. Listen to each sound separately. A split S1 is heard in the tricuspid area.

See Table 12-1 at the end of this chapter.

(text continues on page 232)

Technique and Normal Findings	Abnormal Findings
S2 signals the end of systole and beginning of diastole as the aortic and pulmonic valves close. *S1 > S2 in the mitral and tricuspid areas; S2 > S1 in the aortic and pulmonic areas; and S1 = S2 at Erb's point.*	A split S2 may occur from the pulmonic valve closing slightly after the aortic. (see Table 12-1).
Extra Sounds. When S3 exists, it follows S2 and sounds like "lub dub-dub." It usually is heard best in the apex with the patient lying on the left side. It may be normal in young patients.	S3 is abnormal in patients older than 40 years and results from increased atrial pressure related to *systolic heart failure* or *valvular regurgitation.*
S4 in late diastole, right before S1, sounds like "lub-lub dub." It is usually abnormal.	S4 results from a noncompliant ventricle as a consequence of *hypertension, hypertrophy,* or *fibrosis.*
Listen for the short scratching sound of the pericardial friction rub, high-pitched opening snaps, and ejection clicks. *Normally no extra sounds are heard.*	See Table 12-2 at the end of this chapter.
Murmurs. Describe murmurs according to timing in the cardiac cycle, loudness, pitch, pattern, quality, location, radiation, and position. *Normally no murmurs are heard.*	See Tables 12-3 and 12-4 at the end of this chapter.

Documentation of Normal Subjective and Objective Findings

No chest pain or discomfort. Denies dyspnea, orthopnea, paroxysmal nocturnal dyspnea, cough, fatigue, edema, nocturia, and palpitations. Without JVD, hepatojugular reflux negative. Carotid pulses 2+ bilaterally without bruits. PMI observed and palpated in 5th left ICS at the MCL. No thrills, heaves, or lifts. Heart rate and rhythm regular, without gallops, murmurs, or rubs.

▲ Lifespan Considerations ─────────────

Pregnant Women

Maternal blood volume increases throughout pregnancy, beginning in the first trimester and peaking by the 32nd to 34th week. Increased stroke volume and heart rate elevate cardiac output to keep up with the increased demands of supplying nutrients and oxygen to the developing fetus. Cardiac output is reduced when the pregnant woman is supine, because the uterus impedes venous return. This positioning may be significant enough to reduce blood pressure; thus, a side-lying position is recommended for pregnant women. Cardiac output returns to prepregnancy levels about 2 weeks postpartum.

The left ventricle increases both the wall thickness and muscle mass. Also the uterus enlarges and pushes the diaphragm upward, and the position of the heart shifts more horizontally. Resting pulse rate increases, and blood pressure may rise slightly.

The woman's skin may be slightly redder than normal because of the increased volume and metabolic state. Heart sounds may change because of the increased blood volume. S1 and S2 may be split after 20 weeks. Systolic and diastolic murmurs may be heard over the pre-cordium, although systolic murmurs are more common.

A unique murmur in lactating women is referred to as a *mammary soufflé*. It results from increased blood flow through the internal mammary artery and is best heard in the 2nd to 4th ICS.

Newborns and Infants

At birth, the lungs inflate with air, increasing pulmonary vascular resistance markedly. Along with clamping of the umbilical cord, this forces the pulmonary and systemic circuits to function separately. Within minutes to hours after birth, the atrial septum is pushed to close and right-to-left blood flow is established. Blood flow decreases in the ductus arteriosis, causing it to constrict and close within a few days, separating the pulmonary artery and aorta. Newborn heart rate is increased because the muscle has not yet developed and stroke volumes are lower. The rate may be as high as 180 bpm in response to stress or crying and may decrease to 120 bpm at rest.

Infant blood pressure and arterial resistance increase when the umbilical cord is cut. The left ventricle hypertrophies and becomes more muscular than the right. By 1 year of age, the left ventricle is twice the size of the right, which is similar to adult size.

The heart is positioned more horizontally in infants than in adults, which causes the apex to be in the 4th left ICS slightly lateral to the MCL.

During examination, if possible, place the infant on the parent's lap. Do not undress the baby until necessary, because exposure may be uncomfortable and cold, and assessing a restless baby with high respiratory and cardiac rates is difficult. A bottle or pacifier might help to calm the baby. Observe for cyanosis, especially with crying. Note that the infant's skin may normally be mottled if the examining environment is cool. Inspect for subcostal retractions, left-sided chest prominence, abnormal chest movement, and increased respiratory rates. Because infants have short necks, the jugular veins are not examined. Palpate the faint apical impulse to the left of the xiphoid, at the apex, and in the 2nd ICS at the left sternal border; a prominent pulse is abnormal. Percussion in infants and children is not performed, because related findings do not accurately reflect cardiac size or function. Use a pediatric stethoscope to auscultate the heart.

Children and Adolescents

The heart grows and moves lower as the child's body changes. By 7 years of age, the child's heart is similar to an adult's. Both the left ventricular cavity size and wall thickness increase linearly with age. By 7 years, the apex is palpable in the 5th left ICS at the MCL.

If a child appears likely to cry, auscultate heart sounds before inspecting the precordium. Question older children about exercise, activities, edema, respiratory problems, chest pain, palpitations, fainting, and headaches.

If cardiac disease is suspected, auscultate the heart with the child in different positions, beginning with lying and standing. During auscultation in the pulmonic area, S2 may be closely split in inspiration and single in expiration. Fixed splitting (an important finding) may indicate an atrial septal defect from a patent foramen ovale. In the tricuspid area, S1 may be closely split and S2 will be single; this does not vary with respiration. At the apex, there is a single S1, single S2, and possibly an S3. S3 will be heard best with the bell; it is normal in children because of hyperdynamic circulation and a thin chest wall. If a murmur is heard, it may be innocent, functional, or pathologic. Listen carefully to determine the characteristics, and refer any patients with suspected problems to a physician if previously undiagnosed.

Older Adults

With aging, the left ventricular wall thickens, left atrium increases, and mitral valve closes more slowly. The heart fills more slowly in early diastole but compensates by filling more quickly in late diastole during atrial contraction. Blood flow is approximately equal during early and late diastole. Consequently, the volumes in the heart remain about the same as in younger people.

Because of fibrotic changes and fat deposits on the SA node, older adults have less heart rate variability. Additionally, their hearts respond less to the sympathetic nervous system, with reduced maximum heart rates. Receptors for stress hormones also may become less sensitive.

Cultural Considerations

Heart disease is the leading cause of death in high-income countries and the leading killer across most U.S. racial and ethnic minority communities.

Common Nursing Diagnoses and Interventions for Cardiovascular Conditions

Diagnosis and Related Factors	Nursing Interventions
Decreased cardiac output related to MI, arrhythmia, sepsis, and congenital heart defect	Monitor for symptoms of heart failure. Observe for chest pain or discomfort. Place patient on cardiac monitor. Assess blood pressure carefully.
Impaired tissue perfusion, cardiac related to chest pain, shock, or dysrhythmia	Place patient on cardiac monitor. Administer nitroglycerin with MD order.* Place oxygen.* Ensure that the IV is in place for emergency use.* Notify physician.
Excess fluid volume related to heart failure, excess fluid intake, and excess sodium intake	Monitor edema, intake, and output. Weigh patient daily. Auscultate lung and heart sounds. Administer diuretic with order.* Elevate head of bed for dyspnea.

*Collaborative interventions.

Tables of Reference

Table 12.1   Variations in S1 and S2

Heart Sound	Description

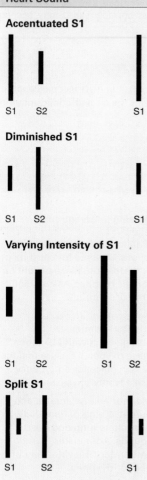

Accentuated S1

S1   S2   S1

S1 is louder when mitral valve leaflets are recessed into the ventricle, as with rapid heart rate, hyperkinetic states, short PR interval, atrial fibrillation, or mitral stenosis.

Diminished S1

S1   S2   S1

S1 is softer with long PR interval, depressed contractility, left bundle branch block, obesity, or a muscular chest.

Varying Intensity of S1

S1   S2   S1   S2

S1 varies in atrial fibrillation and complete heart block when the valve is in varying positions before closing.

Split S1

S1   S2   S1

The first component is heard at the base; the second component is heard at the lower left sternal border. Split S1 accompanies right bundle branch block.

Table 12.1 Variations in S1 and S2 (*continued*)

Heart Sound	Description
Accentuated S2 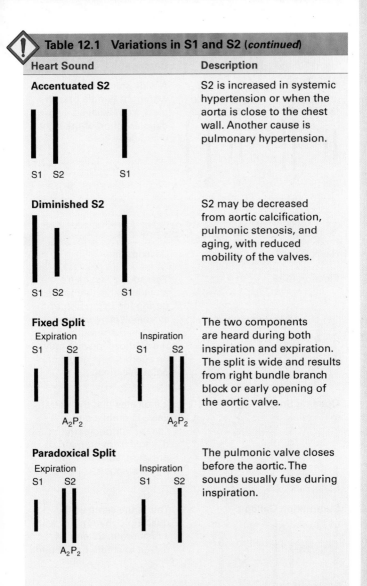 S1 S2 S1	S2 is increased in systemic hypertension or when the aorta is close to the chest wall. Another cause is pulmonary hypertension.
Diminished S2 S1 S2 S1	S2 may be decreased from aortic calcification, pulmonic stenosis, and aging, with reduced mobility of the valves.
Fixed Split Expiration Inspiration S1 S2 S1 S2 A_2P_2 A_2P_2	The two components are heard during both inspiration and expiration. The split is wide and results from right bundle branch block or early opening of the aortic valve.
Paradoxical Split Expiration Inspiration S1 S2 S1 S2 A_2P_2	The pulmonic valve closes before the aortic. The sounds usually fuse during inspiration.

(table continues on page 238)

Table 12.1   Variations in S1 and S2 (*continued*)

Heart Sound	Description
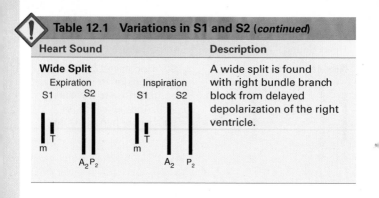**Wide Split**	A wide split is found with right bundle branch block from delayed depolarization of the right ventricle.

Table 12.2   Identifying Extra Sounds

Heart Sound	Description
Ejection Click	This sound results from an open valve that moves during the beginning of systole. It is heard best with the diaphragm of the stethoscope and may be audible over aortic or pulmonic areas.
Opening Snap	It indicates that the mitral valve is mobile and "snaps" during early diastole from high atrial pressure, such as with mitral stenosis.
Summation Gallop	This is the same as the quadruple rhythm but with a faster rate. S3 and S4 merge to create one sound.

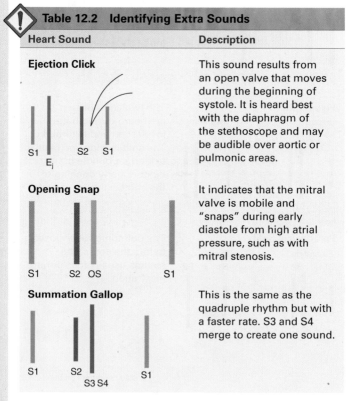

Table 12.2   Identifying Extra Sounds (*continued*)

Heart Sound	Description
Pericardial Friction Rub 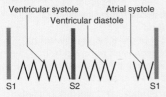	It is triple phased during midsystole, middiastole, and presystole. The scratchy, leathery quality results from the parietal and visceral pleura rubbing together. The sound increases on leaning forward and during exhalation. It is heard best in the 3rd left ICS at the sternal border.
Venous Hum 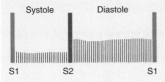	This continuous sound is normal in children and during pregnancy. It is rough, noisy, and occasionally accompanied by a high-pitched whine. It may be louder during diastole. It is low-pitched and heard best with the bell above the medial third of the clavicles.
Quadruple Rhythm with S3 and S4	S3 is generated during early diastolic filling; S4 is generated during atrial contraction late in diastole. Both are present. It is heard best with the bell of the stethoscope over the apex of the heart.

Intensity: Loudness	**I.** Faint; heard only with special effort **II.** Soft but readily detected **III.** Prominent but not loud **IV.** Loud; accompanied by thrill **V.** Very loud **VI.** Loud enough to be heard with stethoscope just removed from contact with the chest wall (Braunwald et al., 2004).
Timing: Point in the cardiac cycle	**Systolic:** Sounds like "swish-dub"; falls between S1 and S2 **Diastolic:** Sounds like "dub-swish," falls after S2 and before the next S1 More specifically murmurs may be labeled as early, mid, or late systolic and early, mid, or late diastolic. **Holosystolic murmurs:** Occur during all of systole **Holodiastolic murmurs:** Occur during all of diastole **Continuous murmurs:** Begin in systole and continue through S2 into part but not necessarily all of diastole
Pitch: High or low tone	**High:** Heard best with diaphragm **Medium** **Low pitch:** Heard best with bell
Pattern: Increasing or decreasing in volume	**Crescendo:** Increasing intensity **Decrescendo:** Decreasing intensity **Plateau:** Remain constant
Quality: Type of sounds	Harsh, blowing, raspy, musical, and rumbling
Location: Site on the precordium	Area of maximum intensity using either the valvular areas or thoracic landmarks
Radiation: Direction it travels	Where the sound radiates, usually in the direction of blood flow in the vessel
Position: Changes with patient position	If the murmur changes depending on patient position, the patient may be turned to the left and right, lie down, sit up, and lean forward. Children may squat.

Table 12.4 Distinguishing Murmurs

Heart Sound	Description
Physiologic Murmur 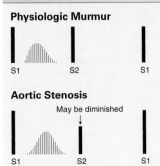	This murmur, caused by a temporary increase in blood flow, has a soft, medium pitch and a harsh quality.
Aortic Stenosis	This midsystolic ejection murmur begins after S1, crescendos, and then decrescendos before S2. It radiates upward to the right 2nd ICS and into the neck. It is soft to loud, with a medium pitch and harsh quality. It is associated with ejection click, split S2.
Pulmonic Stenosis 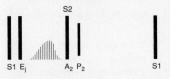	This midsystolic ejection murmur may radiate toward the left shoulder and neck. It is soft-loud, has medium pitch, harsh quality, and is associated with ejection click, split S2.
Mitral Stenosis 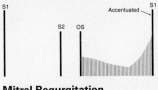	This middiastolic murmur is associated with an opening snap and has a low-pitched, rumbling quality.
Mitral Regurgitation 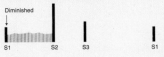	This midsystolic ejection murmur is soft to loud, has medium to high pitch, with a blowing quality. It radiates to the left axilla and is associated with a thrill and lift at the apex.

(table continues on page 242)

Heart Sound	Description
Tricuspid Regurgitation 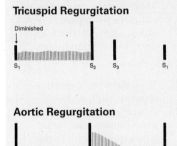	This midsystolic ejection murmur can be holosystolic with elevated right ventricular pressure. It increases with inspiration, with a medium pitch and blowing quality.
Aortic Regurgitation	This early diastolic murmur is decrescendo, soft, high pitched, and blowing.
Pulmonic Regurgitation	This early diastolic murmur may begin with a loud S2. It is a high frequency blowing murmur with a crescendo-decrescendo pattern.
Tricuspid Stenosis	The loudness of this middiastolic murmur increases with inspiration. It has a rumbling quality and is louder during inspiration.

13

Peripheral Vascular with Lymphatics Assessment

Subjective Data Collection

Key Topics and Questions for Health Promotion ———

Questions to Assess Risk Factors	Rationales
Personal/Family History. Do you have a family history of cardiovascular problems? • Who had the illness? • Was it arterial, venous, or lymphatic? • How was it treated? • What was the outcome?	*Cardiovascular disease* has a well-established hereditary component.
Do you have a family or personal history of diabetes? • Who had/has the illness? • How is it treated? • How well is it controlled? • Have there been complications?	Family history of *diabetes* increases a person's risk of developing the same condition. Diabetes significantly increases a patient's risk for lower-extremity peripheral arterial disease (PAD).
Do you have a family or personal history of hypertension? • Who had/has the illness? • How is it treated? • How well is it controlled? • Have there been complications?	Patients with *hypertension* are at increased risk for vascular disease.
Is there a family or personal history of elevated cholesterol? • Who had/has it? • How is it treated? • How well controlled is it?	Increased levels of cholesterol are associated with *athero-sclerosis*, *PAD*, and *abdominal aneurysm*.

(text continues on page 244)

Questions to Assess Risk Factors	Rationales
Have you had any recent trauma to any of your extremities? Provide details.	Monitor for complications of *thromboembolism* and *arterial damage*.
Do you have a family history of lymphedema? (If yes, find out affected person, treatment, outcome, site, when it happened, and any subsequent swelling.)	*Lymphedema* may be familial or result from trauma or excision of lymph nodes.
Tobacco Use • Do you smoke cigarettes, pipes, or cigars? (If yes, find out how many packs per day, for how long, attempts at smoking cessation, and current interest in quitting.) • Are you frequently exposed to smoke? • How do you control exposure?	Smoking is an extremely significant risk factor for lower-extremity *PAD* and *abdominal aneurysm*. Exposure to secondary smoke may affect risk as well.
Activity • Do you exercise regularly? (Describe type, frequency, and duration.) • Do you sit or stand for long periods? • Do you have problems with swelling in your legs because of this?	Regular exercise (four to five times a week) promotes cardiovascular and venous health and decreases risk of diseases.
Oral Contraceptives. Do you use oral contraceptives? If so, for how long? Have you had any side effects?	Oral contraceptives have the side effect of possible deep vein thrombosis (*DVT*).

Health-Promotion Teaching

Controlling Arterial Disease. Modifying risk factors can significantly improve outcomes for patients with PAD. The most controllable risk factors are smoking, high-fat diet, and limited activity. Smoking cessation can delay atherosclerotic progression. Ask patients about readiness to quit; offer resources to assist (eg, individual and group counseling, support groups, medical treatment, and nicotine-replacement therapy). Diet modification includes weight management and decreasing consumption of high-fat foods. Monitoring of cholesterol and triglyceride levels is important. Patients need a thorough understanding of the relationship that diet, activity, and genetic factors have to cholesterol levels and atherosclerosis. Discuss the preventive role of regular exercise. Daily foot assessment is essential for these patients.

Controlling Venous Disease. Patients with venous disease need education about methods to decrease venous pressure. Measures to combat chronic edema include avoiding standing and sitting for long periods and elevating the legs periodically. Some patients benefit from compression stockings. Patients at risk for or with a history of DVT need thorough education on the signs and symptoms of DVT and, in some cases, anticoagulant therapy.

Controlling Lymphatic Disorders. Edema in the extremities is the primary symptom of lymphedema. Thus, management suggestions may include avoiding sitting or standing for long periods, periodically elevating the affected extremity, and applying compression wraps or stockings. Patients with chronic lymphedema may experience disfigurement that affects body image and self-esteem. It is essential to address these areas that affect quality of life.

Focused Health History Related to Common Symptoms

Common Peripheral Vascular and Lymphatic Symptoms

- Pain
- Numbness or tingling
- Cramping
- Skin changes
- Edema
- Decreased functional ability

Questions to Assess Symptoms	Rationales/Abnormal Findings
Pain. Do you have any pain in your arms or legs?	⚠ SAFETY ALERT 13-1 *Determine if pain is acute or chronic before proceeding with the interview.*

(text continues on page 246)

Questions to Assess Symptoms	Rationales/Abnormal Findings
Where is the pain? Can you point to where it hurts? Does it go anywhere?	Location of pain in *PAD* usually closely approximates the affected vessel.
Describe the pain. What does it feel like? How bad is it from 1 to 10, with 10 being worst?	Chronic pain is dull or aching. Acute pain is often described as sharp and stabbing.
What brings on the pain? How long does it last? What makes it worse or better?	Pain brought on by exertion and relieved by rest is called *intermittent claudication*.
Do other symptoms accompany it?	Patients with *PAD* may hang the foot on the affected side over the side of the bed.
Does the pain wake you up at night?	Such pain is termed *rest pain*.
Numbness/Tingling. Have you had changes in sensation in your arms or legs? • Do you have numbness or tingling in your hands or feet? • What makes it worse or better?	*Peripheral neuropathies*, a complication of diabetes, may be painful and result in loss of sensation. Subsequent damage to skin increases risk for wounds.
Cramping. Do you have cramping in your legs? • Are cramps sudden or gradual? • Do they occur with walking or activity? • Can you walk without cramping? • What makes the cramps better?	The area of cramping in arterial disease, termed *intermittent claudication*, closely approximates the level of arterial occlusion.
Skin. Have you had any changes in your skin, hair, or nails? • Any hair loss in your hands or feet? • Are your arms or legs pale or cool? • Have your nails become thicker? • Any color changes in your fingers or toes related to cold weather?	Decreased arterial blood supply may lead to changes in the lower extremities: loss of hair, pallor, cool temperature, or hypertrophic nail changes. *Raynaud's disease* is characterized by color changes in cold weather.

Questions to Assess Symptoms	Rationales/Abnormal Findings
Edema. Have you had swelling in your arms or legs? • Does putting your legs up help? • Is it worse at night or in the morning? • Is swelling accompanied by redness or tenderness?	Vascular causes of swelling in the arms or legs may result from venous occlusion or incompetence of the venous valves.
Functional Ability. Have difficulties with arms or legs affected your daily life? Can you continue activities?	Decreased functional ability may result from arterial insufficiency.

Objective Data Collection

Equipment Needed

- Examination gown
- Nonstretchable measuring tape
- Ultrasonic Doppler stethoscope
- Ultrasonic gel
- Sphygmomanometer
- Tourniquet

Technique and Normal Findings	Abnormal Findings
Arms *Inspection.* Note size and symmetry of arms and hands as well as muscle atrophy or hypertrophy. *Arms and hands are symmetrical with full joint movement.*	*PAD* may result in muscle atrophy. Hypertrophy may result from activity in which the patient uses one arm more than the other.
Assess color of arms and hands; evaluate for venous pattern. *Color is pink, symmetrical, and consistent without prominent venous pattern.*	Pallor indicates arterial insufficiency. Erythema may accompany *thrombophlebitis* or *DVT*.

(text continues on page 248)

BOX 13.1 PITTING EDEMA SCALE

+1: Slight pitting, 2 mm depression
+2: Increased pitting, 4 mm depression
+3: Deeper pitting, 6 mm depression; obvious edema of extremity
+4: Severe pitting, 8 mm depression; extremity appears very edematous

Technique and Normal Findings	Abnormal Findings
Evaluate nail beds for color and angle. *Nail beds are pink. Nail-base angle is 180 degrees without clubbing.*	Capillary refill may be decreased with arterial disease.
Evaluate for edema by pressing the tissue with your fingers. *No indentation remains when you remove your fingers.*	Lymphedema results in unilateral edema. Use the scale in Box 13-1 to document degree of pitting edema.
Evaluate for any ecchymoses or lesions. *These are absent.*	Be alert for signs of abuse or falls. Delayed wound healing occurs with arterial disease.
Palpation. Use the dorsal aspect of your hands to palpate the patient's upper extremities simultaneously. *Arms and hands are warm and equal in temperature.*	⚠ *SAFETY ALERT 13-2* *Coolness of an extremity may indicate arterial occlusion. Assess quickly for the 6 "Ps" (Box 13-2).*
Pinch the skin to assess texture and turgor. *Texture is firm, even, and elastic. Turgor is intact (skin rapidly returns after pinching).*	Rough or dry texture and poor turgor may be noted with *dehydration.*

BOX 13.2 THE SIX Ps

• Pain
• Poikilothermia
• Paresthesia
• Paralysis
• Pallor
• Paralysis

Technique and Normal Findings	Abnormal Findings
Assess capillary refill. Depress and blanch the nail bed, then release. Note the time it takes for color to return (Fig. 13-1). *Capillary refill is <3 seconds.*	Capillary refill of 3 seconds or longer may indicate vasoconstriction, decreased cardiac output, impaired circulation, significant edema, or anemia.

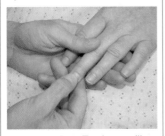

Figure 13.1 Testing capillary refill.

Palpate brachial and radial pulses (Fig. 13-2). Grade them based on the scale in Box 13-3. *A normal pulse is +3/4.*	△ SAFETY ALERT 13-3 *Evaluate any pulse that cannot be palpated with the Doppler stethoscope. If pulselessness persists, quickly evaluate the "Ps" (see Box 13-2). See Table 13-1 at the end of this chapter.*

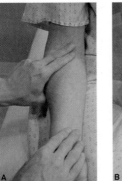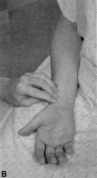

Figure 13.2 Assessing **(A)** radial pulse and **(B)** brachial pulse.

(text continues on page 250)

BOX 13.3 GRADING OF PULSES

+1: Weak and thready
+2: Weak
+3: Normal
+4: Bounding
Document a normal pulse as +3/4.

When indicated, perform the Allen test to assess patency of the collateral circulation of the hands.	Color takes more than 5 seconds to return.
1. Ask the patient to make a fist.	
2. Occlude the radial and ulnar arteries.	
3. Ask the patient to open the hand.	
4. Release pressure on the ulnar artery.	
Color returns within 2 to 5 seconds.	
Palpate for the epitrochlear nodes in the groove between the flexed biceps and triceps muscles. *They are not palpable or are 2 cm or less.*	Enlarged nodes may be noted with regional inflammation, generalized lymphadenopathy, and some cancers.
Auscultation. Evaluate blood pressure (BP) in both arms. Document the arm with the higher pressure and take subsequent BPs in that arm. *Adult SBP is 100 to 140 mm Hg and DBP is 60 to 90 mm Hg.*	Difference >10 mm Hg may indicate arterial disease. See Chapter 3.

Legs

Inspection. Note size and symmetry of legs as well as muscle atrophy or hypertrophy. *Legs are symmetrical with full joint movement.*	Atrophy may occur with arterial disease. See Table 13-2 at the end of this chapter.

Technique and Normal Findings	Abnormal Findings
Assess color of legs; evaluate for venous pattern. *Color is symmetrical and consistent without predominant venous pattern.*	Pallor may indicate arterial insufficiency. Evaluate the "Ps" to determine emergent nature. Erythema, edema, and tenderness may indicate *DVT*. Color change to white in the toes may indicate *Raynaud's syndrome.* Venous insufficiency may result in dilated and tortuous veins. See Table 13-3.
Evaluate nail beds for color and capillary refill. Blanch the nail bed, release, and observe the time it takes for color to return. *Nail beds are pink, with capillary refill less than 3 seconds.*	Delayed capillary refill may be the result of arterial disease.
Evaluate for pitting edema by pressing the tissue with your thumb for at least 5 seconds over dorsum of each foot, medial malleolus, and shin. *No indentation remains when you remove your thumb* (Fig. 13-3).	*Chronic venous insufficiency, DVT,* and *lymphedema* result in edema. Asymmetry between legs should be investigated. Calf or leg swelling, unilateral pitting edema, and localized pain are associated with *DVT.*

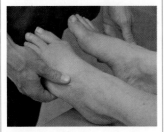

Figure 13.3 Assessing for pitting edema.

Evaluate for ecchymoses or lesions. *These are absent.*	Differentiate ulcers as arterial or venous. See Table 13-4. Assess for *gangrene.*

(text continues on page 252)

Technique and Normal Findings	Abnormal Findings

Palpation. Use the dorsal aspect of your hands to palpate the temperature of the patient's lower extremities. Legs and feet are warm and equal in temperature.

One extremity cooler than the other indicates arterial occlusion. A warm, edematous, and tender extremity indicates *DVT*.

Assess skin texture and turgor by pinching the skin. *Texture is firm, even, and elastic. Turgor is intact (skin rapidly returns).*

Rough or dry texture and poor turgor are found in *dehydration*.

Palpate femoral, popliteal, dorsalis pedis, and posterior tibial pulses (Fig. 13-4). Grade pulses based on the scale in Box 13-3. *A normal pulse is +3/4.* Evaluate any pulse that cannot be palpated with a Doppler.

⚠ *SAFETY ALERT 13-4*
If pulselessness and no Doppler signal are present, quickly assess other "Ps" to determine emergent nature.

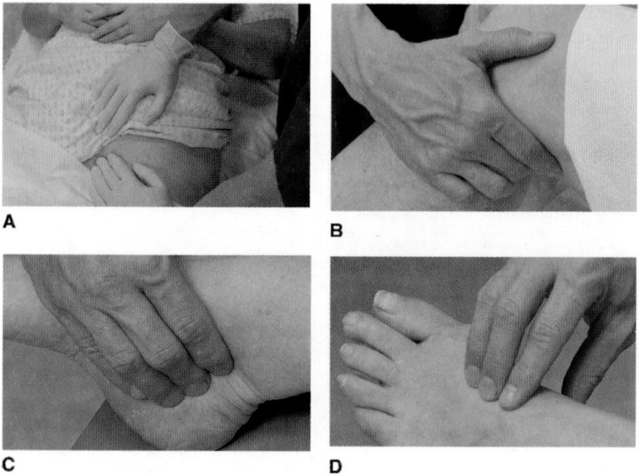

A

B

C

D

Figure 13.4 Assessing **(A)** femoral pulse, **(B)** popliteal pulse, **(C)** posterior tibial pulse, and **(D)** dorsalis pedis pulse.

Technique and Normal Findings	Abnormal Findings

Palpate upper and medial thighs for superficial inguinal lymph nodes. *They may be palpable and up to 2 cm, movable, and nontender.*

Auscultation. The Doppler ultrasonic stethoscope can assess weak peripheral pulses (Fig. 13-5). Apply a drop of ultrasonic gel to the transducer. Place the transducer slightly angled over the artery and turn on the volume.

Nodes >2 cm may be from local (eg, trauma and wounds) or generalized (lymphadenopathy) conditions.

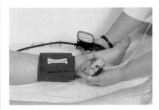

Figure 13.5 Doppler ultrasonic stethoscope.

To assess ankle-brachial index (ABI), assist the patient to a supine position. Take the systolic pressure of the brachial artery. Apply a BP cuff to the ankle; obtain either a dorsalis pedis or posterior tibial artery SBP. *Ankle pressure is slightly higher or equal to brachial pressure.* Divide ankle pressure by highest brachial pressure.

$$\frac{134 \text{ systolic}}{128 \text{ systolic}} = 1.04 \text{ or } 104\%$$
$$\frac{\text{ankle pressure}}{\text{brachial pressure}}$$

Result is 1.0 (100%) or greater.
See Box 13-4.

Arterial sounds should not be confused with the venous sound known as a "venous windstorm." Venous sounds are not rhythmic and should not be mistaken for an arterial signal. An ABI of 0.90 or less is considered to indicate arterial insufficiency.

BOX 13.4 INTERPRETATION OF ABI VALUES

1.0–1.29: Normal
0.91–0.99: Borderline
0.41–0.90: Mild to moderate PAD
0.00–0.40: Severe PAD

Source: ACC/AHA Practice Guidelines, 2005.

(text continues on page 254)

Special Techniques

Color Change. To check for arterial insufficiency, with the patient supine, elevate the legs 12 inches above his or her heart level. Have the patient pump the feet to drain off venous blood (Fig. 13-6). Have the client then sit up and dangle the legs over the side of the table. *Color returns to feet and toes within 10 seconds. Superficial foot veins fill within 15 seconds.*

Return of color taking longer that 10 seconds or persistent-dependent rubor indicates arterial insufficiency.

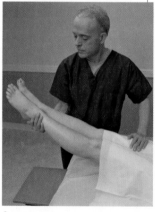
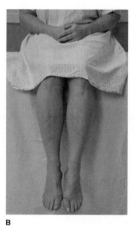

A **B**

Figure 13.6 Testing for color change. **(A)** Elevating the legs. **(B)** Dangling the legs.

Manual Compression Test. To evaluate valvular competence in the patient with varicose veins, have the patient stand. Compress the lower portion of the vein with one hand. Place your other hand 6 to 8 inches higher (Fig. 13-7). *A wave transmission is not palpable.*

A transmission wave indicates that the valves are incompetent.

Technique and Normal Findings	Abnormal Findings

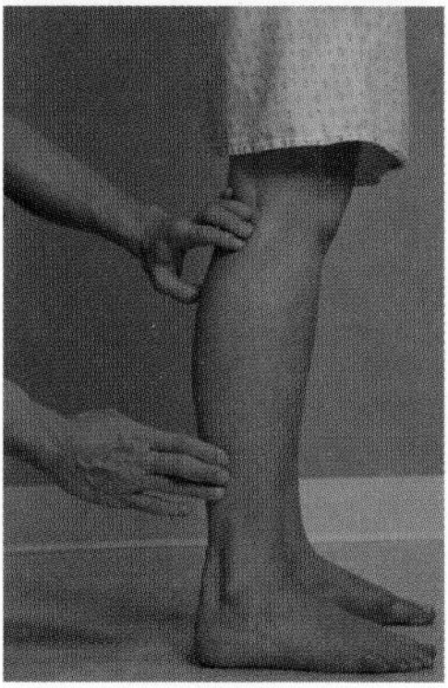

Figure 13.7 Manual compression test.

Trendelenberg Test. For the patient with varicose veins, this test evaluates saphenous vein valves and retrograde filling of superficial veins. With the patient supine, elevate the leg 90 degrees for 15 seconds. Apply a tourniquet to the upper thigh. Assist the patient to stand. Inspect for venous filling. After 30 seconds, release the tourniquet. *Saphenous veins fill from bottom up while the tourniquet is on.*

Filling from above while the tourniquet is on or rapid retrograde filling when the tourniquet is removed indicates that the valves are incompetent.

Documentation of Normal Subjective and Objective Findings

Patient denies upper or lower extremity pain; no claudication, coldness, numbness, pallor, hair loss, or nail changes in the extremity; no color changes related to cold temperatures, swelling, or redness in fingers or toes. Arms and legs are symmetrical with full joint movement. Arms and legs pink and smooth with no ecchymosis or lesions. Skin warm and dry; good turgor. Capillary refill in 2 seconds. Radial and posterior tibial pulses +3/4 bilaterally. No edema. No tenderness or pain.

♠ Lifespan Considerations ——————————

Pregnant Women
A significant increase in maternal blood volume combined with obstruction of the iliac veins and inferior vena cava from fetal growth leads to increased venous pressure. The result may be dependent edema, varicosities in the legs and vulva, and hemorrhoids. An increased venous pattern over the breasts is also common.

Newborns, Infants, and Children
Smoking, hypertension, elevated cholesterol level, obesity, physical inactivity, and high-fat diet are all risk factors that must be evaluated in children and adolescents. Many cigarette smokers begin smoking in their preteen or teen years. Early education and intervention are key.

Older Adults
Calcification of the arteries (*arteriosclerosis*) causes them to become more rigid with aging. Less arterial compliance results in increased SBP, which may be compounded by atherosclerotic disease in arteries supplying the brain, heart, and other vital organs. Incidence of PAD increases dramatically in the 7th and 8th decades of life.

Thickening of the arterial walls decreases nourishment of the tissue and results in classic findings of trophic nail changes, thin shiny skin, and hair loss of the lower extremities. Decreased functional ability (eg, fatigue with walking) may be an indication of PAD.

Older adults often become less active over time, increasing venous stasis and development of DVTs. Decreased activity is also not beneficial to patients with PAD. Venous insufficiency and chronic lymphedema may eventually decrease joint mobility.

◗ Cultural Considerations ——————————

PAD, the most prevalent vascular disease, is highest in African Americans of both sexes and Mexican American women. Hypertension, a significant risk factor for PAD, is increased in African Americans. Smoking, another primary risk factor, also may have environmental effects, such as in the case of secondary smoke inhalation. Genetics play a prominent role in atherosclerosis. Hypertension, diabetes, and hyperlipidemia are cardiovascular risk factors with strong genetic components.

Common Nursing Diagnoses and Interventions for the Peripheral Vascular System

Diagnosis and Related Factors	Nursing Interventions
Altered tissue perfusion, arterial related to reduced blood flow	Assess dorsalis pedis and posterior tibial pulse bilaterally. If reduced or unable to find them, assess with a Doppler and notify physician.
Risk for peripheral neurovascular dysfunction	Perform assessment: Pain, pulses, pallor, paresthesia, and paralysis. Contact physician if present.
Activity intolerance related to pain and claudication with ambulation	Gradually increase activity. Refer to physical therapy as indicated. Allow rest periods before and after activity.

Tables of Reference

⚠ Table 13.1   Variations in Arterial Pulses

Pulse	Characteristics and Causes
Weak Pulse 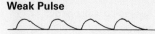	*Characteristics:* Decreased pulse pressure, weak on palpation and easily obliterated, and slow upstroke with prolonged systolic peak *Causes:* Decreased cardiac output
Bounding Pulse	*Characteristics:* Increased pulse pressure, strong and bounding, rapid rise and fall, and brief systolic peak *Causes:* Increased stroke volume and decreased aortic compliance
Pulsus Alternans	*Characteristics:* Alternating small and large amplitude and regular rate *Causes:* Left ventricular failure
Pulsus Bigeminus *Premature contractions*	*Characteristics:* Alternating irregular beats; one normal beat and then one premature beat with alternating strong and weak amplitude *Causes:* Premature ventricular or atrial contractions
Pulsus Bisferiens 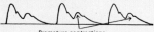	*Characteristics:* Double systolic peak *Causes:* Aortic regurgitation, combined aortic regurgitation and stenosis, less often hypertrophic cardiomyopathy

Pulse	Characteristics and Causes
Pulsus Paradoxus 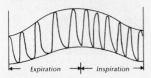 *Expiration* — *Inspiration*	*Characteristics:* Palpable decrease in amplitude on quiet inspiration; with blood pressure cuff, systolic decreases of more than 10 mm Hg during inspiration *Causes:* Pericardial tamponade, constrictive pericarditis, and obstructive lung disease

⚠ **Table 13.2   Abnormal Arterial Findings**

Abdominal Aortic Aneurysm

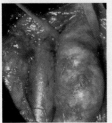

An aneurysm (outpouching of an arterial wall) results from a weakened or damaged medial arterial layer. It may occur in any artery but is most common in the aorta. These critical emergencies are often fatal.

Raynaud's Phenomenon/ Disease

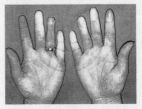

Raynaud's phenomenon is used when the cause is attributed to a connective tissue disorder. When the etiology is unknown (most cases), it is called *Raynaud's disease*. Symptoms include numbness, tingling, pain, extreme pallor, cyanosis, and coolness of the hands.

(table continues on page 260)

Peripheral Arterial Disease

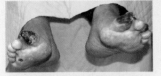

Plaque formation in peripheral arteries limits oxygenated blood from reaching tissues. Resulting ischemia causes cramping pain (*claudication*) in the related area. Severe occlusion may cause ulcers, which turn may lead to gangrene and amputation.

Acute Arterial Occlusion

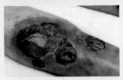

It may result from progression of PAD or thrombus from another source. In the latter case, a thrombus may break off and travel through the arterial system to a smaller vessel that is then occluded.

⚠ Table 13.3   Abnormal Venous Findings

Chronic Venous Insufficiency

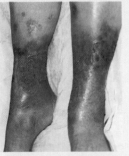

Malfunctioning of the unidirectional valves impairs blood return to the affected extremity. Causes are primary valvular incompetence (which may be congenital), sequeale of DVT, or both.

Neuropathy

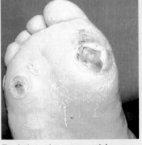

Peripheral neuropathies are most common in patients with diabetes. Paresthesias, burning sensations, and numbness may occur, along with decreased senses of vibration, pain, temperature, and proprioception. Daily foot assessment is critical.

Thrombophlebitis

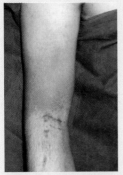

Superficial thrombophlebitis results from thrombus formation in the superficial veins. Assessment findings are unilateral localized pain or achiness, edema, warmth, and redness. In superficial veins, a palpable mass or cord may also be present along the vein.

Deep Vein Thrombosis

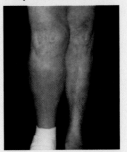

DVT results from thrombus formation in deep veins. They are more common in the lower extremities. Presenting symptoms are unilateral edema of the extremity, redness, pain or achiness, and warmth. Unrecognized DVTs are responsible for most deaths from pulmonary emboli (PE).

Lymphedema

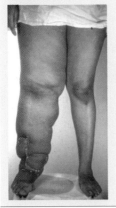

Lymphedema occurs when lymph channels or nodes are obstructed. *Primary lymphedema* is congenital. *Secondary lymphedema* results from injury, scarring, excision of lymph nodes, or, sometimes, trauma or chronic infection. As lymphedema progresses, the skin may thicken, redden, and show nonpitting edema. Small vesicles with lymphatic fluid may develop in more advanced stages. Cellulitis is a frequent complication.

	Arterial	Venous
Location	Toes, metatarsals, malleoli, and heel	Ankle, medial malleolus, and distal third of leg
Borders	Regular	Irregular
Ulcer base	Pale, yellow	Red, pink
Drainage	Minimal	Moderate to large amount
Gangrene	May be present	Not present
Pain	Painful; decreased with dependency	Aching pain, feeling of heaviness; decreased with elevation
Skin	Pale, inflamed, and necrotic	Stasis dermatitis and pigmentation changes
Pulses	Decreased or absent	Normal and may be difficult to palpate because of edema

Table 13.4 Arterial Versus Venous Ulcers

Breasts with Lymphatics Assessment

Subjective Data Collection

Key Topics and Questions for Health Promotion

Key Questions	Rationales
Family History. Do you have a family history of breast cancer? • If so, who had it? • What type of breast cancer was it? • When was the person diagnosed? • How was it treated?	The patient's risk for breast cancer increases if relatives had breast cancer.
Past Medical History. Have you had breast cancer? • If yes, what kind? • At what age were you diagnosed? • Treatment? What and when?	Previous conditions that may increase risk for breast cancer include personal history of *previous breast cancer* or *cancer in situ* and previous atypical epithelial hyperplasia on biopsy.
Have you ever been diagnosed with cysts or benign breast disease (BBD), fibroadenoma, or breast abscess?	See Table 14-1 at the end of this chapter.
Have you ever had breast surgery? • If yes, what kind? • What was the result?	Patients may have difficulty discussing this personal topic. A relaxed but professional demeanor is important.
Have you been treated for a breast infection recently?	Recent breast infection may block ducts, causing a change in breast tissue.

(text continues on page 264)

Key Questions	Rationales
When was your last period?	Breast tissue may be tender in the days before the onset of menses.
Lifestyle/Personal Habits. Do you jog or run? If so, do you wear a sports bra?	Breast movement during sports may put strain on the shoulders or back. Sports bras can reduce movement.
Medications. Are you taking any medications?	Medications that can affect breasts include androgens, antidepressants, antipsychotics, cardiac glycosides, oral contraceptives, and progestins.
Are you taking any natural supplements or over-the-counter medications?	Supplements may interfere with concurrent medications and contribute to side effects.
Breast Examination. Do you know how to perform self-breast examinations (SBEs)? • If yes, how often do you do them? Can you show me how you do your SBEs? • If no, would you like me to show you how to perform an SBE?	Monthly SBE coupled with yearly clinical breast examinations (CBE) by a medical professional increases the chances of detecting cancer in early stages.
Have you ever had a mammogram or ultrasound? When? What were the results?	Annual mammograms should begin at age 40 years; ultrasounds should begin at an earlier age if indicated.

Health-Promotion Teaching

Teach patients how to perform SBEs and alert them to the importance of being diligent about performing them monthly beginning in their early 20s. Although breast cancer is more common in older women, recognizing what normal breast tissue feels like alerts the patient to any changes. Between 20 and 39 years of age, women should also have CBEs performed by a health professional every 3 years; from 40 years onward, patients should have CBEs yearly. They also should begin yearly (or every other year) mammograms at 40 years of age. Women at high risk should get an MRI and a mammogram every year. Women at moderately increased risk should talk with their care providers about the benefits and limitations of adding MRI screening to their yearly mammogram. See Box 14-1.

BOX 14.1   BREAST SBE TEACHING POINTS

- Assist the patient to establish a regular SBE schedule. The best time for SBE is when the breasts are least congested (days 4 to 7 of the menstrual cycle).
- In postmenopausal patients, the time for SBE is irrelevant, because breast size remains stable. Discuss a day of the month that they will remember.
- Starting in their 20s, women should perform SBEs. Although most will never get breast cancer, it is important for them to be aware of how their breasts feel and look so that they can detect any changes.
- Review significant changes (eg, dimpling, bulging, a newly inverted nipple, rash, soreness, swelling, redness). Alert the patient to call a primary care provider for an appointment, should any of these occur.
- Help patients with breast implants to identify the edges of the implants so they can determine what is normal for them.
- Instruct the patient to begin SBE by disrobing and lying down with one arm under the head and a pillow under the side she is going to examine first. The patient should use the pads of the middle three fingers to feel the entire breast in an up-and-down pattern.
- The patient should make sure that she checks the entire breast. Teach her to use all three levels of pressure (soft, medium, and deep). She should repeat the previous steps on her other breast.
- Next, she should look at her breasts in a mirror. Instruct her to keep her shoulders straight and her arms on her hips.
- Instruct the patient to raise her arms over her head to look for equal movement of the breasts. While the patient looks in the mirror, she should squeeze each nipple gently for any drainage. Generally, there is none in the nonpregnant, nonlactating woman.
- From here, the patient should feel each breast in the same manner she did while supine.
- Instruct the patient to examine her underarm while she either stands or sits. It is easiest to feel the armpit with the arm only slightly raised.

Key Topics and Questions for Common Symptoms

Common Breast and Axillary Symptoms

- Breast pain
- Rash
- Lumps
- Swelling
- Discharge
- Trauma

Questions to Assess Symptoms	Rationales/Abnormal Findings
Pain. Do you have breast pain or discomfort? • Where is it? Can you point to where it hurts? Does it stay in one spot or move around? • Can you rate the pain (0–10 scale)? • How long have you had the pain? • Does it fluctuate (worse at certain times of the month)? • Have you had this pain before? When? • Does the pain occur at the same time every month? • Describe the pain (eg, sharp, dull, throbbing, shooting, burning, and tingling). • Do you have other symptoms (eg, warmth, redness, fever, muscle aches, nausea, and vomiting)? • Does anything make the pain worse? • Have you tried anything to treat it (eg, heat, ice, and Tylenol)? Did it work?	When asking questions about pain, it is important to gather all the relevant information. Severe pain (*mastalgia*) is more likely to result from *trauma* or *infection*. Breast pain is common at some point during a woman's life, especially during menstrual years. Pain may occur in one or both breasts. Cyclical pain is common in women who take oral contraceptives or have BBD. Noncyclic pain is sharp or burning; cyclic pain is heaviness. Warmth or redness may indicate local infection; fever, aches, and nausea/vomiting may indicate a systemic infection. Determining remedies the patient has tried will help guide future treatments.
Rash. Do you have a rash? If so, when/where did it start?	Rashes may be from *contact dermatitis*, *eczema*, *Paget's disease*, or allergy.
Lumps. Have you noticed any lumps in your breasts or axillae? • Where is the lump? • When did you notice it? • Has it changed at all? • If you have had previous lumps, does this feel the same or different? • Do you have a history of cystic breast changes or "lumpy" breasts?	Lumps can have many causes. Investigate any lump, especially if new or if patients have noticed changes. Also include information about the axillae—breast tissue and many lymph nodes extend to this area. Single breast masses can indicate benign conditions (eg, *cysts*, *fibroadenoma*, fat necrosis, *lipoma*), or more serious conditions (eg, *cancer*).
Swelling. Do you notice any swelling of the breasts? • Is it cyclical? • Are you breast-feeding?	Cyclical swelling and tenderness on a continuum may correspond with the menstrual cycle. Patients may complain of a

Questions to Assess Symptoms	Rationales/Abnormal Findings
• Is it in one area or does it involve your entire breast? • Has your bra size increased?	"full" feeling in the breasts during menstruation, most often affecting both breasts.
Discharge. Do you have any nipple discharge? • What is the color? • Could you be pregnant?	Spontaneous milky discharge not related to pregnancy or lactation may be from *hyperprolactinemia* or adrenergic medications. Nipple discharge can be associated with a benign *papilloma, ductal ectasia,* and less commonly, cancer.
• What medications do you take?	Clear discharge may be from use of steroids, calcium channel blockers, oral contraceptives, or tranquilizers.
Trauma. Have you had any injuries to your breasts? • When/how did it occur? • Did it cause any break in the skin, residual lumps, swelling, or discoloration?	Injuries to the breast may cause a patient to feel a previously undetected lump or mass. A break in the skin could lead to an infection.

Objective Data Collection

Equipment

- Ruler marked in centimeters
- Small pillow
- Pamphlet or handout for SBE
- Gloves (if drainage is present)
- Adequate lighting

Technique and Normal Findings	Abnormal Findings
Inspection Begin with the patient sitting with arms at the sides (Fig. 14-1).	
Inspect color and texture of the skin. *Skin tone determines color.*	See Table 14-1 at the end of this chapter.

(text continues on page 268)

Technique and Normal Findings	Abnormal Findings

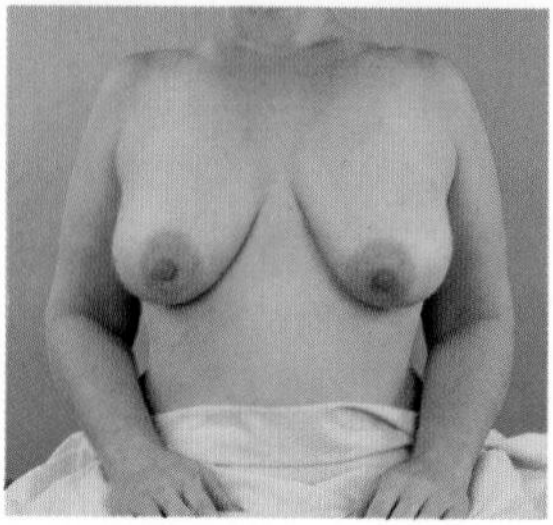

Figure 14.1 Patient sitting with arms at side as breast examination begins.

Striae may be evident after pregnancy or if a woman has gained then lost significant weight.

Inspect the size and shape of the breasts. *Wide variation exists, from small to very large (pendulous).*

Evaluate breast symmetry. *The left breast is often slightly larger.*

Examine the contour of the breasts. *It is uninterrupted on both sides.*

Ask the patient with pendulous breasts to lean forward with her arms on her hips.

One breast is significantly underdeveloped.

Retractions or dimpling may occur with *breast cancer* (Fig. 14-2).

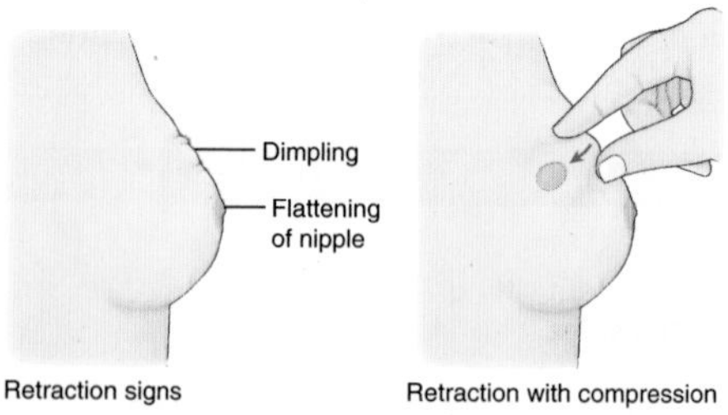

Dimpling

Flattening of nipple

Retraction signs

Retraction with compression

Figure 14.2 Retraction signs.

Technique and Normal Findings	Abnormal Findings
Inspect the appearance of the nipple and areola. *Areola is round or oval and pink to dark brown or black. Most nipples are everted; it may be normal for one or both nipples to be inverted.*	Change from everted to inverted or in angle the nipple points may indicate cancer (see Table 14-2).
An extra nipple **(supernumerary nipple)** along the embryonic nipple line (from axilla to groin bilaterally) is a common variation. It most often appears 5–6 cm below the breast. On initial inspection it looks like a mole, but a tiny nipple and areola are present.	
After inspecting with the arms at the side, reinspect with the patient lifting the arms over the head, pressed firmly on the hips, leaning forward from the waist, and then lying supine. See Figure 14-3. Inspect the axillae with the patient seated. Note any rashes, infection, texture changes, or unusual pigmentation. *There is no rash, edema, or lesions.*	Lifting the arms over the head adds tension to the suspensory ligaments and accentuates any dimpling or retraction. Leaning forward may reveal breast or nipple asymmetry. Rash, edema, or lesion suggests underlying cancer but may also be benign. Velvety axillary skin or deep pigmentation is associated with cancer.

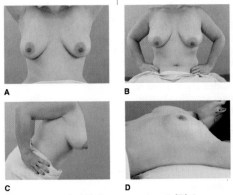

A

B

C

D

Figure 14.3 (A) Arms over head. **(B)** Arms pressed firmly on her hips. **(C)** Leaning forward from the waist. **(D)** Lying supine.

(text continues on page 270)

Technique and Normal Findings	Abnormal Findings

Palpation

Palpate the axillae with the patient seated. Instruct the patient to gently raise the arm. Support the arm and wrist to aid in muscle relaxation. Use the right hand to palpate the left axilla and the left hand to palpate the right axilla (Fig. 14-4).

Firm, hard, enlarged nodes (>1 cm) fixed to underlying tissues or skin suggest malignancy.

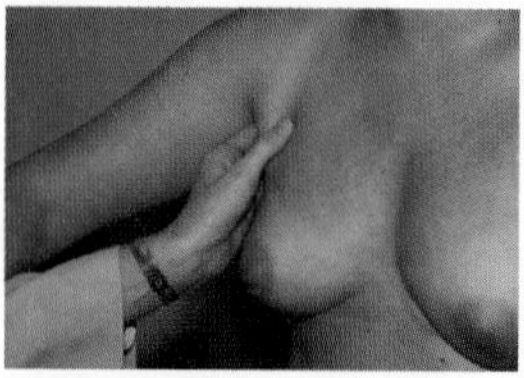

Figure 14.4 Palpation of the axilla.

Point your fingers toward the mid-clavicle, directly behind the pectoral muscles. Feel for the central nodes against the chest wall. *One or more small, soft, nontender nodes are common findings.*

The other axillary lymph nodes are difficult to palpate. Pectoral nodes are inside the border of the pectoral muscle. Lateral nodes are along the upper humerus, high in the axilla. Subscapular nodes are best felt with the examiner standing behind the patient, feeling inside the posterior axillary fold. Adjust the patient's arm in various positions to increase the surface area that can be assessed.

Tender, warm, enlarged nodes suggest infection of the breast, arm, or hand.

Position the patient supine with her arm raised overhead and a small pillow or towel rolled under the side being examined.

Enlarged axillary lymph nodes are sometimes mistaken for nodules in the tail of Spence and vice versa.

Technique and Normal Findings	Abnormal Findings

This will flatten the breast tissue. Palpate the entire breast from clavicle to inframammary fold (bra line) and from midsternum to posterior axillary line, making sure to examine the tail of Spence (Fig. 14-5).

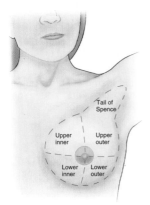

Figure 14.5 Breast with four quadrants and tail of Spence delineated.

Vertical Pattern. The ACS currently recommends using the **vertical pattern** (Fig. 14-6), because some evidence supports that this is the most effective means of examining the entire breast.

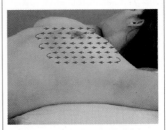

Figure 14.6 Vertical strip pattern.

Using the finger pads of the first three fingers, palpate in small, concentric circles beginning in the axilla and moving in a straight line down toward the bra line

Sliding the fingers along the breast to palpate each section increases the likelihood of palpating the entire breast.

(text continues on page 272)

Technique and Normal Findings	Abnormal Findings

(Fig. 14-7). Apply light, medium, and then deeper pressure at each examining point. Continue in vertical overlapping lines until the sternal edge is met.

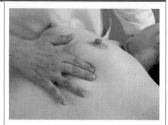

Figure 14.7 Palpation of the breasts with the patient supine.

Consistency. Breast tissue shows wide variations. Nodular masses may be present prior to menses, disappearing when menses has occurred. *The breast of a nulliparous woman feels smooth, elastic, and firm.*

Mammary duct ectasia (dilated, painful mammary ducts) should be suspected when a lump or thickening is palpable.

Prior to menstruation, breasts are often engorged secondary to increased progesterone. The patient may notice nodules, slight enlargement, and tenderness at this time. Lobes may be more prominent with distinct margins. After pregnancy, breasts feel softer and have less tone.

This benign condition may result from hormonal changes, smoking, or lack of vitamin A. An inverted nipple may block the mammary ducts, which can cause inflammation and mammary duct ectasia.

Tenderness. Breasts are often tender during the premenstrual period.

Tenderness or pain in the breast at other times may be from infection or trauma.

Nodules. If a lump is palpated, document the following:

All breast masses require further evaluation and possibly mammogram, ultrasound, aspiration, or biopsy.
The most common site for breast masses is in the upper outer quadrant. See Figure 14-6. Indistinct lumps are more suspicious for breast cancer.

* **Location:** State the quadrant or use clock measurements in centimeters from the nipple.
* **Size:** Measure or judge length × width × depth in centimeters using a ruler as a guide.
* **Shape:** Oval, round, lobular, nodular, or indistinct?

Technique and Normal Findings	Abnormal Findings

- **Consistency:** Smooth, soft, firm, or hard?
- **Mobility:** Movable or immobile?
- **Tenderness:** Tender or not?

Tenderness indicates infection, inflammation, or cancer.

- **Distinctness:** One lump or multiple?

Cancer tends to be single; fibroadenomas may be single or multiple.

- **Skin:** Dimpled, retracted, erythematous?
- **Nipple:** Retracted or displaced?
- **Lymphadenopathy:** Palpable lymph nodes?

Dimpling, retraction, or a retracted or displaced nipple can be signs of cancer.

Breast tissue is soft and homogeneous. No masses or tenderness. No lymphadenopathy.

Lymphadenopathy (swelling of lymph nodes) may occur postmastectomy, from blocked lymph nodes, or from infection.

Palpating the Nipple. Gently compress the nipple between your thumb and index finger. Assess for discharge (Fig. 14-8). If evident, note color, consistency, and amount. Massage the areola if there is discharge to determine where it originates. *Nipple without discharge.*

If discharge is evident, obtain a cytological smear for examination.

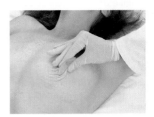

Figure 14.8 Palpating the nipple.

Bimanual Technique. If a patient has pendulous breasts, use the bimanual technique. The patient should sit upright, leaning slightly forward. Place one hand underneath the breast (on the inferior surface) while palpating with the other hand (Fig. 14-9).

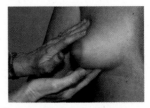

Figure 14.9 Palpating the breasts using bimanual technique.

(text continues on page 274)

Technique and Normal Findings	Abnormal Findings
Examining a Patient Postmastectomy A woman who has had a mastectomy may be self-conscious about being examined. The examiner must be empathetic and sensitive. Malignancy can occur at the scar site or in other areas of the breast.	Masses, inflammation, color changes, and thickening may signify recurrence.
Inspect the scar and axilla for inflammation, rash, color changes, thickening, and irritation. Lymphedema in the axilla and arm may be secondary to impaired lymph drainage. **Palpate** the surgical scar and chest wall with the pads of two fingers to assess for breast changes (lumps, tenderness, thickening, or swelling). Palpate the axilla and supraclavicular lymph nodes; assess for swelling and irritation.	If the patient has undergone breast reconstruction, lumpectomy, augmentation, or reduction, perform the breast examination as described, paying close attention to the scar tissue.
Male Breasts Inspect the nipple and areola for swelling, ulceration, or drainage. Additionally, palpate the areola and breast tissue for nodules or masses.	Firm, glandular tissue (**gynecomastia**) may occur when there is an imbalance of estrogen and androgen. An ulcer or hard, irregular mass suggests cancer. See Table 14-2.

Documentation of Normal Findings

Patient states she is without breast pain, lumps, nipple discharge, rashes, swelling, or trauma. Negative history of breast disease or breast surgery. Reports performing monthly breast exams; routine mammogram 9/10/10, which was "normal." Inspection: (+) Symmetric breasts, everted nipples. Palpation: (−) palpable masses in breast or axilla, nipple discharge, rashes, or dimpling.

⚠ Lifespan Considerations

Pregnant Women

Women experience breast changes as early as the first 2 months of pregnancy, stimulated by placental hormones. Breasts enlarge, feeling tender and nodular. Nipples darken, enlarge, and become more erect. As pregnancy progresses, areolae also become larger, darker, and more prominent. Stretch marks (**striae**) may be evident; these disappear completely when breasts return to the prepregnant size. Small, scattered Montgomery's glands develop within the areolae. Because of increased blood flow, a bluish venous pattern is often evident on the breast tissue.

Breasts may begin to express *colostrum* (milk precursor) during the 4th month of pregnancy. Women continue to produce colostrum through the first few days postpartum. Actual milk replaces colostrum if breast-feeding occurs. During breast-feeding, smooth muscle in the nipple and areola contracts to express milk. Breasts may become larger, reddened, warm, and engorged, especially at this time. Frequent breast-feeding will stimulate milk production, drain the sinuses, and resolve the symptoms. If these symptoms occur at other times during lactation, they could indicate **mastitis**. Nipples often become sore, but generally this resolves spontaneously. If they become cracked and irritated, bleeding may occur.

After completion of lactation, breast glandular tissue shrinks. The nipples and areolae usually remain darker than in the prepregnant state.

Newborns and Infants

Enlarged breast tissue and white discharge ("witch's milk") in newborns of either gender may occur for the first few weeks of life, secondary to the effects of maternal estrogens. If breast enlargement, witch's milk, or both are present, reassure the newborn's parents/caregivers that nothing is wrong and the conditions will resolve spontaneously. At birth, the lactiferous ducts are present in females within the nipples, but alveoli do not develop in females until puberty.

If an examiner finds a supernumerary nipple, he or she should also begin evaluation of the kidneys, because of the association between extra nipples and renal anomalies. Accessory breast tissue (polymastia) is most often seen in the axilla, also along the mammary ridge.

Children and Adolescents

On inspection, the symmetrical nipples of prepubescent children lie between the fourth and fifth ribs just lateral to the midclavicular line. The nipples and areolae are flat and darker than the rest of the breast tissue.

Females begin to develop breasts between 8½ to 10 years of age. Breast tissue may be temporarily asymmetric during growth, which is normal and will resolve on its own. Breast tenderness may also occur. It is important to educate the adolescent female about expected body changes that will occur during this time period.

See Figure 14-10 for a review of Tanner's staging. *Precocious puberty* (before 7 years of age in Caucasians or 6 years in African Americans) may be secondary to endocrine dysfunction or tumor. Delayed development may occur with anorexia nervosa, malnutrition, or hormonal imbalance. Girls may be considered to have a developmental delay if breast development has not occurred by 13 years of age.

The breasts of an adolescent girl are uniform and firm. A mass at this age is most often benign. Adolescence is a good time to introduce patients to what their breasts normally feel like, so that that they will be more likely to perform SBE as they get older.

Older Adults

As women age, glandular, alveolar, and lobular breast tissues decrease. After menopause, fat deposits replace glandular tissue. The inframammary ridge thickens; suspensory ligaments relax, causing breasts to sag and droop. Breasts also decrease in size and lose elasticity. Nipples become smaller, flatter, and less erectile. Axillary hair may stop growing. These changes are more apparent in the eighth and ninth decades of life.

Providers should remind older women to continue monthly SBEs and yearly CBEs. With cessation of menses, hormonal changes no longer affect the breasts. Thus, patients can choose a convenient day of each month to perform SBEs (eg, 1st day of month).

Male Breasts

Male breasts are immature structures with well-developed areolae and small nipples. During midpuberty, one or both male breasts commonly and temporarily enlarge as a result of changing hormone levels, a condition referred to as **gynecomastia**. Pubescent males also may develop breast buds or tenderness, which also is usually temporary. Gynecomastia is physically benign but can cause emotional distress. Reassurance that this is temporary and normal may help alleviate the distress. As males age, gynecomastia may recur from decreases in testosterone.

1) Preadolescents:
   Only a small elevated nipple

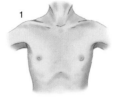

2) The breast bud stage:
   A small mound of breast and nipple develops: the areola widens

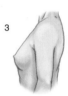

3) The breast and areola enlarge: the nipple is flush with the breast surface

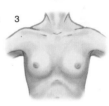

4) The areola and nipple form a secondary mound over the breast

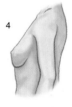

5) Mature breast:
   Only the nipple protrudes; the areola is flush with the breast contour (the areola may continue as a secondary mound in some women)

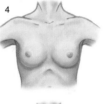

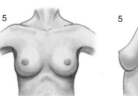

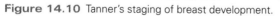

Figure 14.10 Tanner's staging of breast development.

Cultural Considerations

Variations in the color of the skin and nipple relate to ethnic background. Ethnic differences exist in incidence and outcomes of breast cancer. Hispanic, Asian, and American Indian women have a lower risk. African American women experience a lower incidence but higher mortality rate from breast cancer than Caucasian women. Breast cancer is the leading cause of death among Filipino women.

Common Nursing Diagnoses and Interventions Associated with Breasts

Diagnosis and Related Factors	Nursing Interventions
Disturbed body image related to surgery and treatment	Acknowledge feelings as normal when coping with change. Explore strengths. Encourage new clothes or wig in anticipation of changes.
Ineffective coping related to changes in function	Observe causes of ineffective coping. Help identify resources. Discuss changes and previous successful coping strategies. Evaluate suicide risk.
Ineffective role performance related to loss of ability to cook, clean for self	Validate accomplishments. Locate community resources. Suggest physical accommodations.*
Grieving related to the loss of breast, functional ability, and cancer diagnosis	Encourage patient to express feelings and affirm that they are part of the grief process. Refer to spiritual counseling if indicated.

*Collaborative interventions.

Table 14.1   Breast Lumps

Characteristics	Fibroadenoma
Fibroadenoma 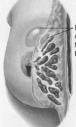 Rubbery, circumscribed, freely movable benign tumor	Oval, round, lobular, and 1–5 cm; firm or rubbery, with well-demarcated, clear margins; usually single, but may be multiple; freely movable and painless
Benign Breast Disease  Cyst Pectoralis muscles Fat Normal lobules	Incidence decreases after menopause; round, lobular; of variable size; firm to soft, rubbery; well demarcated; most often multiple, may be single; movable; painful; breast tenderness, which usually increases before menses; breasts often swollen, usually bilateral
Breast Cancer Skin dimpling Hard Irregularly shaped Immobile, fixed to chest wall Nipple retraction Blood or serous nipple discharge	Irregular, star shaped; variable size; firm to hard consistency; poor definition; usually single and fixed; dimpling, nipple inversion, spontaneous single-nipple bloody discharge, orange-peel texture (*peau d'orange*), axillary lymphadenopathy; may be painful

Carcinoma (Skin, Areola, and Nipple Retraction)

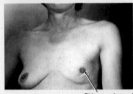

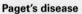

Skin, areola, and nipple retraction

Carcinoma (Bulging of Breast and Skin Changes)

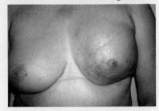

Paget's disease

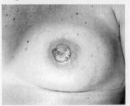

Mastitis

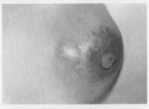

Mastectomy

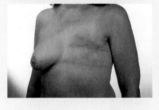

Gynecomastia

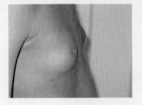

Abdominal Assessment

Subjective Data Collection

Key Topics and Questions for Health Promotion

Key Questions	Rationales
Current Problems. Are you having any abdominal problems now?	This question opens discussion with a general approach.
Have you had any unplanned changes in weight?	These may indicate *cancer, anorexia, bulimia, thyroid disorder,* psychosocial issues, or socioeconomic concerns.
Do you have any special dietary needs?	Special needs may indicate a nutrient imbalance or cause of symptoms.
Have you had a fever or chills?	Fever may indicate an infection.
Have you had any dizziness?	Dizziness may be from possible dehydration.
Family History. Has any first-degree relative had colorectal cancer?	Such family history increases the patient's risk for this disease.
Do you have a family history of gastroesophageal reflux disease (GERD), peptic ulcer disease (PUD), inflammatory bowel disease (IBD), irritable bowel syndrome (IBS), anemia, thalassemia, or celiac disease?	Many of these conditions run in families.
Personal History. How old are you?	Risk of *colorectal cancer* increases with age.

(text continues on page 282)

Key Questions	Rationales
Did you have a blood transfusion before the mid-1980s? Have you been vaccinated against hepatitis B?	Those who received blood transfusions prior to the mid-1980s may be at risk for *hepatitis B*.
Have you had treatments or surgeries for *GERD, PUD, IBD, IBS, anemia, thalassemia*, or *celiac disease*?	Patient history may reveal an exacerbation of a previous condition or a genetic predisposition or familial propensity for a particular disorder.
Do you have a history of previous abdominal or pelvic surgeries?	Previous surgeries increase risk for adhesions, infections, obstructions, and malabsorption.
Have you had any GI tubes?	GI tubes can be a source of infection.
Have you had any recent trauma?	Trauma may cause current symptoms.
Have you recently had mononucleosis?	Mononucleosis can cause hepatosplenomegaly.
Have you had malabsorption disease?	This condition may indicate lactose intolerance, food allergies, or *celiac disease*.
Do you have sickle cell anemia?	Abdominal pain is linked to *sickle cell crisis*.
Have you ever had intestinal polyps?	These increase risk for *colorectal cancer*.
Chewing/Swallowing. Have you had thyroid disease, neck mass, recent infection, vision changes, trouble swallowing, or sore throat?	*Thyroid disease* affects metabolism, weight, and elimination. Neck mass or difficulty swallowing may indicate *cancer* or infection. Infections increase caloric requirements. Visual changes may occur with malnutrition. Throat pain may impede swallowing.
When was your last dental assessment?	Poor dentition affects intake.
Breathing. Do you have a history of breathing problems?	Respiratory problems can diminish energy and decrease food intake.

Key Questions	Rationales
Weight Gain. Do you have cardio-vascular disease, high blood pres-sure, or congestive heart failure?	Weight gain and increased sodium in the diet can exacerbate these problems.
Genitourinary Issues. What color is your urine? Do you have burning, frequency, or urgency?	Dark urine can indicate inad-equate fluid intake or blockage in the biliary system.
Have you had sexually transmit-ted infections?	They may cause lower abdominal pain.
Females: When was your last menstrual period?	Unplanned pregnancy is often a cause of nausea and vomiting.
Do you have any vaginal discharge?	Discharge may indicate an infection.
Males: Do you have a history of prostate problems?	Enlarged prostate may result in urinary difficulty and decreased intake of fluids.
Joint Pain. Do you have a his-tory of fractures, joint pain, or weakness?	Joint pain may result in long-term use of nonsteroidal anti-inflammatory medications, which can cause GI bleeding.
Neurological. How many alco-holic drinks do you have each day?	Excessive alcohol intake is the number one cause of liver disease.
Have you had numbness, back problems, or loss of bowel/bladder control?	Numbness and changes in the bowel or bladder are symptoms of significant spinal injury.
Metabolism. Do you have diabe-tes or thyroid problems?	*Diabetes* is associated with abnormal metabolism and weight changes.
Skin. Have you had any changes in your skin, hair, or nails?	Inadequate or imbalanced nutrition may be exhibited in the skin, hair, or nails.
Do you have rashes, itching, or lesions?	These suggest *liver disease* or malnutrition.
Lymphatic/Hematologic. Have you had any food allergies, infec-tions, or sickle cell anemia?	Food allergies may cause belch-ing, bloating, flatulence, diarrhea, or constipation. Sickle cell anemia may cause significant pain.

(text continues on page 284)

Key Questions	Rationales
Medications. Are you taking over-the-counter or prescribed medications?	Patients will frequently take antacids that may interact with other medications.
Substance Abuse. Use the CAGE questionnaire. See Chap. 10.	
Occupation • What is your profession? • Where do you work? • Do you use personal protective equipment at work?	Health care workers are at high risk for _hepatitis C,_ for which there is no vaccine.
Foreign Travel • Have you traveled to, or lived in, parts of the world where sanitation is less than optimal? • Have you eaten food prepared in places that are not sanitary? • Have you received the hepatitis A vaccine?	_Hepatitis A_ is transmitted by the fecal-oral route, usually within 30 days of exposure. The disease is vaccine-preventable.
Lifestyle • Do you use IV drugs? • How many sexual partners have you had? • Have you had sex with sex workers?	_Hepatitis B_ is transmitted through contact with bodily secretions of infected people. _Hepatitis C_ is transmitted through contact with the blood of infected people. IV drug users are at high risk for hepatitis C.

Health-Promotion Teaching

Immunizations. Be sure to recommend vaccinations against hepatitis A and B to appropriate patients. These include all infants; people whose work may expose them to blood, body fluids, or unsanitary conditions (ie, health care, food services, sex workers); and those traveling to parts of the world where these illnesses are prevalent.

Colorectal Cancer Screening. Risk of colorectal cancer increases with age. Initial screening for all people is recommended at 50 years of age, with serial fecal occult blood and colonoscopy for anyone whose results are positive. Follow-up screening is based on findings and risks, with colonoscopy repeated every 3 to 10 years.

Key Topics and Questions for Common Symptoms

Common Abdominal Symptoms

- Indigestion
- Anorexia
- Nausea, vomiting, hematemesis
- Abdominal pain
- Dysphagia, odynophagia
- Change in bowel function
- Jaundice/icterus
- Urinary/renal symptoms

Questions to Assess Symptoms	Rationale/Abnormal Findings
Indigestion. Have you had heartburn?	Heartburn suggests *gastric acid reflux.*
Do you have excessive gas, belching, abdominal bloating, or distention?	Increased intake of gas-forming foods, chewing gum, carbonated beverages, and motility problems can cause gas.
Are you unpleasantly full after meals?	Gastric-emptying problems, outlet obstruction, and *cancer* can cause fullness.
Do you feel full shortly after eating? Are you unable to eat a full meal?	Early satiety can result from diabetes, anticholinergic drugs, or *hepatitis.*
Anorexia. How is your appetite?	Loss of appetite can be related to stress, difficulty with ingestion, socioeconomic issues, age-related issues, or *dementia.*
Do you deliberately eat small meals?	With *anorexia nervosa* food intake is intentionally limited.
Have you ever vomited after eating?	In *bulimia* patients deliberately vomit.
Nausea/Vomiting/Hematemesis. Do you have nausea or vomiting? Do you vomit blood?	Nausea/vomiting may result from stress, infections, or food poisoning. Hematemesis may indicate *gastric ulcer, gastritis,* or *cirrhosis.*

(text continues on page 286)

Questions to Assess Symptoms	Rationale/Abnormal Findings
Abdominal Pain. Do you have any pain or discomfort? Provide details.	**Visceral pain** may be difficult to localize and described as gnawing, burning, cramping, or aching. **Parietal pain** is usually severe and localized. Patients describe it as steady, aching, or sharp.
Dysphagia/Odynophagia • Do you have difficulty or pain with swallowing? • Does it feel like food gets stuck?	Dysphagia may result from stress, *esophageal stricture*, *GERD*, or tumor.
Change in Bowel Function. What was your normal bowel pattern before symptoms developed?	Normal pattern may range from several times a day to once a week.
Constipation. Are there any changes in your diet, medications, or activity?	Functional constipation results from inadequate fiber and fluids, or medications.
Diarrhea • Is it associated with nausea/vomiting? • Do you get diarrhea with a change in diet or when you eat certain foods? • Does moving your bowels relieve pain?	Diarrhea can result from infection or food intolerances.
Jaundice/Icterus. Have you noticed a change in • The color of your skin and sclera? • The color of your urine or stool?	Jaundice can result from *gallstones* or *pancreatic cancer*. Dark urine is from impaired bilirubin excretion; gray or light stool is common in obstructive jaundice.
Have you recently traveled to, or had meals in, areas of poor sanitation?	Recent travel may indicate exposure to *hepatitis A*.
Have you had any recent exposure to infected blood or body fluids?	Exposure may indicate infection with *hepatitis B or C.*

Questions to Assess Symptoms	Rationale/Abnormal Findings
Urinary/Renal Symptoms Do you have	Patients may perceive these symptoms as abdominal.
• Pain or difficulty on urination (dysuria)?	Pain may be from infection or irritation. Women often report internal pain; men typically feel a burning.
• Urgency or frequency of urination?	Urgency may be from infection.
• Suprapubic pain?	Suprapubic pain is usually from *cystitis*.
• In males, hesitancy or decreased stream?	May be from *benign prostatic hypertrophy (BPH)*.
• Polyuria (how frequent?)?	Polyuria is a symptom of *diabetes*.
• Nocturia (how frequent?)?	Nocturia is usually from *BPH*.
• Hematuria, painful or not painful?	With pain hematuria is usually from bladder infection or renal calculi. Painless hematuria is common with urinary tract infections (UTIs) and *bladder cancer*.
Urinary Incontinence • Do you leak urine? • Are you ever unable to make it to the bathroom fast enough? • Have you ever lost urine before getting to the bathroom?	*Stress incontinence* occurs with coughing, sneezing, or increasing intra-abdominal pressure. *Urge incontinence* is a sudden urge and loss of urine with little warning. *Total incontinence* is an inability to retain urine; ask also about bowel incontinence.
Kidney or Flank Pain. Do you have pain? Is it dull, achy, and steady? Did you have any burning, urgency, or bladder pain prior to its development?	*Renal calculi* and *pyelonephritis* can be causes of flank pain.
Ureteral Colic. Do you have severe, colicky pain in your flank? Is it associated with nausea or vomiting?	Ureteral obstruction by clots or stones causes colicky, cramping pain.

Objective Data Collection

Equipment

- Stethoscope
- Measuring tape
- Pen or marker
- Reflex hammer or tongue blade to ascertain abdominal reflexes
- Pillow placed under the knees to relax the abdominal musculature

Clinical Significance 15-1

Order of abdominal assessment differs from previous systems. Inspection is followed by auscultation for bowel sounds *before* percussion and palpation. Failure to adhere to this order may alter bowel sounds, leading to inaccurate findings.

Technique and Normal Findings	Abnormal Findings
Inspection Look at the abdominal skin, contour, waves, and pulsations (Fig. 15-1). Inspect size, shape, and symmetry. Note the condition of the umbilicus, whether it is inverted or everted, and its position.	Abnormal skin findings include scars, striae, and veins. The umbilicus may have a hernia or inflammation. See also Table 15-1.

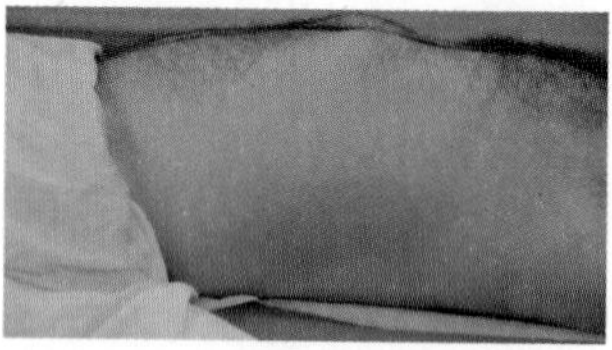

Figure 15.1 Inspecting the abdomen.

Assess for abdominal distention. If present, determine if it is generalized or local.	Several conditions can cause distention.

Technique and Normal Findings	Abnormal Findings

Ask the patient if the abdomen is different from normal. Inspect for visible aortic pulsations, peristalsis, and respiratory pattern. Evaluate for ascites.

Abnormal contours include bulging flanks or a suprapubic bulge. A peristaltic wave may indicate obstruction. Aortic pulsation may signify an *abdominal aortic aneurysm.*

Auscultation

Bowel Sounds. Auscultate all four quadrants. Place the warmed diaphragm of the stethoscope gently in one quadrant (Fig. 15-2). Start at the ileocecal valve (slightly right and below the umbilicus); proceed clockwise. *There are 5 to 30 clicks per minute (one bowel sound every 5 to 15 seconds). Sounds indicate bowel motility and peristalsis. If no sounds are audible, listen for up to 5 minutes.*

Bowel sounds may be hyperactive above and decreased or nonexistent below an obstruction. Increased sounds occur with *diarrhea* and early intestinal obstruction. Decreased sounds occur with *adynamic ileus* and *peritonitis.* High-pitched, tinkling sounds indicate intestinal fluid and air under tension in a dilated bowel. High-pitched, rushing sounds indicate partial intestinal obstruction.

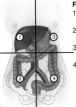

Four quadrants
1 - right upper quadrant (RUQ)
2 - right lower quadrant (RLQ)
3 - left upper quadrant (LUQ)
4 - left lower quadrant (LLQ)

A

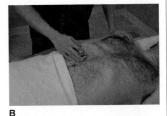

B

Figure 15.2 (A) Division of the abdomen into four quadrants. **(B)** Auscultating the abdomen.

Vascular Sounds. Auscultate with the bell over all four quadrants. Listen over the aorta in the epigastric region and over the renal and iliac arteries for bruits (Fig. 15-3).

Hepatic bruits indicate *liver cancer* or alcoholic *hepatitis.* Bruits over the aorta or renal arteries indicate partial obstruction.

(text continues on page 290)

Technique and Normal Findings	Abnormal Findings

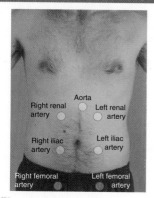

Figure 15.3 Site for auscultating for bruits.

In the epigastric region, near the liver and over the umbilicus, venous hums are best heard (Fig. 15-4).

Venous hums indicate partial obstruction of an artery and reduced blood flow to the organ.

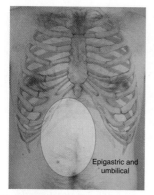

Figure 15.4 Site for auscultating for venous hums.

Lastly, auscultate over the liver and spleen for friction rubs (Fig. 15-5).

These may indicate *liver tumor*, *splenic infarction*, or *peritoneal inflammation*.

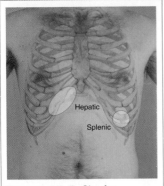

Figure 15.5 Site for auscultating for friction rubs.

Percussion

Percuss all four quadrants for tympany or dullness. Ask the patient if there is pain; percuss painful areas last. Ask the patient to point to the area of maximal tenderness and to suck in the abdomen. Place your hand 15 cm over the abdomen; ask the patient to push the stomach to your hand while coughing. *These maneuvers move peritoneal surfaces without contact. Normal findings include dullness over the liver in the RUQ and hollow tympanic notes in the LUQ over the gastric bubble. Over most of the abdomen, tympanic sounds indicate gas.*

Pain indicates peritoneal inflammation and can indicate a ruptured viscous in the area of the pain, *appendicitis* in RLQ, diverticulum in the LLQ, *cholecystitis* in the RUQ, or *cystitis* over the symphysis pubis. Dullness may be heard over organs, masses or fluid, such as ascites, GI obstruction, pregnant uterus, and an ovarian tumor. See also Tables 15-2 and 15-3.

Kidneys. With the patient sitting, place the palm of your nondominant hand over the costovertebral angle (CVA). Hit that hand with the fist of your dominant hand (Fig. 15-6). Repeat on the other side. *There is slight or no pain.*

Significant pain upon blunt percussion at the CVA can indicate kidney infection (pyelonephritis) or kidney stones.

(text continues on page 292)

| Technique and Normal Findings | Abnormal Findings |

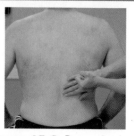

Figure 15.6 Percussing for kidney tenderness at the costovertebral angle.

Liver. To assess liver span, start at the right midclavicular line (MCL) at the third intercostal space (ICS) over the lung tissue. Percuss down until you hear resonance change to dullness over the liver (between the fifth and seventh ICSs) (Fig. 15-7). Mark where the dullness begins. To determine the lower border of the liver, start at the right MCL at the level of the umbilicus and percuss upward until tympany turns to dullness, usually at the sternal border. Mark this area with a pen. Measure the distance between the two marks. *Liver span is 6 to 12 cm. If liver span in the MCL is >12 cm, measure it in the midsternal line. Midsternal liver span is 4 to 8 cm.*

Abnormal findings include hepatomegaly and the firm edge of *cirrhosis.*

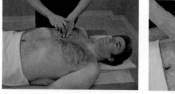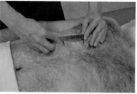

A B

Figure 15.7 **(A)** Percussing the liver. **(B)** Measuring the liver border.

Technique and Normal Findings	Abnormal Findings
Spleen. To assess the approximate size of the spleen: 1. Percuss from the left MCL along the costal margin to the left midaxillary line (MAL). *With tympany, splenomegaly is unlikely.* 2. Percuss at the lowest ICS at the left MAL. Ask the patient to take a deep breath and hold it; percuss again. 3. Percuss downward from the third to fourth ICS slightly posterior to the left MAL, until dullness is heard. *Dullness of the normal spleen is noted around the 9th to 11th rib.*	Dullness at the MAL is indicative of splenomegaly. With splenomegaly, tympany turns to dullness on inspiration.
Bladder. Assess bladder size by percussing for bladder distension. Begin at the symphysis pubis and percuss upward toward the umbilicus. *An empty bladder does not rise above the symphysis pubis.*	Tenderness over the symphysis pubis may indicate a *UTI*.
## Palpation ***Light Palpation.*** Begin with light palpation in all four quadrants for a general survey of surface characteristics and to put the patient at ease. Press down 1 to 2 cm in a rotating motion. Lift your fingertips and move to the next location (Fig. 15-8). Observe for grimacing or guarding. *No tenderness is noted.*	Involuntary guarding is a sign of possible peritoneal inflammation and should be carefully evaluated.

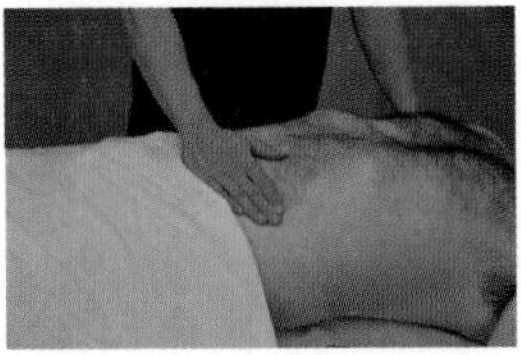

Figure 15.8 Lightly palpating the abdomen.

(text continues on page 294)

Technique and Normal Findings	Abnormal Findings

Deep Palpation. Use single-handed deep palpation to look for organs, masses, or tenderness. With the fingertips depress 4 to 6 cm in a dipping motion in all quadrants (Fig. 15-9). *Tenderness may be noted near the xiphoid process, over the cecum, or over the sigmoid colon.* Use bimanual deep palpation for a large abdomen. Place your nondominant hand on your dominant hand and depress 4 to 6 cm.

If you find a mass, note location, size, shape, consistency, tenderness, pulsation, mobility, and movement with respiration. Refer to Figure 15-10 for the location of abdominal and accessory organs. Size and changes over time offer insight into pathology and the extent of involvement.

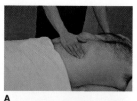

A

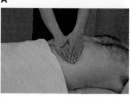

B

Figure 15.9 (A) Single-handed deep palpation. **(B)** Bimanual deep palpation.

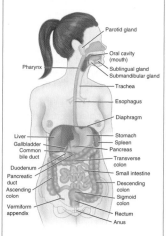

Figure 15.10 Overview of the gastrointestinal system.

Liver. Place your right hand at the patient's right MCL under the costal margin. Place your left hand on the patient's back at the 11th and 12th ribs. Press upward to elevate the liver toward the abdominal wall (Fig. 15-11). Have the patient take a deep breath. Press your right hand gently but deeply in and up during inspiration.

An enlarged liver is palpable below the costal margin. Assess its size as described under "Percussion." An enlarged liver may indicate a *tumor* or *cirrhosis*.

Technique and Normal Findings	Abnormal Findings

The liver edge is palpable against your right hand during inspiration.

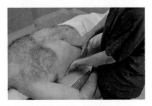

Figure 15.11 Pressing upward to elevate the liver.

With the hooking technique, place your hands over the right costal margin. Hook your fingers over the edge. Have the patient take a deep breath. Feel for the liver's edge as it drops down on inspiration and then rises up over your fingers on expiration (Fig. 15-12).

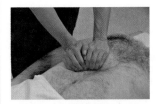

Figure 15.12 Using the hooking technique to assess the liver.

Spleen. Stand on the patient's right side. Place your left hand under the patient's left CVA. Pull upward to move the spleen anteriorly (Fig. 15-13). Place your right hand under the left costal margin. Have the patient take a deep breath; during exhalation, press inward along the left costal margin. Try to palpate the spleen. Alternatively, have the patient turn onto the right side to move the spleen more forward. *A normal spleen is not palpable.*

In an enlarged spleen, you can palpate the spleen tip. Enlarged spleen occurs with *mononucleosis*, *HIV*, *cancers* of the blood and lymph, infectious *hepatitis*, and red blood cell abnormalities of *spherocytosis*, *sickle cell anemia*, and thalassemia.

(text continues on page 296)

Technique and Normal Findings	Abnormal Findings

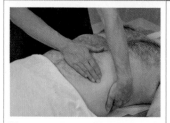

Figure 15.13 Placing the hand under the patient's left CVA to move the spleen.

Kidneys. To assess the left kidney, stand on the patient's right side. Place your left hand on the left CVA. Place your right hand at the left anterior costal margin. Have the patient take a deep breath. Press your hands together to "capture" the kidney. As the patient exhales, lift your left hand and palpate the kidney with your right hand (Fig. 15-14).

Kidneys enlarged from *hydronephrosis* or *tumors* may be palpable.

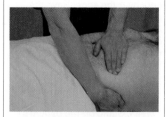

Figure 15.14 Palpating the left kidney.

To assess the right kidney (only palpable if enlarged), remain on the patient's right side. Place your right hand on the right CVA and your left hand on the right costal margin. When the patient exhales, palpate the right kidney (Fig. 15-15). *It is common to be unable to palpate the kidneys except in slender patients.*

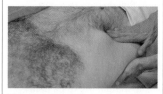

Figure 15.15 Palpating the right kidney.

Abdominal Aorta. To palpate, place your fingers in the epigastric region and slightly toward the left of the MCL.

An enlarged aorta (>3 cm) or one with lateral palpable pulsations can indicate an *abdominal aortic aneurysm.*

Technique and Normal Findings	Abnormal Findings

Palpate for pulsations on either side of the aorta (Fig. 15-16). Assess the width of the aorta by placing one hand on either side. *Pulsations are palpable; the aorta measures 2 cm.*

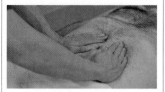

Figure 15.16 Palpating for aortic pulsations.

Bladder. Palpate deeply in the hypogastric area. *The empty bladder is neither tender nor palpable.*

A palpable bladder is either full or enlarged from an underlying mass. A tender bladder usually indicates a *UTI*.

Lymph Nodes. Palpate with the pads of your fingers just below the inguinal ligament for the superficial superior nodes and along the inner aspect of the upper thigh for the superficial inferior nodes. *Inguinal lymph nodes are nontender and slightly palpable.*

If nodes are palpable, note size, shape, mobility, consistency, and tenderness. Enlarged nodes indicate an infection in the regions drained, such as *orchitis* in males, an infection of the lower extremities, or metastatic disease from the anus or vulva.

Assessing for Ascites

Assessing for *ascites*, which is detectable only after 500 mL of fluid has accumulated, is done in two ways: shifting dullness or fluid wave.

Ascites is found in patients with *cirrhosis* or primary or meta-static tumors of the liver.

Shifting Dullness. Percuss in the umbilical area when the patient is supine. Then have the patient lie on the right side and percuss again. Repeat by having the patient turn to the left side.

Dullness moves to the most dependent area.

(text continues on page 298)

Technique and Normal Findings	Abnormal Findings
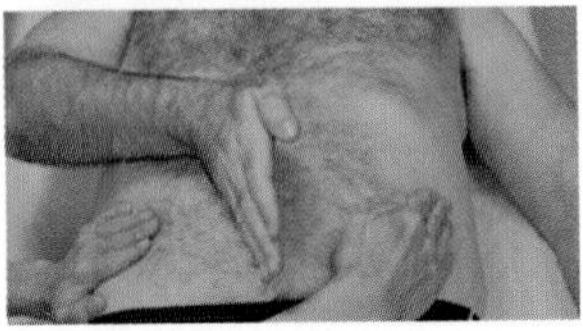 ***Fluid Wave.*** Have the patient place his or her hand vertically in the middle of the abdomen. Place your hands on both sides of the patient's abdomen. Tap one side while palpating the other (Fig. 15-17).	If ascites is present, the tap will cause a fluid wave through the abdomen and you will feel the fluid with the other hand.

Figure 15.17 Assessing for a fluid wave to determine presence of ascites.

### Eliciting the Abdominal Reflex To measure this superficial cutaneous reflex, use a tongue blade or the handle of a reflex hammer to lightly stroke the abdomen in all four quadrants toward the umbilicus. *The umbilicus moves toward the stimulus.*	The abdominal reflex is absent in patients with upper and lower motor neuron diseases. It may be masked and not determinable in obese patients.

Documentation of Normal Subjective and Objective Findings

The patient reports normal appetite, no food intolerance, no excessive belching, no trouble swallowing, no heartburn, and no nausea. Bowel movements are daily, brown in color, and soft. The patient denies changes in bowel habits, no pain with defecation, no rectal bleeding, or black tarry stools. Denies hemorrhoids, passing of gas, constipation, or diarrhea. Denies abdominal pain. No jaundice, no liver or gallbladder problems, and no history of hepatitis. Abdomen is flat with active bowel sounds, soft, and nontender; no masses or hepatosplenomegaly. Liver span is 6 cm in the R MCL; liver edge is smooth and palpable 1 cm below the right costal margin. Spleen and kidneys not palpable. No CVA tenderness.

⚠ Lifespan Considerations

Pregnant Women

During pregnancy, abdominal muscles relax. The uterus protrudes into the abdominal cavity. The rectus muscles separate, increasing the tendency for hernias later. The stomach rises from the increasing size of the uterus and may impinge on the diaphragm. Many women complain of increasing heartburn and indigestion as the pregnancy progresses. The uterus compresses the bowels, which may diminish bowel sounds. The enlarged uterus leads to increased venous pressure in the abdomen, which may result in hemorrhoids and problems with constipation. The appendix is displaced upward and laterally to the right, making it more difficult to diagnose appendicitis. A dark line, the *linea nigra*, may appear midline from symphysis pubis to umbilicus. The umbilicus may evert. Stretch marks (striae) may appear as the abdominal wall and skin stretch to accommodate the enlarging uterus.

Newborns, Infants, and Children

Abdominal musculature is less developed in infants and children, making the abdominal contents more palpable and resulting in a normally protuberant abdomen. The much larger liver proportionately may protrude more than 2 cm below the ribcage. The bladder is found above the symphysis pubis. This situation resolves in adolescence, when abdominal assessment findings become similar to those for normal adults.

Older Adults

Many elders are plagued with poor dentition, which may result in pain when chewing, dramatic changes in diet and weight, and long-term problems. Decreased production of saliva and stomach acid leads to digestive changes. Motility and peristalsis decrease, which may result in more bloating, distention, and constipation. Also contributing is decreased muscle mass and tone. Fat accumulates in the lower abdomen of women and around the waist of men, making inspection more challenging and inaccurate. Liver size is smaller and the liver becomes less functional, resulting in less absorption of medications metabolized by the liver.

◗ Cultural Considerations

- **Obesity** is generally higher in racial and ethnic minorities than in Caucasians.

- African Americans more commonly present with sickle cell anemia, G6PD deficiency, and lactose intolerance. Those with sickle cell disease may have splenomegaly and jaundice on examination. In sickle cell crisis, patients may have acute abdominal pain and vomiting.
- GI cancers, especially stomach cancer, are more often seen in Asian Americans. Asian Americans have a higher incidence of infection with *Helicobacter pylori*.
- Lactose intolerance, inflammatory bowel disease, and colon cancer are more prevalent in Americans of Jewish ancestry.
- Americans of Greek and Italian descent more commonly present with lactose intolerance, thalassemia, and anemia.
- Alcoholism, liver and gallbladder disease, pancreatitis, and diabetes are more common in Native Americans.

Common Nursing Diagnoses and Interventions Associated with the Abdomen

Diagnosis and Related Factors	Potential Interventions
Imbalanced nutrition, less than body requirement related to nausea and vomiting	Provide nutritional supplements, for example, shakes. Administer antiemetics as ordered.*
Diarrhea related to effects of bowel inflammation	Obtain stool specimens to determine infection, for example, *C. difficile* infection.
Constipation related to immobility	Obtain order for stool softener if the patient is on opioids, increase intake of fiber, assist with ambulation, ensure adequate intake of fluids.
Incontinence related to decreased level of consciousness	Review medications that may contribute to incontinence, perform bladder scan to evaluate if residual is present, teach principles of bladder training.

*Collaborative interventions.

Table 15.1   Abdominal Distention

Finding	Description
Obesity 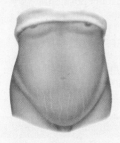	A protuberant abdomen results in a thickened abdominal wall and fat deposits in the mesentery and omentum. Percussion sounds present as normal tympanic sounds.
Gaseous Distention 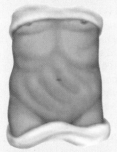	Gaseous distention results from the breakdown of certain foods and fluids, as well as with the altered peristalsis seen in paralytic ileus and intestinal obstruction. It can be found in one area or generalized. Percussion sounds are tympanic over the area of distention.
Abdominal Tumor 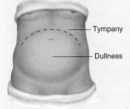 — Tympany / — Dullness	A large abdominal tumor is firm to palpation and dull to percussion. Ovarian and uterine tumors are commonly palpable in the abdominal cavity.

(table continues on page 302)

Table 15.1 Abdominal Distention (*continued*)

Finding	Description
Ascites Tympany Dullness Umbilicus may be protuberant Bulging flank	**Ascites** (fluid accumulation that descends with gravity) results in dullness to percussion in the lowest point of the abdomen based on patient position. Changing the patient's position should shift the fluid to the most dependent point. Ascites occurs in cirrhosis, congestive heart failure, nephrosis, peritonitis, and metastatic neoplasms.

Table 15.2 Common Tests for Abdominal Problems

Problem	Test/Rationale
Acute Abdomen	Apply light and deep palpation. A firm, boardlike abdominal wall suggests *peritoneal inflammation*. Guarding occurs when the patient flinches, grimaces, or reports pain. **Rebound tenderness** (more tenderness when you quickly withdraw your hand from the point of the pain than when you press slowly) also suggests *peritoneal inflammation*.
Appendicitis	The patient reports pain at the umbilicus and moving to the RLQ. When the patient coughs, he or she reports RLQ pain. Local tenderness occurs during palpation in the RLQ, at McBurney's point. A rectal examination or, in women, pelvic examination, may reveal local tenderness. Other peritoneal findings include the following: **Rovsing's sign:** Press deeply and evenly in the LLQ. Quickly withdraw your fingers. The patient reports pain in the RLQ, suggesting *appendicitis*.

Problem	Test/Rationale
	Psoas sign: Place your hand just above the patient's right knee. Ask the patient to raise the thigh against your hand and turn to the left side. Extend the right leg at the hip to stretch the **iliopsoas** muscle. A positive sign is RLQ pain. **Obturator sign:** Flex the patient's right thigh at the hip with the knee bent. Rotate the leg internally at the hip. RLQ pain constitutes a positive obturator sign, suggesting an inflamed appendix or peritoneal inflammation.
Abdominal Aortic Aneurysm	Patients complain of boring, tearing pain and referred pain. Auscultation reveals bruits or exaggerated pulsations. A mass may be palpable. Femoral pulses may be diminished or diffuse. Patients may seem in shock; hypotensive; tachycardic; tachypneic; pale, cool, and clammy skin; and cool extremities.
Acute Cholecystitis	Auscultate, percuss, and palpate the abdomen for tenderness. Bowel sounds may be active or decreased. Tympany may increase with an ileus. There may be RUQ tenderness. Assess for Murphy's sign. Hook your thumb under the right costal margin at the edge of the rectus muscle; ask the patient to take a deep breath. Sharp tenderness and a sudden stop in inspiratory effort constitute a positive Murphy's sign, suggesting cholecystitis.

Table 15.3 Gastrointestinal Diseases

Disease	Signs and Symptoms
Cancer of the Stomach	Epigastric distress, abdominal fullness, anorexia, and weight loss; in late stages, ascites, palpable liver mass, and lymph node enlargement.
Cancer of the Colon	Changes in bowel habits, blood in stool, smaller diameter of bowel movement; in late stages, pain; palpable mass on rectal examination or deep palpation of the LLQ.
Constipation	Diminished bowel sounds on auscultation; feces palpated in the LLQ.
Diverticulitis	Inflammation, possible infection, abscess, and perforation. Severe pain (usually LLQ), diminished bowel sounds on auscultation, nausea, vomiting, and a long history of constipation.
Inflammatory Bowel Disease	Malnutrition and vitamin malabsorption, abdominal pain not relieved with defecation, diarrhea, steatorrhea, bowel perforation, toxic megacolon, mucus in the stool, rectal bleeding.
Irritable Bowel Syndrome	Alternating diarrhea, constipation, or both. Hard compacted stools, abdominal pain relieved by defecation. Range of stools from pebbles to liquid over several days.
Liver Failure	Can develop within 2–8 wk of onset of jaundice; sudden and severe liver impairment.
Pancreatitis	Inflammation of the pancreas; altered flow of digestive enzymes; nausea, vomiting; weight loss; severe boring pain in LUQ; referred pain to the back or shoulder.

Table 15.3 Gastrointestinal Diseases (*continued*)

Disease	Signs and Symptoms
Paralytic Ileus	Lack of peristalsis, usually in the small intestine; may follow surgery, peritonitis, or spinal cord injury; intermittent, colicky pain with visible peristaltic waves on inspection and vomiting. No bowel sounds; abdomen is distended.
Peritonitis	Inflammation of the lining of the abdominal cavity. Presents with fever, nausea, and vomiting; abdominal pain of varying character, rigidity, and guarding; cutaneous hypersensitivity; and diminished bowel sounds.
Pyelonephritis	Active or decreased bowel sounds; tenderness anteriorly over the affected kidney on deep palpation.
Splenic Rupture	Serious abdominal condition resulting in hemorrhage; usually follows trauma but can accompany mononucleosis; severe LUQ pain, radiating to the left shoulder; hemorrhagic shock.
Ulcer	*Gastric ulcer:* Gnawing pain, heartburn, anorexia, vomiting, eructations, and weight loss.
	Duodenal ulcer: Intermittent RUQ pain 2–3 hr after eating.

Musculoskeletal Assessment

Subjective Data Collection

Key Topics and Questions for Health Promotion

Key Questions	Rationales
Demographic Data. Note the patient's age, gender, and ethnic heritage/race.	Some musculoskeletal diseases are age-related or more prevalent by gender or ethnic group. See Table 16-1 at the end of this chapter.
Family History. Do your parents or siblings have muscle, joint, or bone problems? • Who had the problem? • When did it occur? • How was it treated? • What was the outcome?	Musculoskeletal problems with a familial tendency include *osteoporosis*, *bone cancer*, and *rheumatoid arthritis*.
Past Medical History. Have you had musculoskeletal trauma, injury, fracture, stroke, polio, bone or muscle infection, diabetes, or parathyroid disease? • When did it occur? • How was it treated? • What was the outcome?	Following hip replacement, hip dislocation can occur, with hip flexion greater than 90 degrees or adduction of the joint past midline. A person who has had a stroke is at increased risk for shoulder *subluxation* (partial dislocation).
Nutrition/Medications. What is your daily dairy intake?	Calcium and vitamin D are essential for bone health.

Key Questions	Rationales
What medications do you take? • Women: current and past oral contraceptives? • Postmenopausal women: hormone replacement therapy (HRT)? • Calcium and vitamin D supplements? • Pain or anti-inflammatory medications? • Muscle relaxants? • Steroids?	Vitamin D deficiency has been linked to *osteoporosis*. Oral contraceptive use in young women may contribute to *osteoporosis*; HRT may help prevent it. Pain or anti-inflammatory medications and muscle relaxants can mask symptoms. Steroids can affect calcium absorption.
Occupation, Lifestyle, and Behaviors. What work do you do? • Does it involve repetitive motion? Lifting or twisting? • How do you protect yourself from injury at work?	Some occupations increase risk of injury through repetitive movement, twisting, lifting, vibration, exposure to cold, and pushing or pulling heavy objects. Ergonomics and safety equipment can protect workers.
What hobbies and sports do you enjoy? • How do you protect against injury? • Do you consistently use car seats, helmets, and protective gear?	Basketball, baseball, football, and soccer contribute to knee injuries. Skiing increases risk for lower-extremity injuries; skateboarding can lead to upper-extremity injuries. Car seats, helmets, and protective gear decrease injury severity.
What is your weekly or monthly income? How many people live on that income?	Women of lower socioeconomic status are more likely to report activity limitations, *arthritis*, *obesity*, and *osteoporosis*.
Have you ever smoked? • If yes, how many packs per day? • For how many years?	Smoking increases risk for vertebral fracture.
Have you ever consumed alcohol? • If yes, how many drinks per week? • What do you drink?	Alcohol use is associated with risk for *osteoporosis*.

Health-Promotion Teaching

Psychosocial Screening. Problems that limit or compromise movement and mobility can have wide-ranging effects and consequences. If a patient has a musculoskeletal injury, ask how it will affect ability to work, participate in hobbies, or perform routine activities of daily living (ADLs). If a patient cannot work, financial issues may be of concern. Issues to address include whether patients can perform self-care safely, manage pain, avoid isolation and sensory deprivation, and maintain sense of self and healthy body image.

Scoliosis Screening. *Scoliosis* (lateral curvature of the spine) usually affects both the thoracic and lumbar parts, with deviations occurring in opposite directions. Scoliosis may be *structural* (caused by a spinal defect) or *functional* (caused by habits). If not corrected early, scoliosis can progressively worsen. The problem often develops in early adolescence, especially in girls. That is why regular school screening for scoliosis is so important. Because some older people did not undergo such screening, nurses may discover cases in them. Severe cases can interfere with normal functioning of the organs within the chest.

To screen for scoliosis, inspect the patient's back. While the patient stands, look for symmetry of the hips, scapulae, shoulders, and any skin folds or creases. The patient then needs to bend forward with the arms hanging toward the floor. Look for any lateral curves or protrusions on one side. Then, the patient should slowly stand while spine inspection continues. A **scoliometer** may be used to obtain a measurement of the number of degrees that the spine is deviated. During spinal palpation, feel for any abnormal protrusions or deformities.

Nutrition and Weight Management. People of all ages need to learn to maintain a healthy weight and perform weight-bearing exercise at least three times per week.

Safety Measures. Children should alternate the shoulders on which they carry backpacks to help prevent functional scoliosis. Encourage all patients to use good body mechanics with lifting and pushing, use protective equipment with sports and work, and wear seat belts. Exercises to increase strength and flexibility and improve posture decrease the risk of falls.

Bone Density Preservation. Loss of bone density and muscle strength are major age-related concerns that lifestyle modification can help control. Calcium and vitamin D are important for people of all ages, as are weight-bearing exercises. Although there is treatment for osteoporosis, there is no cure. Prevention is very important, especially for women. Current treatment includes bisphosphonates, calcitonin, estrogen and/or HRT, raloxifene, and parathyroid hormone.

Key Topics and Questions for Common Symptoms

Common Musculoskeletal Symptoms

- Pain or discomfort
- Weakness
- Stiffness or limited movement
- Deformity
- Lack of balance and coordination

Questions to Assess Symptoms	Rationales/Abnormal Findings
Pain. Do you have pain or discomfort in your muscles, bones, or joints?	Pain is a subjective experience.
Where is it? Is it only in that area or does it radiate? Do you have pain in different areas at other times? If the pain is in more than one joint, is it symmetrical?	Location and timing of pain may help differentiate if it originates in muscle (*myalgia*), bone, or joint (*arthralgia*).
How bad does it hurt? What does the pain feel like?	Burning pain may be neurological. Bone pain may be aching, deep, and dull. Muscle pain is often cramping or sore.
When do you feel pain? Is it constant? Does it come and go? Is it sudden or gradual?	Arthritic pain may be worse during cold, damp weather. Pain from *rheumatoid arthritis* is often worse in the morning, while pain from *osteoarthritis* is usually worse after rest and at the end of the day.
Is there accompanying weakness, tingling, or numbness?	These indicate pressure on nerves.
What makes it worse? What helps relieve it?	Bone pain does not increase with movement, unless there is a *fracture*. Muscle and joint pain increases with movement.
For patients with chronic pain, what level of pain would you like to achieve?	Patients with chronic pain may never know its absence. The nurse and the patient together need to determine an acceptable level of pain.

(text continues on page 310)

Questions to Assess Symptoms	Rationales/Abnormal Findings
Does pain limit your activities?	Pain can limit ability to perform usual activity.
Weakness. Do you have muscle weakness?	Muscle weakness is associated with certain diseases.
Do all or just certain muscles feel weak?	Weakness may migrate across muscles or muscle groups. Knowing involved muscles helps determine the disease.
When does the weakness occur? How long does it last? What makes it worse? What helps? How bad is weakness on a scale of 1 to 10, with 10 being the worst?	Muscle weakness after prolonged activity may result from *dehydration* or electrolyte imbalance. Grading the degree can help patients see improvement or determine the time of day they can perform better.
Stiffness/Limited Movement. Do you have stiffness or limited movement in any body part?	Stiffness may result from pain in muscles or joints, swelling, or a disease process.
Is the stiffness in one or more joints?	Swelling from *renal failure* affects the entire body, while injury may involve one joint only.
Can you grade stiffness on a scale of 0 to 10, with 10 being the inability to move? Is stiffness constant or intermittent?	Early *rheumatoid arthritis* may cause stiffness that is worse in the morning. Stiffness from *osteoarthritis* is worse at the end of the day.
Did stiffness follow an injury? Was onset gradual?	*Contracture* (shortening of tendons, fascia, or muscles) may result from injury or prolonged positioning.
Deformity. Do you have a deformity? Was it present at birth?	Disuse, including wearing a cast, leads to some wasting or shrinking of the muscle (atrophy).
Does it affect the entire body or is it localized?	Deformities may be general (decreased overall body size) or localized.

Questions to Assess Symptoms	Rationales/Abnormal Findings
Lack of Balance/Coordination. Do you have problems maintaining balance?	Unusual gait or inability to perform ADLs may result from a balance or coordination problem, which may indicate a neurologic disorder.
Have you fallen recently? Have you noticed that your movements are uncoordinated?	_Ataxia_ (irregular, uncoordinated movements) or loss of balance may be from cerebellar disorders, _Parkinson's disease_, _multiple sclerosis_, stroke, brain tumor, inner ear problem, or medications.

Objective Data Collection

Equipment

- Goniometer
- Tape measure

Technique and Normal Findings	Abnormal Findings
Initial Survey **_Posture._** Observe posture while the patient stands with feet together. Observe relationship among the head, trunk, pelvis, and extremities. Assess for symmetry in shoulder height, scapulae, and iliac crests. Also observe posture when the patient sits. _Posture is erect with the head midline above the spine. Shoulders are equal in height._	_Scoliosis_ or low back pain may cause the patient to lean forward or to the side. _Acromegaly_ may result in an enlarged skull and increased length of the hands, feet, and long bones.
Gait/Mobility. Watch the patient walk across the room. Observe from the side and	See Table 16-2 at the end of this chapter for abnormal gait patterns.

(text continues on page 312)

Technique and Normal Findings	Abnormal Findings
behind. Gait can predict risk of falling. *Walking is smooth and rhythmic with arms swinging in opposition to legs. The patient rises from sitting with ease.*	
Balance. Ask the patient to walk on tiptoes, heels, heel-to-toe (tandem walking), and backward. Ask the patient to step to each side and to sit down and stand.	Balance is a function of the cerebellum; however, inner ear problems can also affect it.
To perform the Romberg test, ask the patient to stand with feet together and eyes open. Have the patient close the eyes. If cerebral function is intact, the patient does this without swaying (negative test). *The patient is balanced and has a negative Romberg test.*	The patient sways.
Coordination. Ask the patient to rapidly pat the table or alternate between palm and dorsum of the hand. Ask the patient to perform finger to thumb opposition. To assess gross motor coordination in the legs, have the patient run the heel of one foot up the opposite leg from ankle to knee. *The patient performs all examinations correctly.*	Poor coordination may be from pain, injury, deformity, or cerebellar disorders.
Inspection of Extremities. Look for swelling, lacerations, lesions, deformity, length of long bones, size of muscles, and symmetry.	Asymmetry in bone length may be from injury and in muscle size from neurologic damage. Disuse may lead to muscle atrophy.

Technique and Normal Findings	Abnormal Findings
Size and Shape. Evaluate both extremities at the same time to compare muscle tone and strength. Note size and shape of the extremities and muscles, alignment, and any deformity or asymmetry. Are limbs of equal length?	Swelling or edema may be from of trauma, inflammation, or lymph node resection.
Limb Measurements. Compare arm and leg circumferences. Compare radial length by having the patient place the arms together from elbow to wrist. Observe knee height with the patient sitting. Measure limb circumference on the forearms, upper arms, thighs, and calves. Measure arm length from acromion process to tip of the middle finger. Measure true leg length from anterior superior iliac crest to medial malleolus. Measure apparent leg length from umbilicus to medial malleolus.	Discrepancy in leg length of more than 1 cm may cause gait problems, hip and back pain, and apparent *scoliosis*. Unequal apparent leg length, but equal true leg length is seen with hip and pelvic abnormalities. Unequal arm length does not cause as many problems as unequal leg length. Unequal circumference may be from disuse or neurologic disorders.
Palpation. Palpate joints for contour and size; palpate muscles for tone. Feel for bumps, nodules, or deformity. Ask if there is any tenderness during touch.	Asymmetry may be from disuse or neurological disease. Discomfort on touch may be from inflammation or infection.
Joint Range of Motion (ROM). Simultaneously observe and palpate each joint while the patient performs active ROM. If the patient cannot do so, carefully support the limb on either side of the joint and perform passive ROM. Ask if there is tenderness or discomfort. If ROM is limited, use a goniometer to measure joint angle at its maximum flexion and extension. Listen to or feel the joint while the patient moves. *A healthy joint moves smoothly and quietly.*	Limitation of movement, **crepitus** (cracking or popping), and nonverbal and verbal expressions of discomfort or pain are noted.

(text continues on page 314)

Technique and Normal Findings	Abnormal Findings
Muscle Tone and Strength. Compare one side to the other. *Upper and lower extremity muscle strength is 5/5 bilaterally.*	See Table 16-3.
Temporomandibular Joint (TMJ)	
Inspection. Look for symmetry, swelling, and redness. *Jaw is symmetrical bilaterally.*	Asymmetrical face or joint muscles may indicate facial fractures or surgery.
Palpation. Place your fingerpads in front of the tragus of each of the patient's ears (Fig. 16-1). Ask the patient to open and close the jaw while you palpate. *You feel a shallow depression. Mandible motion is smooth and painless. Muscles are symmetrical, smooth, and nontender.*	Discomfort, swelling, limited movement, and grating or crackling sounds require further evaluation. TMJ dysfunction may present as ear pain or headache. Swelling or tenderness suggests *arthritis* or *myofascial pain syndrome.*

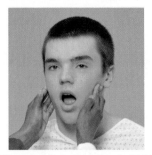

Figure 16.1 Palpating the TMJ.

ROM. Ask the patient to open the jaw as wide as possible, push the lower jaw forward, return the jaw to neutral, and move the jaw from one side to another 1 to 2 cm. *TMJ moves with ease and may have an audible or a palpable click when opened. Mouth opens with 3 to 6 cm between upper and lower teeth.*	Difficulty opening the mouth may be because of injury or *arthritis.* Pain in the TMJ may indicate misalignment of the teeth or arthritic changes.

Technique and Normal Findings	Abnormal Findings

Muscle Strength. Ask the patient to repeat the above movements while you provide opposing force. *Muscle strength is equal and 5/5 on both sides of the jaw; the patient performs the movements against resistance, with no pain, spasms, or contractions.*

Decreased muscle strength may be because of muscle or joint disease.

Cervical Spine

Inspection. With the patient standing, inspect the cervical spine from all sides. It should position the head above the trunk (Fig. 16-2). Observe from the side for the concave cervical spinal curve. *From behind, the patient holds the head erect, and the cervical spine is in straight alignment. From the side, the neck has a concave curve.*

Degenerative joint disease may cause lateral tilting of the head and neck. Lateral deviation of the neck (*torticollis*) may be from acute muscle spasm, congenital problems, or incorrect head posture to correct vision problems. Weight lifting will cause hypertrophy of the neck muscles, resulting in a thickened neck appearance.

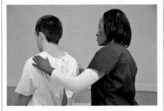

Figure 16.2 Inspecting the cervical spine.

Palpation. Stand behind the patient. Palpate the cervical spine and neck. *C7 and T1 spinous processes are prominent. Paravertebral, trapezius, and sternocleidomastoid muscles are fully developed, symmetrical, and nontender.*

Osteoarthritis, neck injury, disc degeneration, and *spondylosis* can cause decreased ROM, pain, and tenderness. Pain may indicate inflammation of the muscles (*myositis*). Neck spasm may indicate nerve compression or psychological stress.

(text continues on page 316)

Technique and Normal Findings	Abnormal Findings

ROM. Ask the patient to touch the chin to the chest (flexion), look up toward the ceiling (hyperextension), attempt to touch each ear to the shoulder without elevating the shoulder (lateral flexion or bending), and turn the chin to the shoulder as far as possible (rotation) (Fig. 16-3). *Flexion 45 degrees, hyperextension 55 degrees, lateral flexion 40 degrees, and rotation 70 degrees to each side.*

Pain or muscle spasm may impair ROM. Hyperextension and flexion may be limited because of cervical disc degeneration, spinal cord tumor, or osteoarthritis. Pain may radiate to the back, shoulder, or arms. Pain, numbness, or tingling may indicate compression of spinal root nerves.

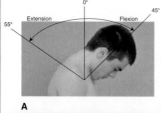
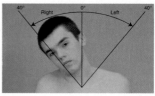

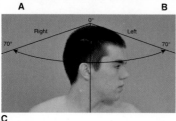

Figure 16.3 Neck ROM.
(A) Flexion. **(B)** Lateral flexion. **(C)** Rotation.

Muscle Strength. Ask the patient to rotate the neck to the right and left, against resistance of your hand. *Muscle strength overcomes resistance.*

Weakness or loss of sensation may result from cervical cord compression.

Clinical Significance 16-1

Following any trauma, do not move patients with neck pain until the neck is stabilized. Moving the patient could cause permanent injury to the spinal cord.

Technique and Normal Findings	Abnormal Findings

Shoulder

Inspection. Compare both shoulders anteriorly and posteriorly for size and contour. Observe the anterior aspect of the joint capsule for abnormal swelling. *No redness, swelling, deformity, or atrophy is present. Shoulders are smooth, bilaterally symmetric, and level. Each shoulder is at an equal distance from the vertebral column.*

Shoulder joints may have some deformity because of *arthritis*, trauma, or *scoliosis*. Redness and swelling may indicate injury or inflammation. Unequal shoulder height may indicate *scoliosis*. See also Table 16-4.

Palpation. Stand in front of the patient. Palpate both shoulders. Note any spasm, atrophy, swelling, heat, or tenderness. Start at the clavicle. Explore the acromioclavicular joint, scapula, greater tubercle of the humerus, subacromial bursa, biceps groove, and anterior aspect of the glenohumeral joint (Fig. 16-4). *Muscles are fully developed and smooth.*

Tenderness may be from inflammation or overuse of muscles or sports injuries.

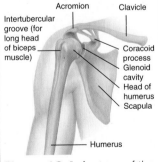

Figure 16.4 Anatomy of the shoulder.

(text continues on page 318)

Technique and Normal Findings	Abnormal Findings

ROM. Ask the person to perform forward flexion, extension, hyperextension, abduction, adduction, and internal and external rotation (Fig. 16-5). Cup one hand over the patient's shoulder during ROM to detect crepitus. *Movement is fluid. Forward flexion 180 degrees, hyperextension 50 degrees, abduction 180 degrees, adduction 50 degrees, internal rotation 90 degrees, and external rotation 90 degrees.*

Limited ROM, pain, crepitation, and asymmetry may be from *arthritis*, muscle or joint inflammation, trauma, or sports injury. Inability to externally rotate the shoulder suggests *rotator cuff injury*.

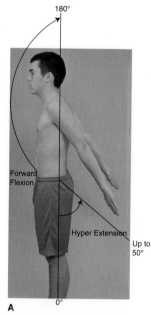
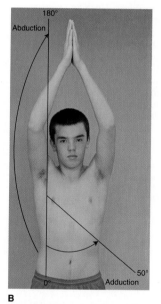

Figure 16.5 Shoulder ROM. **(A)** Extension. **(B)** Abduction/ adduction. **(C)** External rotation. **(D)** Internal rotation.

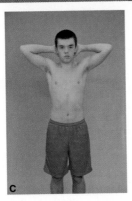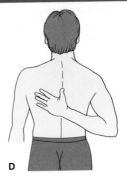

Figure 16.5 (*continued*).

Muscle Strength. Ask the patient to shrug both shoulders, flex forward and upward, and abduct against resistance. *The patient performs full ROM against resistance.*	Decreased ability to shrug the shoulders against resistance may indicate compressed spinal cord root nerve or spinal accessory cranial nerve (CN XI).
Elbow	
Inspection. Inspect size and contour in both extended and flexed positions. Check the olecranon bursa for swelling. *Elbows are symmetrical with no swelling.*	Subluxation shows the forearm dislocated posteriorly. Swelling and redness of the olecranon bursa are easily observed. Effusion or synovial thickening is observed as a bulge on either side of the olecranon process and indicates *gouty arthritis.* See also Table 16-4.
Palpation. Support the forearm. Passively flex the elbow to 70 degrees. Palpate the olecranon process and medial and lateral epicondyles of the humerus (Fig. 16-6). Check for synovial thickening, swelling, nodules, or tenderness. *Elbows are smooth with no swelling or tenderness.*	Epicondyles and tendons are common sites for inflammation and tenderness. Soft, boggy swelling occurs with synovial thickening or effusion. Local heat or redness may indicate inflammation. Subcutaneous nodules at pressure points may indicate *rheumatoid arthritis.*

(text continues on page 320)

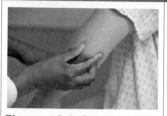

Figure 16.6 Palpation of the elbow.

ROM. Ask the patient to bend and straighten the elbow and to pronate and supinate the forearm by laying the forearm and ulnar surface of the hand on a table. Have the patient touch the palm and then the hand dorsum to the table (Fig. 16-7). *Flexion 150 to 160 degrees, extension 0 degrees. Some people cannot extend the elbow fully; some can hyperextend the elbow −5 to −10 degrees. Pronation and supination of 90 degrees is normal.*

Decreased ROM, pain, or crepitation may be from *arthritis*, inflammation, trauma, or sports injury. Redness, swelling, and tenderness of the olecranon process may be *bursitis*. *Lateral epicondylitis* (tennis elbow) is inflammation of the forearm extensor and supinator muscles and tendons, causing disabling pain that radiates down the lateral forearm. *Medial epicondylitis* (golf elbow) is the same, except that it affects the flexor and pronator muscles and tendons.

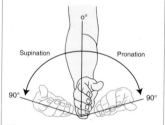

Figure 16.7 Supination and pronation of the elbow.

Muscle Strength. While supporting the patient's arm, apply resistance just proximal to the wrist. Ask the patient to flex and extend both elbows (Fig. 16-8). *The patient performs full ROM against resistance.*

Decreased strength may be from pain, nerve root compression, or arthritic deformity. People may compensate for weakened biceps or triceps muscles by using the shoulder muscles.

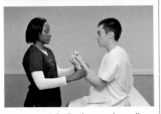

Figure 16.8 Assessing elbow muscle strength.

Wrist and Hand

Palpation. Hold the patient's hand in your hands. Use your thumbs to palpate each joint of the wrist and hand (Fig. 16-9). *Surfaces are smooth with no nodules, edema, or tenderness.*

Painful joints are common in *osteoarthritis.* A firm mass over the dorsum of the wrist may be a *ganglion. Rheumatoid arthritis* may cause edema, redness, and tenderness.

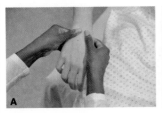 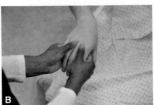

Figure 16.9 Palpating the joints of the **(A)** wrists and **(B)** hands.

ROM. Observe wrist and hand ROM (Fig. 16-10). *Wrist flexion (90 degrees), extension (return to 0 degrees), hyperextension (70 degrees), and ulnar (55 degrees) and radial (20 degrees) deviation. Meta-carpophalangeal joint ROM flexion (90 degrees), extension (0 degrees), and hyperextension (up to 30 degrees). Proximal and distal intraphalangeal*

Joint or muscle inflammation may cause decreased or unequal ROM. Previous trauma may limit ROM.

(text continues on page 322)

joints perform flexion, extension, and abduction. Thumb performs opposition with each fingertip and base of the little finger.

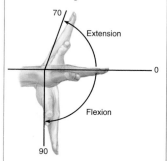

Figure 16.10 Wrist and hand flexion and extension.

Muscle Strength. Perform each motion above against resistance. Ask the patient to grasp your first two fingers tightly while you pull to remove them. *Muscle strength is equal bilaterally and sufficient to overcome resistance.*

Weak muscle strength may be because of arthritic changes or fractures.

Hip

Inspection. While standing, assess the iliac crest, size and symmetry of the buttocks, and number of gluteal folds. With the patient supine and legs straight, look for swelling, lacerations, lesions, deformity, muscle size, and symmetry. Look at the hips from the anterior and posterior views. *Hips are rounded, even, and symmetrical.*

When lying supine, external rotation of the lower leg and foot indicates a fractured femur. Unequal gluteal folds or height of iliac crests may indicate uneven leg length or *scoliosis*.

Technique and Normal Findings	Abnormal Findings
Palpation. Palpate the hip joints, iliac crests, and muscle tone. Feel for any bumps, nodules, and deformity. Ask if there is any tenderness with touch. Feel for crepitus when moving the joint. *Buttocks are symmetrical. Iliac crests are at the same height on both sides.*	Asymmetry, discomfort, or crepitus with movement may occur with hip inflammation or *degenerative joint disease.*
ROM. Observe for full active ROM of each hip: • Flexion (lift straight leg to 90 degrees or draw knee to chest to 120 degrees) • Extension (standing position or lying with the leg straight) • Abduction (lift, if standing, or slide, if lying, foot and straight leg to the side, away from body to 45 degrees) • Adduction (swing foot and straight leg in front and past the other leg to 30 degrees) • Internal and external ROM (with the hip and knee flexed, move the leg medially 40 degrees and then laterally 45 degrees). Have the patient stand or position prone to test hyperextension. Ask the patient to move the straight leg backward, away from the body (15 degrees). Circumduction while standing or lying on one side moves the foot and leg in a circle beside the body in all movements. *The patient can perform full ROM without discomfort or crepitus.*	Straight leg flexion that produces back and leg pain radiating down the leg may indicate a *herniated disc.* When lying down, one leg longer than the other or limited internal rotation may indicate a hip fracture or dislocation.

(text continues on page 324)

Technique and Normal Findings	Abnormal Findings
Muscle Strength. With the patient lying down, apply pressure to the top of the leg while the patient flexes the hip. *Apply pressure to the side while the patient abducts the hip. The patient performs full ROM against resistance.*	Asymmetry of strength may be from pain, or a muscle or nerve disease.
## Knee ***Inspection.*** Inspect contour and shape while the patient stands and sits. Look for any swelling, lacerations, lesions, deformity, muscle size, and symmetry. When the patient stands, is one hip higher than the other? When seated, is one knee higher? Does one knee protrude further? *Hollows are on each side of the patella. Knees are symmetrical and aligned with thighs and ankles.*	Knee swelling indicates inflammation, trauma, or *arthritis.* Atrophy may accompany disuse or chronic disorders. Part of a limb twisted toward and out from midline is labeled *varus* and *valgus* respectively. Asymmetry in muscle size may be from disuse or injury. See also Table 16-4.
Palpation. With the knee flexed, palpate the quadriceps muscle for tone. Palpate downward from approximately 10 cm above the patella; evaluate the patella and each side of the femur and tibia (Fig. 16-11). Palpate the tibiofemoral joints with the leg flexed 90 degrees. Assess tibial margins and lateral collateral ligament. Feel for any bumps, nodules, or deformity. Ask if there is any tenderness. Feel for crepitus when moving the joint. *Quadriceps and surrounding tissue are firm and nontender. Suprapatellar bursa is not palpable. Joint is firm and nontender.*	Pain, swelling, thickening, or heat may indicate synovial inflammation, *arthritis,* or meniscus tear. Painless swelling may occur with *osteoarthritis. Bursitis* causes swelling, heat, and redness.

Technique and Normal Findings	Abnormal Findings

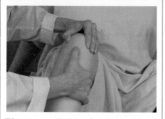

Figure 16.11 Palpating the knee.

ROM. Observe for full active ROM of each knee with the patient seated. Flex the knee to 130 degrees; return to extended position. *Knees perform full ROM without discomfort or crepitus.*

Inability to perform full ROM may be from contractures, pain associated with trauma or inflammation, or neuromuscular disorders.

Muscle Strength. With the patient seated, apply pressure to the anterior lower leg while the patient extends the leg. Also, with the leg bent, ask the patient to maintain that position while you pull the lower leg as if to straighten it. *Muscle strength is equal bilaterally and able to overcome resistance.*

Injury or deconditioning may lead to asymmetry of strength.

Ankle and Foot

Inspection. Inspect feet with the patient standing and sitting. Look for swelling, lacerations, lesions, deformity, muscle size, symmetry, and toe alignment. *Feet are of the same color as the body and symmetrical, with toes aligned with the long axis of the leg. No swelling is present. When the patient stands, weight falls on the middle of the foot.*

See Tables 16-4 and 16-5.

(text continues on page 326)

Technique and Normal Findings	Abnormal Findings
Palpation. Palpate for muscle tone. Feel for any bumps, nodules, or deformity. Holding the heel, palpate the anterior and posterior aspects of the ankle, Achilles tendon, and metatarsophalangeal joints in the ball of the foot (Fig. 16-12). Palpate each interphalangeal joint; note temperature, tenderness, and contour. Ask if there is any tenderness during touch. Feel for crepitus when moving the joint. *Ankle and foot joints are firm, stable, and nontender.*	Pain or discomfort may indicate *arthritis* or inflammation. Pain and tenderness along the Achilles tendon may be from *bursitis* or *tendonitis*. Small nodules on the tendon may occur with *rheumatoid arthritis*. Cooler temperature in the ankles and feet may be from vascular insufficiency (see Chapter 13).

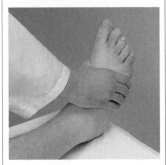

Figure 16.12 Palpating the ankle.

ROM. Observe for full active ROM of the ankle (Fig 16-13). • Dorsiflexion: The patient raises toes toward the knee. • Plantar flexion: The patient points toes downward toward the ground. • Inversion: Sole of the foot is turned toward the opposite leg. • Eversion: Sole of the foot is turned away from the other leg.	Limited ankle or foot ROM without swelling indicates *arthritis*. Inflammation and swelling with limited ROM indicate trauma.

Technique and Normal Findings	Abnormal Findings

Ask the patient to curl the toes and return them to straight position, to keep the soles on the ground and raise the toes upward, to spread the toes as far apart as possible, and to return toes to their original position. *Dorsiflexion 20 degrees, plantar flexion 45 degrees, inversion 30 degrees, and eversion 20 degrees. Toes flex, extend, hyperextend, and abduct.*

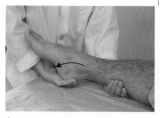

A

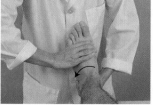

B

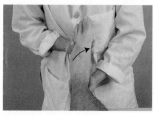

C

Figure 16.13 (A) Plantar flexion. **(B)** Foot inversion. **(C)** Foot eversion.

Muscle Strength. Ask the patient to perform dorsiflexion and plantar flexion against resistance. Then ask the patient to flex and extend the toes against resistance. *Muscle strength is equal bilaterally and overcomes resistance.*

Asymmetry of strength may be from pain, inflammation, deconditioning, or chronic disease.

(text continues on page 328)

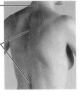

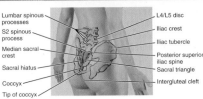

A   **B**

Figure 16.14 Assessing the spine and upper back. **(A)** Side view. **(B)** Posterior view.

Thoracic and Lumbar Spine

Inspection. With the patient standing, look from the side for the normal S pattern (Fig. 16-14). From behind, note whether the spine is straight (Fig. 16-15). Observe if the scapulae, iliac crests, and gluteal folds are level and symmetrical. Ask the patient to bend forward. Reassess that vertebrae are straight and scapulae are equal in height. *Spine is aligned both standing and sitting.*

Kyphosis, forward bending of the upper thoracic spine, may accompany *Paget's disease, osteoporosis,* and *ankylosing spondylosis.* *Lordosis* is common in late pregnancy and obesity. A flattened lumbar curve may occur with lumbar muscle spasms. *List* (leaning of the spine to one side) may occur with paravertebral muscle spasms or herniated disc.

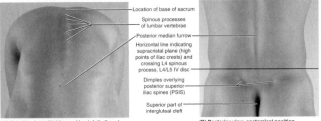

(A) Anterior view with hips and back fully flexed   (B) Posterior view, anatomical position

Figure 16.15 Lower back.

Palpation. Palpate the spinous processes for bumps, nodules, or deformities. Ask if there is any tenderness during touch.

Pain on palpation may indicate inflammation, disc disease, or *arthritis.* Unequal spinous processes may indicate subluxation.

Technique and Normal Findings	Abnormal Findings
Feel for crepitus when the spine bends. *Spinous processes are in a straight line. The patient denies tenderness. Paravertebral muscles are firm. There is no crepitus.*	
ROM. Observe for full active ROM. Ask the patient to stand and bend forward to 75 to 90 degrees and lean backward to 30 degrees (Fig. 16-16). Include lateral flexion (abduction) to 35 degrees on either side. Ask the patient to slide a hand on one side down the thigh and bend away from the midline toward the side. Do this on both sides. To perform rotation of the spine, ask the patient to keep legs and hips forward facing while the shoulders move turn to the side (30 degrees). Repeat to the other side. *The patient performs full ROM without crepitus or discomfort.*	Pain, back injury, *osteoarthritis*, and *ankylosing spondylitis* may result in limited ROM.

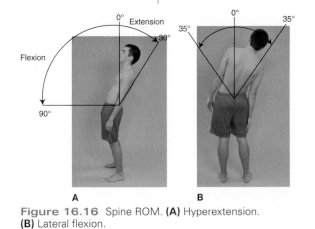

Figure 16.16 Spine ROM. **(A)** Hyperextension. **(B)** Lateral flexion.

Documentation of Normal Subjective and Objective Findings

The patient denies discomfort, weakness, or stiffness and reports no musculoskeletal difficulties with work, hobbies, or ADLs. When standing, trunk and head are erect with weight distributed equally on both feet. Head is midline and aligned with spine. Shoulders, hips, scapulae, and iliac crests are level. Feet are under the hips and knees. Toes and knees point forward. Extremities are symmetrical and in proportion to the body. Arm span is equal to height. When sitting, both feet are flat on the floor with toes pointed forward. Head and trunk are perpendicular to the floor. Walking is smooth and rhythmic with the patient erect. Arms swing freely at the sides and in the opposite direction of the moving legs. The patient transfers from standing to sitting and sitting to standing with ease. Muscles are well formed, firm to touch, and symmetrical.

TMJ: Symmetrical bilaterally. Muscles smooth with strength of 5/5. TMJ moves smoothly through all ROM without pain. A slight popping sound is heard when the jaw is widely opened. Teeth align correctly.

Cervical Spine: From behind, neck is straight and holds the head in alignment with the spine. From the side, neck is slightly concave. Muscle size is symmetrical bilaterally. Neck has full ROM and moves smoothly and painlessly. Muscle strength is 5/5. The patient denies tenderness on palpation. C7 and T1 spinous processes are prominent and palpable. Muscles are fully developed. No nodules, swelling, crepitus, or muscle spasms are noted.

Shoulders: Equal height and equidistant from spinal column. Muscle size is symmetrical bilaterally. Both have full ROM and move smoothly and painlessly. Muscle strength is 5/5. The patient denies tenderness during palpation. No nodules, swelling, crepitus, or muscle spasms are noted.

Elbows: Equal in size and shape. Muscle size is symmetrical bilaterally. Both have full ROM and move smoothly and painlessly. Muscle strength is 5/5. The patient denies tenderness during palpation. No nodules, swelling, crepitus, or muscle spasms are noted.

Hip: Muscles are well formed, firm to touch, and symmetrical. Joints have full active ROM through flexion, extension, hyperextension, abduction, adduction, circumduction, and internal and external rotation. Muscle strength is 5/5. The patient denies discomfort while still or moving.

Knees: Aligned with the long axis of the leg. Muscles well formed, firm to touch, and symmetrical. Joints have full active ROM through flexion and extension. No bulging or swelling. Muscle strength is 5/5. The patient denies any discomfort while still or moving.

Ankles and Feet: Symmetrical and same color as the rest of the body. Muscles are well formed, firm to touch, and symmetrical. Ankles have full active ROM through dorsiflexion, plantar flexion, inversion, and eversion. Toes abduct, flex, and extend. Muscle strength is 5/5. The patient denies any discomfort while sitting, standing, or walking.

Spine: Muscles are well formed, firm to touch, and symmetrical. Spinous processes are straight and nontender. Thoracic and lumbar spines have full active ROM through flexion, extension, hyperextension, lateral flexion (or abduction), and rotation. Muscle strength is 5/5. The patient denies discomfort while still or moving.

▲ Lifespan Considerations

Pregnant Women

Pregnant women have increased joint mobility from progesterone and relaxin. Increased mobility in the sacroiliac, sacrococcygeal, and symphysis pubis joints contributes to changes in posture. *Lordosis* (increased lumbar curvature) compensates for the enlarging uterus, shifting weight to the lower extremities and causing lower back strain. Anterior neck flexion and shoulder slumping compensate for lordosis. Upper back changes may put pressure on the ulnar and median nerves during the third trimester, leading to aching, numbness, and upper-extremity weakness in some pregnant women.

Newborns, Infants, and Children

At birth, newborns are assessed for congenital hip dislocation. The examiner performs either a Barlow-Ortolani maneuver or a test for Allis' sign. See Chapter 22 for more information. Examiners assess newborn muscle tone by observing flexion of the arms and legs and by holding the infant under the arms. With good muscle strength, the shoulders support the weight of the infant. Infants with poor muscle tone slide through the examiner's hands.

The spinal column undergoes changes in contour as the child becomes more active. At birth the spine has a C-shaped curve.

The cervical curve develops by age 3 to 4 months as the child begins raising the head. The lumbar curve develops when the child stands, usually between 12 and 18 months.

Bones grow through infancy and childhood by depositing new bone around the shaft to increase width. They elongate by increasing cartilage at epiphyses (growth plates) at the ends of long bones. The cartilage later calcifies. This lengthening continues until approximately 21 years, when the epiphyses close. Any injury to the epiphyses before closure may result in bone deformity.

All muscle fibers are present at birth, but lengthen throughout childhood. During the adolescent growth spurt, muscle fibers grow following increased secretion of growth hormone, adrenal androgens, and, in boys, testosterone. Muscles vary in size and strength because of genetic factors, nutrition, and exercise. Throughout life, muscles strengthen with use and atrophy with disuse. Weight lifting can cause enlarged muscles, called hypertrophy.

Older Adults

Examiners should allow extra time for older adults to complete each activity. They may divide the assessment into portions if an older patient appears fatigued.

With aging, bone resorption occurs more rapidly than deposition, termed *osteoporosis*. Osteoporosis is most evident in women with small bone frames. Bone mass is related to race, heredity, hormonal factors, physical activity, and calcium intake. Smoking, calcium deficiency, high salt intake, alcohol intake, and physical inactivity increase bone loss.

Postural changes and decreased height occur. Loss of water content in the intervertebral discs contributes to height loss from 40 to 60 years. Shortening after 60 years results from osteoporosis, which compresses the vertebrae.

Joints become less flexible because of changes in cartilage. Tendons and ligaments shrink and harden, decreasing ROM. Muscle mass also decreases as a result of atrophy and loss in size. This involuntary loss of muscle function increases the risk of falls and disability in older adults. Exercise training and adequate nutrition are successful in improving muscle mass and strength.

Subcutaneous fat distribution changes with aging. Men and women usually gain weight after 40 years, predominantly in the abdomen and hips. After 80 years, subcutaneous fat continues to decrease, causing bony prominences to be more obvious.

Cultural Considerations

Curvature of the long bones results from both ethnicity and body weight. African Americans have straight femurs, while Native Americans have anteriorly curved femurs. The femoral curve in Caucasians is intermediate. Thin people of all cultures have less curvature than obese people. Caucasians, Mexican Americans, and African Americans have no difference in metabolism of vitamin D; however, conversion of active metabolites by sunlight is less efficient in African Americans.

Common Nursing Diagnoses and Interventions Associated with the Musculoskeletal System

Diagnosis and Related Factors	Nursing Interventions
Impaired physical mobility (differentiate from impaired bed and wheelchair mobility)	Use footwear that facilitates walking and prevents injury. Use assistive devices. Screen for mobility skills (eg, transitions to sitting or standing).
Activity intolerance	Determine cause of intolerance. Promote reconditioning. Gradually increase activity according to symptoms.
Self-care deficit: specify bathing/ hygiene, dressing/ grooming, feeding, and toileting	Observe the patient's ability to perform skill. Ask for input on habits and preferences. Encourage the patient to do as much independently as possible. Use adaptive devices such as Velcro or elastic versus buttons or ties.
Impaired walking	Follow weight-bearing restrictions.* Use assistive devices such as a cane or walker. Obtain appropriate number of people to assist with walking the patient. Limit distractions during ambulation.

*Collaborative interventions.

Tables of Reference

Table 16.1 Musculoskeletal Problems: Onset, Gender, and Ethnicity

Amyotrophic lateral sclerosis	**Age at Onset:** Median age 55–66 years **Gender:** More common in men **Ethnicity:** Most common in Caucasians
Ankylosing spondylitis	**Age at Onset:** Women 17–35 years; men 20–30 years **Gender:** Three times more common in men **Ethnicity:** Common in Native Americans
Bursitis	**Age at Onset:** Older than 40 years **Gender:** Occurs in men and women, related to chronic stress or acute injury
Carpal tunnel syndrome	**Age at Onset:** 25–50 years **Gender:** Three times more common in women; especially prevalent in pregnant and menopausal women **Ethnicity:** Most common in Caucasians
Dupuytren's contracture	**Age at Onset:** After 40 years **Gender:** More common in men **Ethnicity:** Most common in Caucasians of north European ancestry
Gout	**Age at Onset:** Older than 70 years **Gender:** Three times more common in men **Ethnicity:** Slightly more common in African Americans
Low back pain	**Age at Onset:** 30–50 years **Gender:** More common in men **Ethnicity:** Affects all ethnicities

Multiple sclerosis

Age at Onset: Average age 18–35 years but can occur at any age
Gender: Twice as common in women
Ethnicity: Most common in Caucasians, but the more aggressive form occurs more frequently in African Americans

Multiple myeloma

Age at Onset: Older than 50 years
Gender: More common in men
Ethnicity: Two to four times more common in African Americans

Myasthenia gravis

Age at Onset: Women 18–25 years; men older than 60 years
Gender: Twice as common in women
Ethnicity: Occurs in all ethnicities

Osteoarthritis

Age at Onset: Older than 50 years in women; 40–50 years in men
Gender: More common in women, although hip osteoarthritis is similar
Ethnicity: Most common in Caucasians

Osteoporosis types I and II

Age at Onset: Postmenopausal women; 50–70 years in men
Gender: Type I more common in women
Ethnicity: Type I most common in Caucasians

Osteosarcoma

Age at Onset: Younger than 20 years and also 50–60 years
Gender: Slightly more common in men
Ethnicity: Slightly more common in African Americans

(table continues on page 336)

Paget's disease
Age at Onset: Older than 40 years
Gender: More common in men
Ethnicity: Most common in Caucasians

Polymyalgia rheumatica
Age at Onset: Over 50 years
Gender: More common in women
Ethnicity: Most common in Caucasians

Rheumatoid arthritis
Age at Onset: 20–40 years
Gender: Two to three times more common in women
Ethnicity: Most common in North American Indians

Scleroderma
Age at Onset: 30–50 years
Gender: Two to eight times more common in women
Ethnicity: Most common in Choctaw Indians, followed by African, Hispanic, Caucasian, and then Japanese Americans

Scoliosis
Age at Onset: 10–15 years
Gender: Eight times more common in girls
Ethnicity: Found in all ethnicities

SLE
Age at Onset: 20–30 years
Gender: Ten times more common in women
Ethnicity: Most common in non-Caucasians

Table 16.2 Abnormal Gait Patterns

Gait and Description	Associated Pathological Condition
Antalgic: The patient walks with a limp to avoid pain. The gait is characterized by a very short stance phase.	Degenerative knee or hip disease
Ataxic: The patient shows unsteady, uncoordinated walking with a wide base, feet thrown out, and a tendency to fall to one side.	Cerebellar lesion
Short leg: The patient limps with walking unless he or she wears adaptive shoes.	Discrepancy in length of one leg, flexion contracture of hip or knee, congenital hip dislocation
Footdrop or Steppage: The patient lifts the advancing leg high so that the toes may clear the ground and places the sole on the floor at one time, instead of placing the heel first. This problem may be unilateral or bilateral.	Peroneal or anterior tibial nerve injury, paralysis of dorsiflexor muscles, lower motor neuron damage, damage to spinal nerve roots L5 and S1
Apraxic: The patient has difficulty initiating walking. After starting, gait is slow and shuffling. Motor and sensory systems are intact.	Frontal lobe tumors, Alzheimer's disease
Trendelenburg: The trunk lists toward the affected side when weight bearing is on that side. A waddling gait may develop if both hips are affected.	Developmental hip dysplasia, muscular dystrophy

Other gait abnormalities are described in Chapter 17.

Table 16.3   Rating Scale for Muscle Strength

5/5 (100%)	Normal	Complete ROM against gravity and full resistance
4/5 (75%)	Good	Complete ROM against gravity and moderate resistance
3/5 (50%)	Fair	Complete ROM against gravity
2/5 (25%)	Poor	Complete ROM with the joint supported; cannot perform ROM against gravity
1/5 (10%)	Trace	Muscle contraction detectable, but no movement of the joint
0/5 (0%)	Zero	No visible muscle contraction

Muscle strength can be described on a 0–5 scale, with 5 being the strongest, as percentage or by words.

Table 16.4   Common Musculoskeletal Conditions

Rheumatoid Arthritis

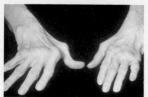

In this chronic, systemic disease, inflammation causes thickening of synovial membrane, fibrosis, and eventual bony ankylosis. Characteristics include bilateral and symmetrical heat, redness, swelling, and painful motion of affected joints. Associated symptoms include fatigue, weakness, anorexia, weight loss, low-grade fever, and lymphadenopathy.

Osteoarthritis

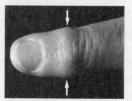

This localized, progressive, noninflammatory disease results in deterioration of articular cartilage and bone and deposition of new bone at joint surfaces, commonly the hands, knees, hips, and lumbar and cervical vertebrae. Manifestations include stiffness, swelling, hard bony protuberances, pain with motion, and limited motion.

Epicondylitis

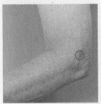

Epicondylitis

With this inflammation of the lateral epicondyle of the elbow, pain radiates down the extensor surface and increases with resisting extension of the hand. It results from activities combining excessive forearm supination with wrist extension.

Polydactyly

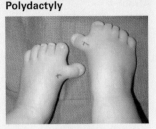

This congenital deformity results in extra fingers, usually at the thumb or fifth finger.

Joint Dislocation

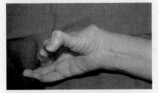

The ends of bones slip out of the usual position, usually from a sports-related injury, trauma, or a fall. Manifestations include swelling, pain, and immobility of the affected joint.

Carpal Tunnel Syndrome

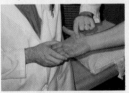

Carpal tunnel syndrome occurs from repetitive motion. Symptoms include burning, pain, and numbness from compression of the median nerve inside the carpal tunnel of the wrist. Atrophy of the thenar eminence at the base of the thumb is common.

(table continues on page 340)

Atrophy

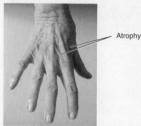

Atrophy

Hand of an 84-year-old woman

Decreased size can occur in any muscle. Causes include nerve damage, disuse, and nerve or muscle damage.

Ulnar Deviation

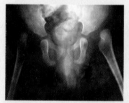

Stretching of the articular capsule and muscle imbalance in rheumatoid arthritis cause fingers to point in the ulnar direction.

Rotator Cuff Tear

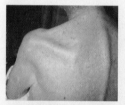

Manifestations include a hunched shoulder and limited arm abduction. A positive drop arm test (arm is passively abducted, person cannot maintain position, and arm falls to side) is diagnostic. This condition may result from trauma while arm is abducted, falling on shoulder, throwing, or heavy lifting.

Congenital Hip Dislocation

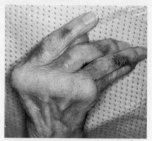

The head of the femur is displaced from the acetabulum. Signs include asymmetric gluteal creases, uneven limb length, and limited abduction of flexed thigh. Diagnosis for newborns is a positive Barlow-Ortolani sign. Older children will have a positive Trendelenburg's sign.

Syndactyly

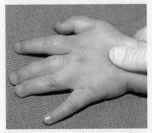

In this congenital deformity of webbed fingers, the metacarpals and phalanges are unequal in length and the joints do not align, which limits flexion and extension. Toes may also be webbed.

Heberden's and Bouchard's Nodes

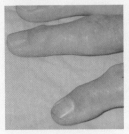

Hard, nontender bony growths on the distal (Heberden's) and proximal (Bouchard's) intraphalangeal joints. Frequently occurs with deviation of the fingers.

Joint Effusions

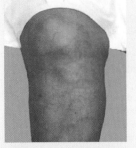

Inflammatory processes from trauma, joint overuse, and rheumatoid arthritis can cause synovial fluid to accumulate in a joint, which can eventually cause the joint to appear swollen.

Osteoporosis

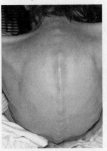

Osteoporosis occurs when bone resorption is faster than deposition. The weakened bone increases risk for fractures, especially in vertebrae, wrist, and hip.

(table continues on page 342)

Acute Rheumatoid Arthritis

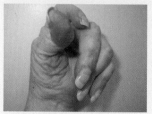

Inflammation results in painful, reddened, swollen joints, and limited function. The condition is common in proximal intraphalangeal joints.

Ganglion Cyst

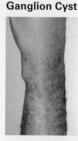

A soft, nontender, round nodule on the dorsum of the wrist that becomes more prominent during flexion. It is a benign tumor.

Bursitis (Olecranon Bursitis)

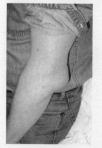

Bursitis (inflammation of bursa) can follow injury, infection, or a rheumatic condition. Shoulders, elbows, and hip are common sites; however, bursitis can occur in any joint. Characteristics include swelling, tenderness, and pain that increase with movement.

Dupuytren's Contracture

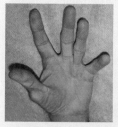

Hyperplasia of the palmar fascia causes painless flexion contracture of the digits, which impairs function. Incidence increases with age, diabetes, epilepsy, family history of Dupuytren's contracture, and alcoholic liver disease.

Genu Valgum ("Knock Knee")

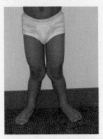

Many children have a temporary period of this condition, but persistent knock knee may be genetic or the result of metabolic bone disease. The patient may need to swing each leg outward while walking to prevent striking the planted limb with the moving limb. The strain on the knee frequently causes anterior and medial knee pain.

Herniated Nucleus Pulposus

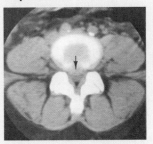

The intervertebral discs may slip out of position following trauma or strain. Rupture of the nucleus pulposus (soft inner portion) may put pressure on the spinal nerve root. Symptoms include sciatic pain radiating down the leg, numbness, parasthesia, listing from the affected side, decreased mobility, low back tenderness, and decreased motor and sensory function in the affected leg.

(table continues on page 344)

Talipes Equinovarus ("Club Foot")

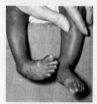

The foot is turned to the side; the involved foot, calf, and leg are smaller and shorter than the normal side. One or both feet may be affected. This condition is not painful; if left untreated, significant discomfort and disability will develop.

Swan Neck and Boutonnière Deformity

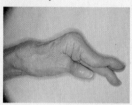

Fingers have a "swan-neck" appearance resulting from flexion contracture of the metacarpophalangeal joint with hyperextension of the distal joint. Boutonnière deformity causes flexion of the proximal interphalangeal joint with hyperextension of the distal joint. Both conditions occur with chronic rheumatoid arthritis.

Ankylosing Spondylitis

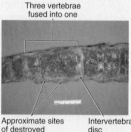

Three vertebrae fused into one

Approximate sites of destroyed intervertebral discs

Intervertebral disc

This chronic, progressive inflammation of the spine and sacroiliac and large joints in the extremities affects men 10 times more than women. It is characterized by bony growths. Muscle spasms pull the spine forward and eliminate the cervical and lumbar curves.

Table 16.5 Abnormalities of the Ankles and Feet

Problem	Signs, Symptoms, Findings
Gouty arthritis	Enlarged, swollen, hot, red metatarsophalangeal joint and bursa of the great toe
Ankle sprain or strain	Pain on palpation and ROM
Fracture	Crepitus
Hallux valgus (bunion)	Great toe that angles away from midline
Hammertoe	Flexion of the proximal interphalangeal joint with hyperextension of the distal joint
Flatfoot (pes planus)	Flattened arch of the foot that touches the floor; may only be visible when the person is standing
Pes varus	Foot that is turned inward toward the midline
Pes valgus	Foot turned outward from the midline
Pes cavus	Exaggerated arch height
Corn	Conical area of thickened skin from pressure; may be painful and can occur between toes
Callus	Thickened skin from pressure; usually occurs on the sole of the foot and is usually not painful
Plantar fasciitis	Pain in the heel early in the morning or with prolonged sitting, standing, or walking; inflammation of the plantar fascia where it attaches to the calcaneus
Talipes equinovarus (club foot)	Inward turning foot

17

Neurological Assessment

Subjective Data Collection

Key Topics and Questions for Health Promotion

Key Questions	Rationales
Obtain from the chart the patient's age, heredity, gender, date and result of last blood pressure reading, and date and result of last cholesterol level.	Increased age, male gender, and family history of stroke increase risk for *stroke*. African Americans are at increased risk for death from stroke.
Have you ever been diagnosed with a neurological problem (eg, seizure)? • When? How often? • Seizure history? • How was the seizure treated? • Was the treatment effective?	Various scales have been developed to identify *seizure* severity.
Have you ever had a head injury? • When? • How was it treated? • What were the outcomes?	Suspect *head injury* if there is a witnessed loss of consciousness for more than 5 minutes, history of amnesia of more than 5 minutes, abnormal drowsiness, more than three vomiting episodes, suspicion of nonaccidental injury, or seizure in a patient with no history of epilepsy.
Have you ever had a stroke? • When did you have it? • How was it treated? • What were the outcomes?	Exact time of onset, definite focal symptoms, neurological signs, and ability to lateralize signs to the left or right side of the brain suggest a *stroke*.

Key Questions	Rationales
Have you ever had any infectious or degenerative diseases?	Symptoms of *meningitis* include high fever, stiff neck, drowsiness, and photosensitivity. Symptoms of *degenerative disease* include weakness, tingling or numbness, difficulty seeing, and elimination-control problems.
Have you had health-related changes in your emotional state or coping strategies?	Pay attention to functional health patterns. Relationships and socioeconomic background provide valuable clues to support systems and independence.
Do you have high blood pressure? • When was it diagnosed? • How is it being treated?	Systolic blood pressure above 140, diastolic blood pressure above or equal to 90, or both are a risk factor for *stroke*.
Do you have diabetes mellitus, coronary artery disease, atrial fibrillation, or sickle cell disease?	These conditions increase risk for stroke.
Which of the following place you at risk for neurovascular disease: smoking, high-fat diet, obesity, inactivity?	Risk factors for *stroke* are the same as for cardiovascular disease (see Chapter 12).

Health-Promotion Teaching

Stroke Prevention. Patients should control blood pressure through weight reduction, healthy diet, and use of prescribed antihypertensive medications. At every visit, ask patients about smoking and, for those with a positive response, about the desire for cessation. Provide all patients with information about a diet low in saturated fat and high in fruits and vegetables. Ask overweight and obese patients about willingness to reduce calories. Also, advise all patients to exercise aerobically three to seven times a week for 20 to 60 minutes per session.

Injury Prevention. Provide information about prevention of traumatic injury. Recommend use of protective helmets and gear to patients who engage in sports involving physical contact. During assessment of driving, advise patients about the importance of seat belts; discourage use of alcohol and drugs. Provide teaching materials to reinforce concepts, especially for adolescents and young adults.

Key Topics and Questions for Common Symptoms

History of present illness or problem should elucidate a detailed account of each symptom, its nature (location, quality, and severity), date of onset, precipitating factors, and duration. Note what, if anything, makes the symptom worse or better and the general pattern of progression.

During neurological assessment, inquire about common symptoms in all patients to screen for the early presence of disease. If a patient is concerned about specific neurological problems, assess these focused areas with follow-up questions.

Common Neurological Symptoms

- Headache or other pain (see Chapter 7)
- Weakness of single limb or one side of body
- Generalized weakness
- Involuntary movements or tremors
- Difficulty with balance, coordination, or gait
- Dizziness or vertigo
- Difficulty swallowing
- Change in intellectual abilities
- Difficulties with expression or comprehension of speech/ language
- Alteration in touch, taste, or smell
- Loss or blurring of vision in one or both eyes, diplopia (double vision)
- Hearing loss or tinnitus (ringing in the ears)

Questions to Assess Symptoms	Rationales/Abnormal Findings
Limb/Unilateral Weakness. Do you have weakness on one side or in one limb? • How long does it last? • Is there a speech problem?	Unilateral weakness, disturbed speech, and symptoms longer than 10 minutes increase risk of *stroke*.

Questions to Assess Symptoms	Rationales/Abnormal Findings

Generalized Weakness. Do you have generalized weakness?
- Is it mostly in the hands and feet or core muscles?
- Do repetitive actions lead to weakness?
- Are there associated symptoms such as rash or joint inflammation?

Neuropathy primarily occurs in distal muscles. Rash is a sign of *lupus*. Repetitive actions exacerbate *myasthenia gravis.* Common neurological causes include *demyelinating disorders, amyotrophic lateral sclerosis, Guillain-Barré syndrome, multiple sclerosis, myasthenia gravis,* and *degenerative disc disease.*

See Tables 17-1 and 17-2 at the end of this chapter.

Involuntary Movements/ Tremors. Have you noted any shaking or tremors? Do they occur at rest? With movement? While maintaining a fixed position?

Balance/Coordination Problems. Do you have difficulty with balance, coordination, or walking?

Multiple sclerosis, Parkinson's disease, stroke, and *cerebral palsy* are neurological causes of impaired gait. See Table 17-3.

Dizziness or Vertigo. Have you had periods of dizziness?
- Can you describe what it feels like without using the word dizziness?
- Is there nausea and vomiting?
- Does changing positions make it better or worse?

Common causes include *multiple sclerosis, Parkinson's disease, cerebellar ischemia or infarction, benign or malignant neoplasms,* and *arterial-venous malformation of blood vessels in the brain.* Position changes usually worsen dizziness associated with the inner ear.

Difficulty Swallowing. Have you had difficulty swallowing? Are any foods or liquids especially difficult to swallow?

Dysphagia, associated with cranial nerve dysfunction, is a common symptom of *stroke* or *neuromuscular disease.*

Intellectual Changes. Have you had difficulty with concentration, memory, or attention?

Common causes of memory loss are *stroke, dementia, Alzheimer's disease, depression, some medications,* and *metabolic imbalances.*

Speech/Language Difficulty. Do you notice any difficulty with expression or comprehension?
- Difficulty understanding speech?
- Difficulty forming words?
- Difficulty finding words and putting sentences together?

Aphasia is a common symptom of *stroke,* especially when it affects the speech centers in the left hemisphere. Neuromuscular disease also affects the speech center.

(text continues on page 350)

Questions to Assess Symptoms	Rationales/Abnormal Findings
Changes in Taste, Touch, or Smell. Any alterations? Numbness, tingling, or hypersensitivity? Where?	**Paresthesia** (abnormal prickly or tingly sensations) is most common in the hands, arms, legs, and feet. Causes include *neurological disease* or traumatic nerve damage.
Lost or Blurred Vision. Have you had a loss or blurring of vision in one or both eyes, or double vision?	Central causes of **diplopia** include *stroke, vascular malformation, tumor, mass, trauma, meningitis, hemorrhage,* and *muscular sclerosis.*
Hearing Loss or Tinnitus. Have you noticed any hearing loss or tinnitus (ringing in the ears)? • Do you have a history of hearing loss? • Was it a sudden or slow onset? • Is it in one or both ears?	Common causes include noise, *autoimmune disorders, Meniere's disease, ototoxic medications,* and *head trauma.* See Chapter 9 for more information.

Objective Data Collection

Equipment

- Penlight or flashlight
- Tongue blade
- Cotton swab

- Optional: Tuning fork, reflex hammer, supplies for cranial nerve testing

Technique and Normal Findings	Abnormal Findings
Level of Consciousness (LOC) People visibly express LOC through degree of response to stimulus, with the highest level being spontaneous alertness. Apply stimulus in the correct order (Box 17-1). Description of specific response to stimulus provides the best chance of identifying changes that may initially be subtle. *The patient is alert and opens the eyes spontaneously.*	The Glasgow Coma Scale (Box 17-2) has facilitated assessment of patients with impaired consciousness. It determines the degree of conscious impairment by evaluating (1) motor responses, (2) verbal responses, and (3) eye opening. The minimum score is 3; the maximum is 15.

BOX 17.1 ASSESSMENT OF CONSCIOUSNESS: APPLYING STIMULATION

- *Spontaneous*: Enter room and observe arousal.
- *Normal voice*: State the patient's name; ask him or her to open eyes.
- *Loud voice*: Use loud voice if no response to normal voice.
- *Tactile (touch)*: Touch patient's shoulder or arm lightly.
- *Noxious stimulation (pain)*: Apply nail bed pressure to elicit pain response, telling the patient that you will be applying pressure.

Cognitive Function

If the patient can interact, evaluate cognitive function (many components may have been done during history taking). Components are basic

BOX 17.2 GLASGOW COMA SCALE

The GCS is a tool for assessing a patient's response to stimuli. Scores range from 3 (deep coma) to 15 (normal).

Eye opening response	Spontaneous	4
	To voice	3
	To pain	2
	None	1
Best verbal response	Oriented	5
	Confused	4
	Inappropriate words	3
	Incomprehensible sounds	2
	None	1
Best motor response	Obeys command	6
	Localizes pain	5
	Withdraws	4
	Flexion	3
	Extension	2
	None	1
Total		3–15

Source: Teasdale, G. & Jennett, B. (1974). Assessment of coma and impaired consciousness. A practical scale. *Lancet*, *304*, 81–84.

(text continues on page 352)

Technique and Normal Findings	Abnormal Findings
orientation, concentration, attention span, and more complex functions (ie, memory, calculation ability, abstract thinking, reasoning, and judgment).	
Test complex cognitive function informally whenever you interact with the patient, especially when teaching, establishing goals and priorities, and planning for home care. See Chapter 5.	Ask patients about items related to functional ability: telling the time using a clock face and counting change.
Orientation. Directly question the patient about person, place, and time. *The patient is "oriented."*	Asking "What month (year, season) is it?" may be more reasonable than asking "What day is it?" if the patient has been hospitalized. Asking about place through yes or no questions may be necessary for patients with *aphasia*. Regarding person, as well as identifying self, ask the patient to identify visitors or family pictures. Also ask the patient about his or her age.

Communication (Speech/Language)

Observe clarity and fluency of speech through basic conversation. Ask the patient to repeat words or phrases with multiple combinations of consonants and vowels to test articulation. Formal testing includes assessment of comprehension, repetition, naming, reading, and writing (see Chapter 10). *Speech is clear and articulate.*	Deficits in articulation are **dysarthria**. In some cases, distinguishing speech/language deficits from confusion is difficult. Those with speech/language deficits behave appropriately to situation and environment, especially to visual cues. Patients with a language deficit might be unable to express needs but usually follow commands.

Pupillary Response

Basic assessment of pupils includes size, shape, and reactivity to light. See Chapter 8 for techniques.	Causes of *nystagmus* (jerking movement of the eye) include *medications, cerebellar disease, weakness in the extraocular*

Technique and Normal Findings	Abnormal Findings
Test accommodation by having the person shift the gaze from a distant to near object. *PERRLA* (see Chapter 8).	*muscles*, and *damage to cranial nerve III*. See Tables 8-3 in Chapter 8 and Table 17-4 at the end of this chapter.
Assess gaze for eye contact and drifting. If the eyes deviate, assess if it is conjugate or dysconjugate. *Gaze is purposeful and conjugate.*	

Abnormal Movements

Inspect for abnormal movements or posturing. *Movements are smooth and symmetric.*

See Tables 17-1 and 17-2 at the end of this chapter.

Cranial Nerve Testing

Aside from a thorough screening assessment for a suspected problem, it is rarely necessary to assess complete CN function. For selected testing:

See Table 17-5.

• Observe functional near and far vision; assess pupil constriction and extraoculomotor movements (EOMs); assess corneal reflexes if LOC is acutely impaired.
• Observe facial expression, facial strength and sensation, uvula rise with "ah"; test gag reflex and observe tongue movement when assessing for dysphagia. Alertness and attention span are also relevant.

PERRLA, EOMs intact. Positive gag and corneal reflexes. Facial strength 4+ with intact sensation bilaterally.

(text continues on page 354)

Technique and Normal Findings	Abnormal Findings
Motor Function ***Muscle Bulk and Tone.*** Observe and palpate muscle groups to check for any atrophy. *The relaxed muscle shows some muscular tension.* To further assess tone, determine the degree of resistance of muscle groups to passive stretch. Instruct the patient to relax totally and to let the examiner move the limbs. Commonly tested groups include deltoids, biceps, triceps, hamstrings, and quadriceps. *Findings are good muscle bulk and tone.*	See Box 17-3.
Muscle Strength. Assess muscle strength (pyramidal motor system) by asking the patient to move extremities or selected muscle groups both independently and against resistance.	Motor strength of 0 to 3+ indicates weakness.

BOX 17.3 MUSCLE TONE DEFINITIONS

- *Flaccid or atonic*: Absolutely no resistance to movement
- *Hypotonia:* Tone seems only decreased or "flabby"
- *Hypertonia:* Increased resistance of the muscles to passive stretch
- *Spasticity*: Increased resistance to rapid passive stretch, especially in flexor muscle groups in the upper extremities, resulting from hyperexcitability of the stretch reflex
- *Clasp-knife spasticity:* Resistance is strongest on initiation of the movement and "gives way" as the examiner slowly continues the movement. Describes hypertonicity noted in patients with Parkinson's disease.
- *Rigidity*: Steady, persistent resistance to passive stretch in both flexor and extensor muscle groups.
- *Cogwheel rigidity*: Seen in patients with Parkinson's disease and is manifested by a ratchetlike jerking noted in the extremity on passive movement.

Technique and Normal Findings	Abnormal Findings
Evaluate strength by hand grasp, pronator drift, dorsiflexion, and plantar flexion. Grade strength on a scale of 0 to 5+: 0: No muscle contraction 1: Barely detectable, flicker 2: Active movement with gravity eliminated 3: Active movement against gravity 4: Active movement against some resistance 5: Active movement against full resistance *Strength is 4 to 5+.*	
During conversation, observe for ptosis or palsy. Observe for pronator drift. Ask the patient to close the eyes and outstretch the arms straight ahead with palms upward for 10 seconds (Fig. 17-1). *The patient extends the hands for 10 seconds without drifting.*	Pronation of the hands and downward drift of the arm indicate weakness.

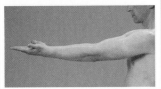

Figure 17.1 Assessing for pronator drift.

If possible, ask the patient to walk down a corridor. Points to observe include smoothness of gait, position of feet, height and length of step, and symmetry of arm and leg movement. Ask the patient to walk on heels and toes, then tandem-walk (ie, heel-to-toe in a straight line) (Fig. 17-2). *The patient walks smoothly without swaying.*	See Table 17-2 at the end of this chapter.

(text continues on page 356)

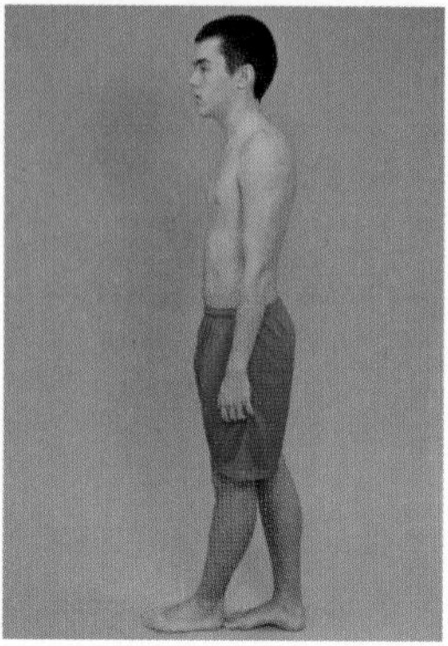

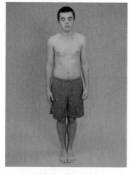

Technique and Normal Findings	Abnormal Findings
Figure 17.2 Assessing the tandem walk to evaluate gait and posture.	
In the **Romberg test,** ask the patient to stand with feet together and arms at sides (Fig. 17-3). Note any swaying. Ask the patient to close the eyes for additional testing. Slight swaying may be normal, because visual cues help humans maintain balance. *The patient can maintain position without opening the eyes.*	Moderate swaying with eyes open and closed indicates *vestibulocerebellar dysfunction.* Pronounced increase in swaying (sometimes with falling) with the eyes closed usually indicates a *lesion in the posterior columns of the spinal cord.*
Figure 17.3 Positioning for the Romberg test.	

Technique and Normal Findings	Abnormal Findings

Cerebellar Function

Ask the patient to touch the tip of the examiner's finger with the tip of his or her forefinger (test each hand separately), then to touch his or her own nose, and to repeat this maneuver several times while the examiner's finger is moved each time (Fig. 17-4).

Ataxia is unsteady, wavering movement with inability to touch the target. During rapid alternating movements, lack of coordination is **adiadochokinesia**. Deficits in any of these maneuvers indicate an *ipsilateral cerebellar lesion*. Note any tremor. See Table 17-1.

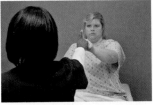
A

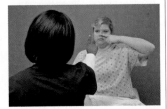
B

Figure 17.4 Assessing cerebellar function. **(A)** The patient touches the examiner's finger with her forefinger. **(B)** The patient touches her own nose.

- To assess rapid alternating movements, instruct the patient to slap his or her thigh with first the palm of the hand and then the back as fast as possible (Fig. 17-5).
- To assess lower extremities, ask the seated or supine patient to take the heel of one foot and, without deviation, move it steadily down the shin of the other leg.

Normal responses are good coordination of movements.

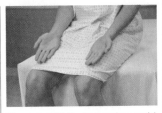

Figure 17.5 Assessing rapid alternating movements.

Sensory Function

It is important for the patient's eyes to be closed to prevent visual cues from influencing responses. Have the patient

This testing includes peripheral nerves, sensory tracts, and cortical perception. Consider the clinical situation and whether the problem is generalized or

(text continues on page 358)

Technique and Normal Findings	Abnormal Findings
identify where he or she feels the sensation. Avoid asking "Do you feel this?" which cues the patient to respond. Allow 2 seconds between each stimulus. Begin with light stimulation; increase pressure until the patient reports a sensation. Stronger stimulation is needed over the central torso and back than on the more sensitive hands. Observe areas of sensory decrease or loss. Compare findings between sides.	specific. *Spinal cord injury* generally follows the pattern of the dermatome, while sensory loss in *diabetic neuropathy* is distal.

Light Touch. Pull the end of a cotton swab so that it is wispy. Ask the patient to close the eyes. Apply light touch to the skin with the swab (Fig. 17-6).

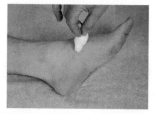

Figure 17.6 Applying a cotton swab to assess light touch sensation.

Ask the patient to state where he or she feels the sensation. *The patient correctly identifies light touch.*

Hyperesthesia refers to increased touch sensation. **Anesthesia** refers to absent touch sensation. Reduced touch sensation is **hypesthesia**.

Superficial Pain Sensation. Break a tongue blade or cotton swab so that the end is sharp. Ask the patient to close the eyes; lightly touch the patient's skin with the sharp end. Ask the patient to state where he or she feels the sensation. *Pain sensation is intact.*

Hyperalgesia refers to increased pain sensation. **Analgesia** refers to absent pain sensation. Reduced pain sensation is **hypalgesia**.

Technique and Normal Findings	Abnormal Findings
Temperature Sensation. Test temperature sense only if pain or touch is abnormal. Use one prong of a tuning fork that has been warmed with the hands or test tubes containing warm and cold water. Ask the patient to close the eyes. Touch the skin with warm or cold objects. Have the patient identify when he or she feels warm or cold. *Temperature sensation is intact.*	Abnormal temperature sensation is common in *neuropathies.*
Point Localization. Ask the patient to close the eyes. Using a finger, gently touch the patient's hands, lower arms, abdomen, lower legs, and feet. Have the patient identify where he or she feels the sensation. Don't cue the patient by asking, "Do you feel this?" Observe areas of sensory loss. Compare side to side. *Point localization is intact.*	Observe the pattern of sensory loss. "Stocking-glove" distribution suggests peripheral nerves; dermatomal distribution suggests isolated nerves or nerve roots; reduced sensation below a certain level is associated with the spinal cord. A crossed face-body pattern suggests the brainstem, and hemisensory loss suggests a stroke.
Vibration Sensation. Strike a low-pitched tuning fork on the side or heel of the hand. Ask the patient to close the eyes. Hold the fork at the base; place it over body prominences, beginning at the most distal location (Fig. 17-7). If the sensation is felt at the most distal point, no further testing is necessary. Ask the patient to state where the sensation is felt and when it disappears. To stop, dampen the tuning fork by pressing on the tongs. *Vibration sense is intact.*	*Peripheral neuropathy* is more severe distally and improves centrally and is a consequence of *peripheral vascular disease* and *diabetic neuropathy.* Often, vibration sense is the first lost. With damage to a specific dermatome, the line of sensory loss is usually marked and specific.

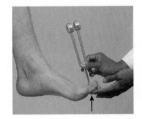

Figure 17.7 Testing vibration sensation.

(text continues on page 360)

Technique and Normal Findings	Abnormal Findings
Motion and Position Sense. Ask the patient to close the eyes. Move the distal joints of the patient's fingers and then the toes up or down. If the patient cannot identify these movements, test the next most proximal joints. *Motion and position sense are intact.*	Involuntary writhing, snakelike movements of a limb (athetosis) result from loss of position sense.
Stereognosis. Ask the patient to close the eyes and identify a familiar object (eg, coin, key) placed in the palm (*stereognosis*) (Fig. 17-8). *The patient correctly identifies the object.*	Inability to identify objects correctly (**astereognosis**) may result from damage to the sensory cortex caused by *stroke*.

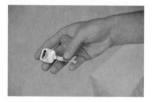

Figure 17.8 Testing stereognosis.

Graphesthesia. Use a blunt object to trace a number (eg, "8") on the patient's palm. Ask the patient to identify the traced number (*graphesthesia*) (Fig. 17-9). *The patient correctly identifies the number.*	Cortical sensory function may be compromised following a *stroke*.

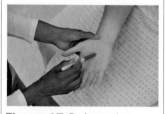

Figure 17.9 Assessing graphesthesia.

Technique and Normal Findings	Abnormal Findings
Two-point Discrimination. Ask the patient to close the eyes. Hold the blunt end of two cotton swabs 2 inches apart and move them together until the patient feels them as one point. The fingertips are most sensitive, with a minimal distance of 3 to 8 mm, while the upper arms and thighs are least sensitive, with a minimal distance of 75 mm. *There is more discrimination distally than centrally.*	Cortical sensory function may be lost with a *stroke*.
Extinction. Ask the patient to close the eyes. At the same time, touch a body area on both sides. Ask the patient to state where he or she perceives the touch. *Sensations are felt on both sides.*	Cortical sensory function may be lost with a *stroke*.

Reflex Testing

Deep Tendon Reflexes (DTRs). DTRs tested include biceps, triceps, brachioradialis, patellar, and Achilles (Table 17-6). These reflexes are observed for symmetry when tested bilaterally and for briskness of movement. DTRs are graded as follows:

- 4+ Very brisk, hyperactive with clonus
- 3+ Brisker than average
- 2+ Average, normal
- 1+ Diminished, low normal
- 0 No response

Reflex response depends on the force of the stimulus, accurate location of the striking area over the tendon, and the patient's relaxation level. To ensure accuracy, have the patient flex the muscle to find the tendon and then relax it for testing. *DTRs are 2+ bilaterally without clonus.*

Pathologic reflexes are primitive responses and indicate loss of cortical inhibition (see Table 17-7). **Clonus** is characterized by alternating flexion/extension movements (jerking) in response to a continuous muscle stretch. In unconscious patients, DTRs may be tested in the usual manner; however, depth of coma alters the response. Deep coma is associated with loss of all reflexes, as well as loss of muscle stretch and tone.

(text continues on page 362)

Technique and Normal Findings	Abnormal Findings
Superficial Reflexes. Elicit superficial reflexes by stimulation of the skin. Record the response to stimulation as present, absent, or equivocal.	
Plantar Response. Stroke the sole of the foot with a blunt instrument (eg, edge of a tongue blade). Apply the stimulus firmly but gently to the lateral aspect, beginning at the heel and stopping short of the base of the toes. *The toes flex (a flexor-plantar response).*	With abnormal plantar reflexes, the great toe extends upward and the other toes fan out (*Babinski's sign*) (Fig. 17-10). *Triple flexion* describes reflex withdrawal of the lower extremity to plantar stimulus through flexion of ankle, knee, and hip.

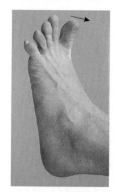

Figure 17.10 Babinski's sign.

Upper Abdominal. To identify the integrity of T8 to T10, stroke the upper quadrants of the abdomen with a tongue blade or reflex hammer. *The umbilicus moves toward each area of stimulation symmetrically.*	Depression or absence of this reflex may result from a *central lesion*, *obesity*, lax skeletal muscles, or *spinal cord injury*.
Lower Abdominal. To identify the integrity of T10 to T12, stroke the upper abdominal quadrants with a tongue blade or reflex hammer. *The umbilicus moves toward each area of stimulation symmetrically.*	Abnormal findings are the same as for the upper abdominal region.

Technique and Normal Findings	Abnormal Findings
Cremasteric (Male). To identify the integrity of L1 to L2 in male patients, stroke the inner thigh. *The testicle and scrotum rise on the stroked side.*	Response is diminished or absent.
Bulbocavernous (Male). To identify the integrity of S3 to S4 in male patients, apply direct pressure over the bulbocavernous muscle behind the scrotum. *The muscle should contract and elevate the scrotum.*	Response is diminished or absent.
Perianal. To identify the integrity of S3 to S5, scratch the tissue at the side of the anus with a blunt instrument. *The anus should pucker.*	Response is diminished or absent.
Carotid Arteries Auscultation over the carotid artery may elicit a bruit. Refer to Chapter 12 for technique. *No bruit is heard.*	A bruit is associated with an increased risk of *stroke*.

Documentation of Normal Subjective and Objective Findings

The patient is without headache, weakness, and tremors; has no difficulty with balance, coordination, or gait. Denies dizziness, vertigo, dysphagia, and intellectual changes; denies difficulty with concentration, memory, attention span, and expression or comprehension of speech/language; no alteration in sense of touch, taste, or smell. No loss, blurred vision, or diplopia; no hearing loss, tinnitus, altered sensation, numbness, or paresthesia. Well-groomed and relaxed; good eye contact. A&O X3; good attention span and judgment. Speech clear and appropriate. Immediate and recent memory intact. Cranial nerves II to XII grossly intact. PERRLA with L5 → 3 and R5 → 3; EOMs intact without ptosis or nystagmus. Can correctly identify light touch on face, arms, and legs; strength 5+ bilaterally. Gait smooth and coordinated; no tremors.

▲ Lifespan Considerations ─────────────────

Newborns, Infants, and Children

The neurological system develops dramatically during the first 2 to 3 years. At birth, newborns have protective reflexes including sucking and swallowing. Depressed or hyperactive reflexes may indicate a disorder of the CNS. Refer to Chapter 22 for more information. Spontaneous motor activity is noticeable, especially during crying. Transient tremors are normal and should disappear by 1 month of age. Muscle tone and strength are usually related. Depressed LOC may result from maternal sedation and should be differentiated from hypoglycemia or CNS disorders.

Variations in consciousness for infants are called *sleep-wake states* and range from deep sleep to extreme irritability. Infants use purposeful behavior to maintain the optimal arousal state by withdrawing, fussing, and crying. A weak or high-pitched cry may indicate CNS abnormality.

Persistent tremors, increased tonicity or spasticity, or twitching of the facial muscles may indicate seizures and should be evaluated. Birth trauma may cause nerve damage that results in asymmetry or paralysis.

Myelination, incomplete at birth, develops from head to toe and centrally to peripherally. It is nearly complete by 2 years, as manifested by children's ability to walk unassisted and to move purposefully in space. By the end of the first year, all brain cells are present; however, they continue to increase in size. Various brain areas develop as children gain intellectual capacity. Postural control continues to develop as the functions are integrated.

Children and Adolescents

Cognitive abilities and speech articulation develop during preschool and early childhood. Fine and coarse motor skills follow developmental milestones. Expected motor function by 2 to 3 years includes grasping, sitting, crawling, standing, and walking. Further investigation is warranted with reduced amount of rotation during crawling, delayed balance, and delayed onset and poor quality of early walking behavior. See Chapter 22 for more information.

School-age children are steadier on their feet than preschoolers, more coordinated, and have better posture that enables them to climb, ride bikes, and play games. Head circumference is decreased in relation to height. The skull and brain grow very slowly during this period; most of the growth has been completed. Adolescence is a period of cognitive growth and completion of myelinization of nerve fibers.

Older Adults

Normal changes in neurological function accompany aging. Examples include lost nerve cell mass, atrophy in the CNS, decreased brain weight, and fewer nerve cells and dendrites. Such changes lead to slower thought, memory, and thinking; however, plasticity enables the lengthening and production of dendrites to accommodate for this loss. Demyelinization of nerve fibers leads to delayed impulse transmission. An increased latency period (period before next stimulation) causes slowed reflexes, which may produce mobility and safety issues. Fewer cells are in the spinal cord, although this does not appear to reduce function. Peripheral nerve conduction slows. Therefore, assessment techniques, interpretation of findings, and linked interventions may require adjustments as appropriate. Refer to Chapter 23 for more information.

Common Nursing Diagnoses and Intervention Associated with the Neurological System

Diagnosis and Related Factors	Nursing Interventions
Impaired verbal communication related to aphasia	Observe behavioral cues for needs. Maintain eye contact. Ask yes and no questions. Anticipate patient's needs. Use touch as appropriate.
Acute confusion related to stroke	Perform mental status examination. Provide environmental cues (eg, large clock and calendar). Orient to time, place, and person frequently.
Impaired memory related to dementia and stroke	Encourage patient to use a calendar, keep reminder lists, set alarm watches, and make signs for room number or bathroom.

(table continues on page 366)

Diagnosis and Related Factors	Nursing Interventions
Unilateral neglect related to left-sided muscle weakness	Provide safe, well-lit, and clutter-free environment. Set up environment so that most activity is on unaffected side. Encourage patient to compensate for neglect.
Risk for aspiration related to muscle weakness and impaired swallowing	Auscultate lungs before and after feeding. Request swallowing evaluation by speech therapy. Elevate head of bed when eating.
Risk for intracranial adaptive capacity related to potential increased intracranial pressure	Keep head and neck in midline. Avoid suctioning. Reduce environmental stimuli. Adjust sedation. *Provide adequate oxygen.
Ineffective brain tissue perfusion related to stroke	Monitor neurological status using neurological flow sheet. Notify physician for changes in condition. Prevent injury.

*Collaborative interventions.

Tables of Reference

⚠ Table 17.1 Abnormal Postures

Posture	Description
Abnormal Extension	Very stiff, spastic movements may persist after noxious stimulation. Upper extremities are extended, adducted, and internally rotated; palms are pronated. Lower extremities are extended, back is hyperextended, and there is plantar flexion. It occurs with damage to the midbrain or upper pons; it is more serious than abnormal flexion, because the patient is posturing toward rather than away from a noxious stimulus.
Abnormal Flexion	With damage to the cerebral cortex, very stiff, spastic movements may persist after noxious stimulation. Upper extremities are flexed and arms are adducted. Lower extremities are extended, internally rotated with plantar flexion.
Hemiplegia	With stroke, sensation and motor strength are lost unilaterally.
Flexion Withdrawal	Gross movements of all body parts are away from the noxious stimulus. Rather than localizing pain to one side, the patient may withdraw both arms when nail bed pressure is applied.
Flaccid Quadriplegia	With a nonfunctional brainstem, sensation and muscle tone are completely lost.

Picture	Description
Paralysis 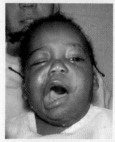	Loss of motor function resulting in flaccidity over the area of damage; may be total, one-sided (hemiplegia), in all four extremities (quadriplegia), or in only the legs (paraplegia) *Common Associations:* Stroke, spinal cord injury, chronic neuromuscular diseases, Bell's palsy
Resting Tremor 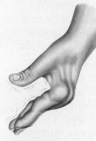	Prominent at rest, may decrease or disappear with voluntary movement *Common Association:* Parkinson's disease
Intention Tremor	Absent at rest; increase with movement; may worsen as movement progresses *Common Associations:* Multiple sclerosis with damage to the cerebellar pathways, or essential tremor

Picture	Description
Tic 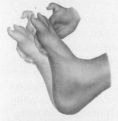	Brief, repetitive, similar but irregular movements, such as blinking or shrugging shoulders *Common Associations:* Tourette's syndrome, use of psychiatric medications, and use of amphetamines
Clonus/Myoclonus 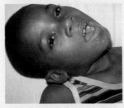	Rapid, sudden clonic spasm of a muscle that may occur regularly or intermittently *Common Associations:* Seizures, hiccups, or just prior to falling asleep
Dystonia 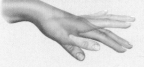	Slow involuntary twisting movements that often involve the trunk and larger muscles; may be accompanied by twisted postures *Common Associations:* Use of psychiatric medications
Choreiform Movements	Brief, rapid, jerky movements that are irregular and unpredictable; commonly affect the face, head, lower arms, and hands *Common Association:* Huntington's disease

(table continues on page 370)

Table 17.2 Abnormalities of Movements (*continued*)

Picture	Description
Athetoid Movements 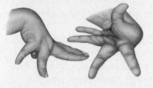	Slow involuntary wormlike twisting movements that involve the extremities, neck, facial muscles, and tongue; may be associated with drooling and dysarthria *Common Association:* Cerebral palsy

Table 17.3 Abnormal Gaits

Picture	Description
Spastic Hemiparesis 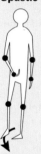	One side is normal. The other side is flexed from spasticity. The elbow, wrist, and fingers are flexed; the arm is close to the side. The affected leg is extended with plantar flexion of the foot. When ambulating, the foot is dragged, scraping the toe, or it is circled stiffly outward and forward. It accompanies *stroke*.
Scissors 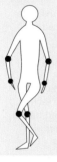	Moves the trunk to accommodate for the leg movements. Legs are extended and knees are flexed. Legs cross over each other at each step, similar to walking in water. It is common with *spastic diplegia* associated with bilateral leg spasticity.

Picture	Description
Parkinsonian 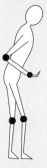	Stooped posture, head and neck forward, and hips and knees flexed in patients with *Parkinson's disease*. Arms are also flexed and held at waist. There is difficulty in initiating gait, often rocking to start. Once ambulating, steps are quick and shuffling. Has difficulty stopping once started.
Cerebellar Ataxia 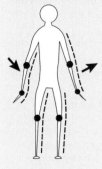	Wide-based gait. Staggers and lurches from one side to another. Cannot perform Romberg because of swaying of the trunk. Common in *cerebral palsy*.
Sensory Ataxia 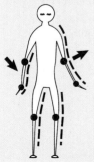	Wide-based gait. Feet are loosely thrown forward, landing first on the heels and then on the toes. The patient watches the ground to help guide the feet. Positive Romberg from loss of position sense. Common in *cerebral palsy*.

(table continues on page 372)

Table 17.3 Abnormal Gaits (*continued*)

Picture	Description
Dystrophic (waddling)	In patients with weak hip abductors, gait is wide. Weight is shifted from one side to another with stiff trunk movement. Abdomen protrudes and lordosis is common.

Table 17.4 Pupils in Comatose Patients

Pupil	Pathological Indication	Description
Unequal pupil size, physiological	Physiological anisocoria, not associated with any disease	May be congenital in 20% of the population
Unequal pupils size, abnormal	Anisocoria related to compression of the optic nerve	One pupil is 0.1 mm different from the other.
Constricted and fixed (pinpoint)	Miosis related to hemorrhage in the pons or opiate narcotics	Pinpoint pupils (<0.1 mm) or small pupils (1–2.5 mm) suggest damage to the sympathetic pathways or metabolic encephalopathy.
Dilated and fixed	Anoxia, sympathetic effects, atropine, tricyclics, amphetamines, or pilocarpine drops for glaucoma treatment; when associated with a head injury, prognosis is poor.	Pupils are >6 mm bilaterally.

Pupil	Pathological Indication	Description
Horner's syndrome	Preganglionic, central, or postganglionic lesion	Miosis (small pupil), ptosis (lid droop), anhydrosis (lack of sweat), and apparent enophthalmos (affected eye appears to be sunken)
Adie's pupil	Denervation of the nerve supply from diabetic neuropathy or alcoholism	Both the pupillary response and accommodation are sluggish or impaired in one eye.
Argyll Robertson pupil	Neurosyphilis, meningitis	Virtually no response to light, but brisk response to accommodation bilaterally. Pupils are small and frequently irregular in shape.
Third nerve palsy	Third nerve palsy	Sudden ptosis, diplopia, and pain are some of the symptoms. Pupil is fixed and dilated, and extraocular motility is restricted.

For more on abnormal pupils, see Chapter 8.

Table 17.5   Summary of Cranial Nerve Assessment

Cranial Nerve	Technique	Abnormal Findings
I. Olfactory (sensory)	Assess patency by closing off one nostril and asking the patient to inhale. Perform the same technique on the opposite side. Occlude one naris. Tell the patient to close the eyes, place a familiar scent near the open naris, and ask the patient to inhale and identify the scent. Repeat on the opposite side.	Only a few neurological conditions are linked with deficits. An olfactory tract lesion may compromise the ability to discriminate odors (anosmia).
II. Optic (sensory)	Ask the patient to identify how many fingers you are holding up. Use the Snellen chart to evaluate far vision and small print for near vision. Test visual fields using confrontation. See Chapter 8.	Visual acuity is <20/20.
III. Oculomotor (motor), IV. trochlear (motor), and VI. abducens (motor)	Assess pupils for size, shape, and equality. Assess six cardinal positions of gaze. Observe for nystagmus. See Chapter 8.	**Nsytagmus** may manifest as quick and jerky movements or slow pendulous movements. Check the plane of movement.
V. Trigeminal (sensory and motor), includes corneal	Using a cotton swab and broken tongue blade or swab, ask the patient to identify sharp or dull sensations. Be sure to evaluate	Decreased or dulled sensation, weakness, and asymmetric movements are abnormal findings.

Table 17.5 **Summary of Cranial Nerve Assessment** (*continued*)

Cranial Nerve	Technique	Abnormal Findings
	all three divisions of the nerve at the scalp (ophthalmic), cheek (maxillary), and chin (mandibular) on each side. Evaluate motor function by observing the face for atrophy, deviation, and fasciculations. Ask the patient to tightly clench the teeth; palpate over the jaw for masseter muscle symmetry. Ask the patient to open the jaw against resistance. To assess the corneal reflex, have the patient remove any contact lenses. Instruct him or her to look up. Inform the patient that you will touch the eye with a cotton swab wisp. Bring the swab in from the side and lightly touch the cornea, not the conjunctiva.	Weakness may result from paralysis of CN V or VII. A depressed or absent corneal response is common in contact lens wearers.
VII. Facial (sensory and motor)	Place sweet, sour, salty, and bitter solutions on the anterior two thirds of the tongue on both sides; also test the posterior one third of the tongue. The patient	Fasciculations or tremors are abnormal. Asymmetric movements may be noted with the lower eyelid sagging, loss of

(table continues on page 376)

Cranial Nerve	Technique	Abnormal Findings
	should properly identify the taste. Evaluate motor function by observing facial movements during conversation. Ask the patient to raise the eyebrows, squeeze the eyes shut, wrinkle the forehead, frown, smile, show teeth, purse lips, and puff out cheeks.	the nasolabial fold, or mouth drooping.
VIII. Acoustic (sensory)	Evaluate hearing during normal conversation using a simple whisper test or with an audiometer. Refer to Chapter 9 for more information.	Inability to hear conversation is abnormal; note the presence of a hearing aid.
IX. Gloss-opharyngeal (sensory and motor)	Evaluate sensory function with CN VII. Evaluate motor function with CN X upon swallowing.	Impaired taste or swallowing is common following a stroke.
X. Vagus (sensory and motor), includes gag reflex	Ask the patient to open the mouth and stick out the tongue, which should be symmetric. Place a tongue blade on the middle of the tongue and have the patient say "ah"; observe the uvula and soft palate for symmetry. Evaluate the sensory	Injury to the vagus or glossopharyngeal nerve causes the uvula to deviate from midline. Asymmetry of the soft palate or tonsillar pillars is also abnormal. An impaired gag reflex, coughing

Table 17.5   Summary of Cranial Nerve Assessment
(*continued*)

Cranial Nerve	Technique	Abnormal Findings
	component by stimulating the gag reflex. Inform the patient that you will be touching the posterior pharyngeal wall, and it may cause gagging. Observe for upward movement of the palate and contraction of the pharyngeal muscles with the gag reflex.	during oral feeding, and changes in voice after swallowing are all associated with aspiration.
XI. Spinal Accessory (motor)	Evaluate the sternomastoid and trapezius muscles for bulk, tone, strength, and symmetry. Ask the patient to press against resistance on the opposite side of the chin. Also ask the patient to shrug the shoulders against resistance.	Weakness or asymmetry in movement accompanies neurological and musculoskeletal problems.
XII. Hypoglossal (motor)	First inspect the tongue; then ask the patient to stick out the tongue and observe for symmetry. Ask the patient to say, "light, tight, dynamite" and note that the letters l, t, d, and n are clear and distinct.	Fasciculations, asymmetry, atrophy, or deviation from midline may occur with general neuromuscular conditions or lesions of the hypoglossal nerve.

Deep Tendon Reflex: Level Tested	Technique
Biceps: C5 and C6 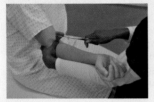	Have the patient partially flex the elbow and place the palm down. To assist with relaxation, the patient may rest the arm against the nurse's. Place one finger or thumb on the biceps tendon. Strike the finger or thumb with the reflex hammer briskly so that the impact is delivered through the digit to the biceps tendon. Observe for flexion at the elbow and contraction of the biceps muscle. If the patient's reflexes are symmetrically diminished or absent, ask the patient to clench the teeth or squeeze one hand tight with the opposite hand to aid in detection (reinforcement).
Triceps: C6, C7, and C8 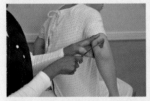	Have the patient flex the arm at the elbow and turn the palm toward the body if supine. If the patient is seated, it may be easiest for the nurse to hold the patient's arm in a relaxed dangling position. Palpate the triceps muscle and strike it directly just above the elbow. Observe for extension of the elbow and contraction of the triceps muscle.

Deep Tendon Reflex: Level Tested	Technique
Brachioradialis: C5 and C6 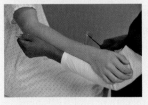	Have the patient flex the arm (up to 45 degrees) and rest the forearm on the nurse's arm with the hand slightly pronated. Palpate the brachioradial tendon approximately 1–2 in above the wrist and strike it directly with the reflex hammer. Observe for pronation of the forearm, flexion of the elbow, and contraction of the muscle.
Patellar: L2, L3, and L4 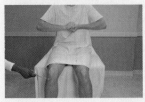	Have the patient flex the knee at 90 degrees, allowing the lower leg to dangle. Support the upper leg with the hand. Palpate the patellar tendon directly below the patella. Observe for extension of the lower leg and contraction of the quadriceps muscle. If the patient's reflexes are symmetrically diminished or absent, ask the patient to lock the fingers in front of the chest and pull one hand against the other (reinforcement).
Achilles: S1 and S2 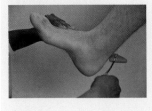	With the patient sitting and legs dangling, hold the patient's foot. (The patient may also kneel on a stool with the feet dangling.) Palpate the Achilles tendon; strike the tendon directly near the ankle malleolus. Observe for plantar flexion of the foot and contraction of the gastrocnemius muscle.

Table 17.7 Pathological (Primitive) Reflexes

Procedure	Abnormal Findings in Adults
Grasp reflex. Apply palmar stimulation.	A grasping response is associated with dementia and diffuse brain impairment.
Snout reflex. Elicit by tapping a tongue blade across the lips.	The snout reflex is present if tapping causes the lips to purse.
Sucking reflex. Touch or stroke the lips, tongue, or palate.	Observe sucking movement of the lips; this reflex also may be noted during oral care or oral suctioning.
Rooting reflex. Stroke the lateral upper lip.	The rooting reflex is present if the patient moves the mouth toward the stimulus.
Palmomental reflex. Stroke the palm of the hand.	It is present if stroking of the palm causes contraction of the same-sided muscle of the lower lip.
Hoffman's sign. Tap the nail on the third or fourth finger.	A positive Hoffman's sign is if tapping elicits involuntary flexion of the distal joint of the thumb and index finger.
Glabellar sign. Tap the forehead to cause the patient to blink.	Normally, the first five taps cause a single blink and then the reflex diminishes. Blinking continues in patients with diffuse cerebral dysfunction.

Male Genitalia and Rectal Assessment

Subjective Data Collection

Key Topics and Questions for Health Promotion

Key Questions	Rationales
Family History. Is there a family history of testicular cancer?	Risk for testicular cancer is greater in men whose brother or father had the disease.
Is there a family history of prostate cancer?	Prostate cancer in a first-degree relative increases the patient's risk. African American men have the highest incidence. Prevalence is highest in North America and Europe.
Is there a history of penile cancer in your family?	Some studies suggest a link between penile cancer and human papillomavirus (HPV).
Is there infertility in siblings?	Encourage the patient to review his family tree for signs of infertility, especially if he is having problems conceiving.
Is there a history of hernia in your family?	Congenital weakness may predispose the patient to *hernia*.
Personal History • Do you have diabetes, hypertension, neurologic impairment, asthma, chronic obstructive pulmonary disease (COPD), chronic bronchitis, or cardiovascular disease?	Men with these illnesses are at increased risk for erectile dysfunction. *(text continues on page 382)*

Key Questions	Rationales
• Was surgery ever performed on your penis, scrotum, or rectum? • What type of procedure, year/ date? • How has this procedure affected you?	Surgery is used to treat enlarged prostate, *testicular cancer, hydrocele, varicocele,* undescended testicle, *hemorrhoids, anorectal fissures,* and *carcinoma of the rectum and anus.* Some men choose vasectomy.
• Have you ever been treated for a sexually transmitted infection (STI)? • Where and when? • What type of STI? • How was it treated? • Did you have a test of cure afterward?	STIs are sensitive but important subjects. Tactful direct questioning is an essential part of the assessment.
• Have you ever had an injury to or other problems with your scrotum, penis, or testes? • Have you had benign prostatic hyperplasia or prostatitis?	Examples include *testicular torsion, hydrocele, spermatocele,* and *varicocele.* Identification of previous problems may help when documenting current health concerns.
• Do you have a history of cancer? • When was the diagnosis? • What treatment did you have?	Even with removal of a cancerous testicle, cancer can recur in the other testicle.
Sexual History • When was your first sexual intercourse? • Was this by choice? • Do you have sex with men, women, or both? • In what type of sex do you engage? • How frequently do you have intercourse? • Do you have sex with multiple partners? • How many partners have you had in the last 6 months? • Do you or your partner frequently use drugs or alcohol before sexual intercourse? • Are you satisfied with your sexual relationship? • Do you use contraceptives? Do you always use protective barriers?	Conversation about sexual history is important to help identify high-risk sexual practices, establish patient norms, and provide education. Sexual dysfunction can present as anxiety, anger, or depression. Physical problems can lead to sexual problems.

Key Questions	Rationales

- Have you ever gotten someone pregnant?
- What was the outcome of this situation?
- Have you ever been pushed, slapped, or had something thrown at you?
- Have you ever been kicked, bit, or hit?

⚠ SAFETY ALERT 18-1
Men can be victims of abuse. Often it is difficult for men to admit that they are being victimized.

Medications. What medications, herbal supplements, recreational drugs, and over-the-counter (OTC) drugs do you take?

Many medications and supplements can affect the genitourinary tract and its function.

Additional Risk Factors. Do you wear protective gear during contact sports?

Lack of protection can lead to injury of sensitive genitalia.

Have you received a hepatitis A or B vaccine?

⚠ SAFETY ALERT 18-2
The Centers for Disease Control and Prevention (CDC) recommend hepatitis A vaccine for unimmunized men who have sex with other men. The CDC recommends hepatitis B vaccine for all unimmunized people at risk for STIs.

Do you perform self-genital examination?

This question serves as an excellent teaching opportunity.

Do you have regular clinical examinations by a health professional?

Primary prevention helps patients maintain health. Age-appropriate screenings should be discussed during the appointment.

Health-Promotion Teaching

Testicular Self-examination (TSE). The purpose of performing TSE is not to find something currently wrong. By performing monthly self-examinations, men older than 14 years become familiar with what is normal for them. Once "normal" is established, changes are easier to identify. Thus, testicular cancer can be detected at an early (and most often curable) stage. Steps for TSE are as follows:

1. TSE is best after a warm shower or bath. Heat relaxes the scrotum, making TSE easier.
2. Examine each testicle one at a time with both hands. Place the index and middle fingers under the testicle; place the thumbs on top. Roll the testicle gently from one side to another. You should not feel the pain. One testicle may normally be larger (Fig. 18-1).
3. Cancerous lumps usually are on the sides, but can show up on the front. Become familiar with the location of the epididymis (soft, tubelike structure behind the testes that collects and carries sperm) so that you won't mistake it for a lump.
4. Make an appointment with a physician, preferably a urologist, as soon as possible if you find a lump, enlarged testes, pain or discomfort, scrotal heaviness, a dull ache in the groin, significant loss of size of one testicle, or a sudden collection of fluid in the scrotum.

Screening for Prostate Cancer. Evidence is insufficient to conclude whether screening for prostate cancer with prostate-specific antigen (PSA) or digital rectal examination (DRE) reduces mortality from prostate cancer. The PSA screening test can detect cancer earlier, but

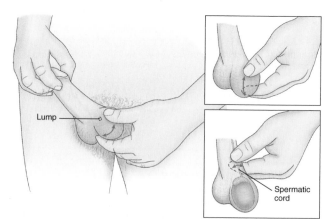

Figure 18.1 The testicular self-examination.

it remains unclear if this leads to any change in natural history and outcome of the disease.

Key Topics and Questions for Common Symptoms

Common Symptoms of the Male Genitalia, Prostate, and Rectum

- Pain
- Problems with urination
- Erectile dysfunction
- Penile lesions, discharge
- Scrotal enlargement

Key Questions	Rationales/Abnormal Findings
Pain. Point to the painful area. • Do you feel pain anywhere else? • When did it begin? How long have you had it? Have you ever had it before? • Can you rate your pain on a scale of 0 to 10, with 10 being the worst ever? • What does the pain feel like? • Do you also have nausea, vomiting, fever, abdominal distention, and burning on urination? Is urine of a different color? • What makes the pain worse or better? What have you done to help the pain, if anything? How well did this help? • What is your pain goal?	Sudden distention of the ureter, renal pelvis, or bladder may cause flank pain. Pain around the costovertebral angle may be from renal distention. *Kidney-stone* pain may radiate down the spermatic cord and present as testicular pain. Pain in the groin or scrotum may be from a *hernia* or problems in the spermatic cord, testicles, or prostate. Testicular pain can occur secondary to any problem of the testes such as *epididymitis, orchitis, hydrocele, spermatic cord torsion,* and *tumor.* Understanding what interventions the patient does to relieve pain assists with developing a treatment plan.
Have you ever had a prolonged painful erection *(priapism)*?	*Priapism* can occur with *leukemia* or *hemoglobinopathies* (eg, sickle cell anemia).
Are you experiencing rectal or anal pain?	*Perianal abscess, rectal fissure,* and *hemorrhoids* are among the most painful problems of the anus and rectum.

(text continues on page 386)

Key Questions

Rationales/Abnormal Findings

Problems with Urination

- Do you have trouble starting a stream?
- Is there a change in the flow?
- Do you have sudden urges to urinate?
- Can you estimate how much urine is passed with each void or urination?
- Do you need to urinate at night?
- Are you straining to urinate?
- Are you drinking more fluids than usual?
- Do you involuntarily lose urine?
- What color is your urine? Do you ever notice red urine?

Urgency and frequency may be from *UTI*, *prostatitis*, *STI*, or *bladder cancer*. Prostate enlargement, common in older men, can affect urine flow. The following are signs of partial prostate obstruction: recurrent acute UTIs, sensation of residual urine, decreased caliber of the urine stream, hesitancy, straining, and terminal dribbling.

Blood in the urine is associated with benign disease, eating red-colored food, or life-threatening malignancy.

Male Sexual Dysfunction

- Do you have persistent erections unrelated to sexual stimulation?
- With an erection do you have a curvature of the penis in any direction?
- Do you have difficulty with erection? Is there pain associated with it?
- When you have sexual stimulation or intercourse, how often do you ejaculate (color, consistency, and amount)?
- How strong is your sex drive? Over the last month how would you rate your ability to keep and maintain an erection?
- If you were to spend the rest of your life with your sexual function the way it is now, how would you feel?

The main types of sexual dysfunction include premature ejaculation, erectile dysfunction (difficulty achieving or maintaining erection), low libido, delayed orgasm, and penile physical abnormalities. Erectile dysfunction is important to address. Many men welcome the opportunity to discuss it. Presenting the topic in a nonthreatening, nonjudgmental manner encourages the patient to talk about matters of concern.

Penile Lesions, Discharge, or Rash

- When did you first note the lesion? Is there more than one?

Direct, tactful questions about history of exposure to STIs are important. A lesion raises the

Key Questions	Rationales/Abnormal Findings
• Is pain, itching, burning, or stinging associated with the lesion? • Is there discharge? When did it begin? Is there an associated odor or color? • If you are sexually active, does your partner have the same symptoms? Have you changed sexual partners?	possibility of STI. Ask if the patient has had *genital warts*, *syphilis*, *gonorrhea*, *trichomoniasis*, or other STIs. Assess if discharge is continuous or intermittent. Bloody penile discharge is associated with *urethritis* and *neoplasm*. Tactfully explore if the patient has been with a new partner recently or if there has been a change in sexual habits.
Scrotal Enlargement • When did you notice the enlargement? • Is there pain associated? Is it constant or intermittent? • Has there been any recent groin trauma? • Have you ever had a hernia? Do you use a truss or any treatment? • Have you had fertility problems?	Although rarely fatal, scrotal enlargement and pain carry a risk of morbidity from testicular atrophy, infarction, or necrosis. Any patient with scrotum pain should be presumed to have testicular torsion until this diagnosis can be proven otherwise. Assess the patient for *varicoceles*, which are often linked with infertility.

Objective Data Collection

Equipment

- Latex gloves
- Water-soluble lubricant
- Flashlight or penlight (for transillumination)
- Stethoscope (to listen for bowel sounds if hernia is suspected)

- Measurements of the nurse's index finger, which can be used as a ruler to measure the patient's penis, testes, and prostate gland

Technique and Normal Findings	Abnormal Findings

Groin

With the patient supine, inspect the groin and genital hair distribution. *Skin is clear, intact, and smooth. Hair is diamond shaped or in an escutcheon pattern, appears coarser than at the scalp, and has no parasites.*

Abnormal findings are no hair, patchy growth, and distribution in a female or triangular pattern. Look for inflammation, lesions, dermatitis, or infestations. *Candidiasis* causes crusty, multiple, red, round erosions and pustules. *Tinea curis* ("jock itch") is a fungal infection with large red, scaly, and extremely itchy patches.

Penis

Observe surface characteristics and color. Look for lesions or discharge. Inspect the posterior side. *The dorsal vein is apparent on the dorsal surface. Penis has no edema, lesions, discharge, or nodules.*

See Table 18-1 at the end of this chapter.

In the uncircumcised penis, the prepuce covers the gland. Ask the patient to retract it. *It retracts easily. Smegma (thin, white, cheesy substance) may surround the corona.*

In the circumcised penis, the glans and corona are visible, lighter in color than the shaft, and free of smegma. *Circumcised penises have varying lengths of foreskin: some have folds of skin, while others have no extra foreskin.*

Glans. Inspect the glans. *It is glistening pink, smooth in texture, and bulbous.*

See Table 18-1.

Shaft. Inspect and palpate. *The shaft feels smooth without lesions or pain. Normal variations include ectopic sebaceous glands that appear as tiny, whitish-yellow papules.*

Technique and Normal Findings	Abnormal Findings
External Urethral Meatus. Inspect and palpate (Fig. 18-2). *It is located centrally on the glans. The orifice is slitlike and millimeters from the penis tip. The external urethral meatus has no discharge, stenosis, or warts.* The glans can be opened by pressing it between thumb and forefinger. The patient can be instructed to do this. Next, strip or milk the penis from the base toward the glans or head. Note color, consistency, or odor of any discharge. *The glans is smooth and pink with no discharge.*	See Table 18-2 at the end of this chapter.

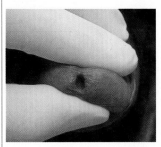

Figure 18.2 Inspecting and palpating the external urinary meatus.

Scrotum Ask the patient to hold the penis out of the way. Inspect the scrotal septum and anterior and posterior scrotum. *It is divided into two sacs. The scrotum could hang asymmetrically, with the left side lower than the right. Sebaceous cysts or glands may be noted on the sac. The anterior and posterior skin appears darker with a rugous or wrinkled surface.*	See Tables 18-1 and 18-3 at the end of this chapter.

(text continues on page 390)

Technique and Normal Findings	Abnormal Findings

Sacrococcygeal Areas

Inspect for surface character-istics and tenderness. *Skin is clear and smooth with no palpable masses or dimpling.*

A dimple with an inflamed tuft of hair or a tender palpable cyst suggests a *pilonidal cyst* or *sinus*. Generally, the patient is asymptomatic unless the area becomes infected, when red-ness, tenderness, and a cyst can be palpated. A ruptured cyst drains purulent mucus.

Perineal Area

With the patient on his side, spread the buttocks and inspect the perineal area. *Skin sur-rounding the anus is coarse and dark. The anal sphincter is closed.*

See Table 18-4 at the end of this chapter.

Inguinal and Femoral Areas

Instruct the patient to stand. Ask him to bear down. While he does so, inspect the inguinal canal and femoral areas for bulges or masses.

Bulges or masses suggest a **hernia.** See Table 18-5 at the end of this chapter.

Advanced Techniques

Testicles

Inspect the scrotal sac. Palpate each testicle separately. *Note the smooth, rubbery consis-tency of each testicle; no nod-ules should be felt.*

Irregularities in texture or size may indicate an infection, tumor, or cyst.

Palpate the epididymis on the posterolateral surface of each testicle. *It feels smooth and nontender.*

Note the site of any unusual findings and if the condition resolves when the patient is supine.

Vas Deferens

Palpate the vas deferens, located in the spermatic cord (Fig. 18-3). *It feels smooth and cordlike. No nodules or lesions are palpable.*

See Table 18-4.

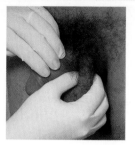

Figure 18.3 Palpating the vas deferens.

Transillumination of the Scrotum

To assess for a mass or fluid, transilluminate each scrotal pouch. *The testes and epididymides do not transilluminate. The sac does not contain additional fluids or contents.*

See Table 18-3.

Hernias

Palpate the inguinal canal. With the patient relaxed, insert your finger into the scrotal sac; follow upward along the vas deferens. For a child, the little finger is appropriate; for an adult, the middle finger is used. Palpate the oval external ring. If a hernia is present, you should feel the sudden presence of a viscus against your finger (Fig. 18-4). *There is no bulging or pain.*

Hernias occur when a loop of intestine prolapses through the inguinal wall or canal or abdominal musculature. The patient reports pain on exertion or lifting. On examination, pain increases when maneuvers or positioning increases intra-abdominal pressure.
See Table 18-5.

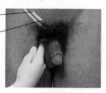

Inguinal ligament
External inguinal ring

Figure 18.4 Palpating for a hernia.

(text continues on page 392)

Technique and Normal Findings	Abnormal Findings

Perianal and Rectal Examination

A standing position allows for visualization of the anus and palpation of the rectum. Rectal examination can also be performed with the patient on his left side with the right leg flexed and left leg semi-extended (Sims' position). Have the standing patient place both feet together, slightly flex both knees, and bend forward over the examination table (Fig. 18-5).

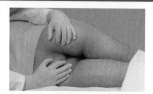

Figure 18.5 Sims's positioning for rectal examination.

Anus. Spread the buttocks apart. Inspect the anus with a penlight. Have the patient bear down. Observe for lesions, warts, tags, hemorrhoids, fissures, and fistulas.

Apply lubricant to the index finger of the gloved hand. Explain to the patient that lubricant is used for comfort but might feel cool. Add that initially he may feel like he is going to have a bowel movement, but that this will not happen. Have the patient take a deep breath while you insert the finger into the rectum. Assess rectal tone. *Full closure around the finger is palpable.* Rotate your index finger around the anal ring. *It feels smooth without nodules, masses, or irregularities.*

Look for thrombosed hemorrhoids, rectal fissures, or hard stool.

Continue to advance your index finger into the anal canal. *The lateral and posterior rectal walls feel smooth and uninterrupted. Internal hemorrhoids are usually not felt.*

A hypotonic or lax sphincter could be from rectal surgery, neurological deficit, or trauma from anal sex. Hypertonic or tight sphincter may be from inflammation, scarring, or anxiety.

Note nodules, masses, irregularities, or polyps. Pay attention to any discomfort felt by the patient.

Patients complain of pain with *anal fissures* or *fistulas.* Local anesthesia may be necessary to complete the examination.

Technique and Normal Findings	Abnormal Findings
Rotate your index finger to palpate the anterior rectal wall, repeating the above process. *There are no nodules, masses, irregularities, or polyps.*	Extreme rectal pain is associated with local disease. Abnormalities may be related to *BPH, prostatitis,* and *prostate cancer.* See Table 18-4 at the end of this chapter.
Prostate. At this point, the posterior surface of the prostate gland can be felt (Fig. 18-6). Explain to the patient that it may feel like he is going to urinate, but he will not. Note prostate size, contour, consistency, and mobility. *The prostate has the consistency of a rubber ball. It is nontender, firm, smooth, and slightly moveable. The diameter is approximately 4 cm; less than 1 cm protrudes into the rectum.* The lateral lobes should feel symmetric and divided by the median sulcus. The sulcus may be obliterated when the lobes are neoplastic or hypertrophied. The DRE of the prostate allows palpation of the posterior surfaces, which is the area where cancer often starts.	Prostate enlargement is classified by the amount of projection into the rectum (Table 18-6). A hard prostate may indicate *carcinoma, prostatic calcui,* or chronic fibrosis. A rubbery or boggy consistency may suggest benign prostatic hyperplasia (*BPH*), a common finding in men older than 60 years. Signs and symptoms of BPH are urine retention, hesitancy, urgency, dribbling, nocturia, and straining to void. If the problem becomes chronic, the patient can develop overflow incontinence.

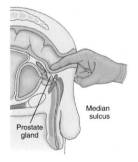

Median sulcus

Prostate gland

Figure 18.6 Palpating the prostate.

Upon completion of the examination of the rectum, explain to the patient that you are going

(text continues on page 394)

Technique and Normal Findings	Abnormal Findings
to remove your finger. Offer the patient a cleansing wipe and a private few minutes to redress.	
Stool. Upon removing your finger from examining the rectum, inspect the gloved finger for consistency and color of the stool. *Stool is brown and soft.*	Abnormal findings include stools with an unusual color, blood, purulent drainage, or mucus. Black tarry stool raises suspicion of upper GI bleeding. Very light tan or gray stool could indicate obstructive jaundice.

Documentation of Normal Subjective and Objective Findings

The patient denies pain, discomfort, and problems with urination. States that he has no premature ejaculation, erectile dysfunction, low libido, delayed orgasm, or physical abnormalities of the penis. No lesions, discharge, or scrotal enlargement. Skin is clear, intact, and smooth. No masses or lesions noted. Foreskin intact. No phimosis or paraphimosis. Penis size is appropriate to age and smooth without lesions or pain. No discharge, edema, or redness.

🔺 Lifespan Considerations

Infants and Children

Rectal examination is not performed routinely. Indications for such examination include bowel abnormalities, abdominal distention, pelvic pain, mass or tenderness, bleeding, bladder discomfort, pain, or distention. If examination is necessary, prepare the patient and guardian before starting. Explain every step. Use your little finger. It is not unusual for the infant or child to have a small amount of bleeding directly following. The patient should be in the lithotomy position. Hold the feet together and flex the knees and hips on the abdomen. Routinely inspect the perineum, anus, and surrounding areas for masses, redness, or ecchymosis. Inspect the anus for abscess, perirectal tears, or fistulae.

When determining rectal patency, assess whether the infant has passed meconium. If the infant has not passed stool in the first 48 hours after birth, suspect rectal atresia.

If perirectal redness or excoriation is noted, check for enterobiasis. Candida and other irritants can produce perineum excoriation.

Rectal prolapse may be from constipation, diarrhea, or severe coughing. Hemorrhoids are rare; if present, they suggest portal hypertension. Inspect the rectum for small flat skin flaps—these may be evidence of syphilitic condylomas. Finally, inspect the coccyx area for dimpling, sinuses, and tufts of hair in the pilonidal area, which indicate lower spinal deformities. Lightly touching the anal area should produce an anal contraction. If no contraction is noted, assess for lower spinal cord lesion.

Assess rectal tone. It should feel tight but not loose. A lax sphincter could indicate neurological lesions. Bruises, scars, anal tears, and anal dilation could indicate sexual abuse and must be investigated. Lastly, feel for stool in the rectum; note if the stool is hard or soft. Following examination, test any stool on the examination glove for occult blood.

Infants commonly have a stool after each feeding because of the gastrocolic reflex. Between 12 and 18 months, they gradually achieve control of the external anal sphincter.

There is much debate over routine circumcision. Recent evidence suggests fewer urinary tract infections (UTIs) in circumcised males. Observational studies presented strong evidence of an association between male circumcision and reduced risk of acquiring HIV through vaginal intercourse. Nonetheless, these benefits are not significant enough to recommend that all males be circumcised. Because circumcision has potential benefits and risks, parents should determine what is in the best interest of the child. Often the decision is based on family tradition, culture, religion, and ethnic traditions.

Adolescents

With puberty, testicular growth begins. Scrotal skin thins and becomes pendulous. Testes become active and begin to secrete testosterone, which promotes bone maturation and epiphyseal closure. Genital hair appears at the base of the penis, darkens, and extends over the entire pubic area; at this time, the prostate gland enlarges. When maturation is complete, genital hair is curly, dense, and coarse, with a diamond shape from umbilicus to anus. Growth and development of the scrotum and testes are complete and the length and width of the penis are increased. See Table 18-7 for the Tanner's Stages.

Older Adults

Pubic hair may be thin and gray. Testes may be smaller and softer. The scrotal sac has less ruggae and appears to droop. Rectal tone is intact, but strength of the rectal reflex may be reduced slightly.

Older men may have rectal distention from degeneration of afferent neurons. This may contribute to fecal incontinence.

Testosterone levels decline with aging, which may affect both libido and sexual function. Erection becomes more dependent on tactile stimulation and less responsive to erotic cues. The penis may decrease in size. Fibromuscular prostate structures atrophy. Ironically, benign hyperplasia of the glandular tissue often obscures the atrophy of aging.

◗ Cultural Considerations

Patients with darkly pigmented skin may have darker pigmentation in the scrotal and anal area. The pubic hair may also be darker and coarser.

Common Nursing Diagnoses and Interventions Associated with the Male Genital System

Diagnosis	Interventions
Ineffective sexuality pattern related to erectile dysfunction	After establishing a relationship, give the patient permission to discuss issues by asking, "Are you concerned about sexual function because of changes in your health?"
Risk for infection	Teach safe sexual practices, warning signs of genital tract infections. Remove urinary catheters as soon as possible.
Urinary retention related to obstruction	Obtain a postvoid bladder ultrasound. Teach double voiding and to avoid OTC cold medications with decongestant.
Risk for urge incontinence related to irritation of bladder	Assess the patient for functional barriers to continence; teach spacing of fluids in consistent quantities over the day. Avoid fluid late in the evening.

Table 18.1 Abnormal Conditions of the Penis

Genital Piercing

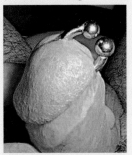

The most common issue associated with piercing is infection. Other complications include bleeding and difficulty urinating.

Phimosis

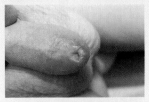

A prepuce that cannot be retracted may be congenital or follow recurrent infections or inflammation. Barrowed foreskin may obstruct urinary flow.

Paraphimosis

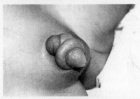

The retracted prepuce cannot be placed back over the glans. Paraphimosis may be severe enough to restrict circulation to the glans. An uncircumcised male would always have the foreskin pulled toward the urethral opening.

Balanitis or Balanoposthitis

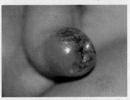

Inflammation of the glans and prepuce may be from poorly controlled diabetes. Scars and narrowing of the urethral opening may cause inflammation, infections, and foul discharge.

(table continues on page 398)

Hypospadias

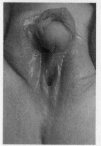

The urethral meatus opens
on the ventral side of the
penis, making urination
difficult while standing.
Physical appearance of the
penis is altered, causing
body image issues.

Epispadias

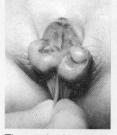

The urethral meatus
opens on the dorsal penile
surface. Epispadias may be
associated with underlying
congenital anomalies. The
lower urinary tract may be
exposed in severe cases.

! Table 18.2   Sexually Transmitted Infections

STI	Findings and Clinical Implications
Scabies Infection 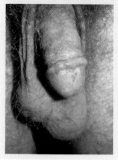	This highly communicable skin condition caused by an arachnid ("itch mite") is transmitted by direct skin contact and is associated with papules, vesicles, pustules, and intense itching.

STI	Findings and Clinical Implications
Chlamydia 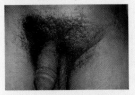	This most frequently reported bacterial STI in the United States is **reportable in every state.** In men the urethra has a mucopurulent discharge. There is burning on urination. Commonly, Chlamydia can present asymptomatically.
Gonorrhea 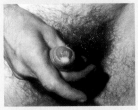	Transmission results from intimate contact; incubation period is 2–7 days. **This STI is reportable in every state.** Men may present with dysuria, urethral discharge, rectal pain, or discharge. Common sites of infection are the urethra, epididymis, prostate, rectum, and pharynx.
Syphilis 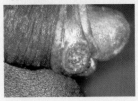	*T. pallidum* penetrates intact skin or mucous membrane during sexual contact, multiplies, and rapidly spreads to regional lymph nodes. Primary incubation period for acquired syphilis is about 3 weeks, but can occur 10–90 days after exposure. Secondary syphilis develops 6–8 weeks later. Latent and tertiary syphilis can occur years later. **Report all cases of syphilis to the public health department.**

(table continues on page 400)

Table 18.2 Sexually Transmitted Infections (*continued*)

STI	Findings and Clinical Implications
Human Papillomavirus 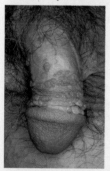	HPV produces epithelial tumors of the skin and mucous membranes. Incubation period can range from 3 months to several years. Most men with HPV never develop genital warts.
Herpes Simplex Virus (HSV) Type 1 and 2 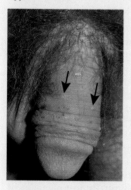	Transmission of HSV-1 and HSV-2 is only by direct contact with active lesions or virus-containing fluid such as saliva. Incubation period is 2–14 days. HSV-1 is associated with infection of the lips, face, buccal mucosa, and throat. HSV-2 is associated with genitalia. Usual sequence is painful papules followed by vesicles, ulceration, crusting, and healing.

Spermatocele

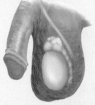

This benign scrotal mass or cyst develops on the head of the epididymis or testicular adnexa. Patients may report a lump in the scrotal sac or edema. Upon palpation a mobile, cystic nodule usually less than 1 cm is noted superior and posterior to the testis. The mass will transilluminate with a pink or red glow.

Epididymitis

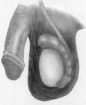

Acute infection of the epididymis, commonly by Chlamydia, gonorrhea, or other bacterial infection, is often linked to prostatitis, especially after surgical intervention/urethral instrumentation. Scrotal pain is severe, accompanied by swelling and fever.

Testicular Torsion

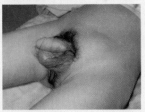

Sudden twisting of the spermatic cord, usually on the left side, is rare after 20 years. It results from faulty anchoring of the testis on the scrotal wall. Impaired blood supply results in ischemia and venous engorgement. Because the testis can become gangrenous within a few hours, *this is a surgical emergency*.

(table continues on page 402)

Varicocele

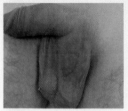

Dilated, tortuous varicose veins are common in young males but rare before 10 years. Screen for varicocele in early adolescence, because this *is the most common cause of infertility*. No visual abnormality may appear, but a bluish tinge of the scrotum may be seen in light-skinned patients. When the patient is upright, a soft, irregular mass feels distinctly like a "bag of worms" posterior and superior to the testis.

Hydrocele

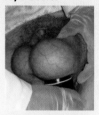

This circumscribed collection of serous fluid develops in the tunica vaginalis surrounding the testis. In *noncommunicating hydrocele*, fluid collects only but persistently in the scrotum. *Communicating hydrocele* has a patent process vaginalis, so fluid can move from abdomen to scrotum. The patient presents with unilateral and intermittent edema but no pain. On palpation a large scrotal mass is noted and can be transilluminated.

External Hemorrhoids

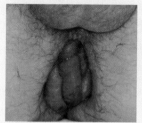

These varicose veins originate below the pectinate line and are covered by anal skin. They are usually not visible at rest but become visible on standing or defecation. Patients have rectal itching, pain, or burning.

Internal Hemorrhoids

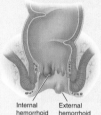

Internal   External
hemorrhoid   hemorrhoid

These can be painless unless thrombosed, infected, or prolapsed. They occur above the pectinate line and are covered by anal mucosa. They create soft swelling and are difficult to palpate unless prolapsed. They can bleed daily with or without defecation, leading to anemia.

Anorectal Fissure

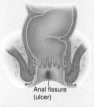

Anal fissure
(ulcer)

This tear in anal mucosa can occur midline, posterior, or anterior. It usually follows passage of large, hard stool. A sentinel skin tag may be seen at the lower end of the fissure. Ulcerations may appear at the site. The patient has bleeding, pain, and itching.

Anal Fistula

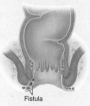

Fistula

This inflammatory tract or tube opens at one end in the anus/rectum and at the other onto the skin surface. It originates in the anal crypts and can occur spontaneously or from perirectal abscess. Drainage may appear, with the area raised, red, and granular.

(table continues on page 404)

Rectal Polyp

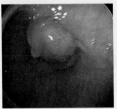

Polyps can occur anywhere in the intestinal tract. They can be adenomas or inflammatory, single or clustered. They can cause rectal bleeding and be seen protruding through the rectum. Polyps can be felt as soft nodules and either be pedunculated or sessile.

Carcinoma of the Rectum and Anus

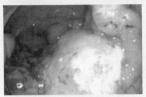

The most common cause is anal intercourse, especially if associated with chronic irritation. Symptoms include constant discharge, bowel changes, blood in the stool, and weight loss. A stony, irregular, sessile polypoid mass is felt. It is nodular with areas of ulceration.

Rectal Prolapse

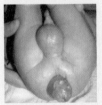

This problem usually occurs with defecation; rectal mucosa, with or without muscular wall, prolapses through the anal ring. A prolapse may present like a doughnut. A complete prolapse includes the muscular wall and is larger with circular folds.

Prostatitis

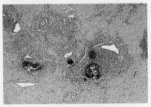

Prostate inflammation or infection can be acute or chronic. Manifestations of both are fever, chills, malaise, dysuria, hematuria, frequency, low back and perineal pain, inhibited urinary voiding, and suprapubic discomfort. Patients may complain of pain during sex or defecation. The prostate is tender, warm, swollen, and boggy.

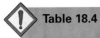

Table 18.4   Conditions of the Anus, Rectum, and Prostate (*continued*)

Prostate Cancer

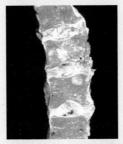

This second most common cancer is usually very slow growing and asymptomatic in early stages. As the prostate enlarges, patients may develop hesitancy, dribbling, frequency, urgency, nocturia, retention, slow stream, or feeling of bladder fullness. Diagnosis is made with a PSA blood test and rectal examination.

Table 18.5   Types of Hernias

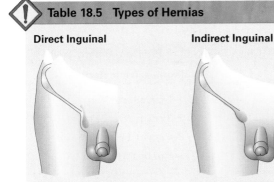

Direct Inguinal	Indirect Inguinal
Occurs in middle-aged and elderly men. Bilateral in 55% of cases. Develops above the lingual ligament, directly behind and through external ring. Scrotal involvement is rare.	Occurs across all age groups. Bilateral in 30% of cases. Occurs above the inguinal ligament, with the hernial sac entering the inguinal canal at internal ring and exiting at external ring. Scrotum is commonly involved.

(table continues on page 406)

Table 18.5 Types of Hernias (continued)

Femoral

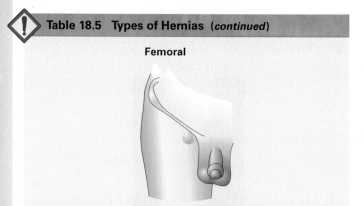

Least common type, occurring more often in women. Rarely bilateral. Develops below the inguinal ligament; never involves the scrotum in men.

Table 18.6 Classifications of Prostate Enlargement

Grade	Protrusion into Rectum
Grade I	1–2 cm or ⅜ to ¾ in
Grade II	2–3 cm or ¾ to 1⅛ in
Grade III	3–4 cm or 1⅛ to 1¾ in
Grade IV	>4 cm or 1¾ in

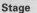

Table 18.7 Tanner's Stages: Male Development

Stage	Male Development
1	There is no pubic hair. Testes and penis are small (prepubertal). Apparent in boys younger than 10 years.
2	Sparse thin hair is at base of the penis. Testes enlarge. Scrotal skin becomes coarser and redder. Age range is 10–13 years.
3	Scrotum and testes continue to grow. Penis lengthens, with diameter increasing slowly. Pubic hair increases, becoming darker, coarse, curly, and extending laterally. Age range is 12–14 years.
4	Penis and testes continue to grow. Pubic hair extends across pubis but spares the medial thighs. Age range is 13–15 years.
5	Penis is at its full size. Pubic hair is diamond shaped in appearance with adult color; texture extends to surface of medial thighs. Age range is 14–17 years.

Tanner, J. (1962). *Growth at adolescence*. Oxford: Blackwell.

19

Female Genitalia and Rectal Assessment

Key Topics and Question for Health Promotion

Key Questions	Rationales
Family History. Tell me about your family history (two generations) of diabetes, heart disease, cancer, thyroid problems, gynecologic conditions, asthma, hypertension, allergies, maternal DES use, multiple pregnancy, and congenital anomalies.	History of these conditions poses risks for the patient's current reproductive health.
Menstrual History. How old were you when you got your first period? • What was the 1st day of the last period? • What is your flow like? • For how many days do you experience flow? • How many pads or tampons do you use per day? • For how many days is there heavy, moderate, or light flow?	Menarche usually begins around 12 years of age; if a girl has not had menarche by 16 years, an endocrine evaluation is recommended. Calculate menstrual cycle from the 1st day of the last period to the 1st day of the next period. Usual cycle is 28 to 32 days. Flow is approximately 25 to 60 mL per menstrual period. Normal length is 2 to 8 days.
Obstetrical History • Have you ever been pregnant? • If so, how many times? • How many living children do you have? • Were births vaginal or cesarean?	**Gravida:** Number of pregnancies a woman has had, including if she is presently pregnant. **Para:** Number of births a woman has had after 20 weeks even if the fetus died at birth.

Key Questions	Rationales
• Were there any complications? • Have you ever had a miscarriage? • Have you ever had an abortion? Was it elective, spontaneous, or incomplete?	**Term:** Infant born after 37 weeks' gestation. **Preterm:** Infant born after 20 weeks but before 37 weeks. **Abortion:** Pregnancies that ended spontaneously or for therapeutic reasons. **Living:** Number of living children either delivered or adopted.
Menopause • Have you stopped having periods? • Are menstrual cycles irregular? • Do you experience any irregularity or absence of menses?	**Menopause** is the cessation of menstrual periods for 12 months or more. **Perimenopause** is irregularity of menstrual cycles and accompanying symptoms in women of age 40 to 55 years.
Gynecologic History • Have you ever had a Papanicolaou (Pap) smear? When? • Have Pap results been normal? If not, did you receive treatment? When? • Have you had previous surgeries? • Have you been treated for vaginal infection? • Do you have frequent vaginal infections? • Do you use over-the-counter (OTC) vaginal medication? • Have you ever had pelvic infections? • Do you use scented vaginal products? • Do you douche? How often?	**Pap smear** is cytologic evaluation of cervical cells to screen for pre-cancerous lesions. It does NOT screen for sexually transmitted infections (STIs) or any cancers other than cervical cancer. A patient with recurring yeast infections should be evaluated for *diabetes* and *HIV*. Frequent use of OTC creams or suppositories can mask other more serious infections. Use may result in *contact dermatitis*. Douching can cause vaginal infections or *pelvic inflammatory disease (PID)*.

(text continues on page 410)

(text continues on page 410)

Key Questions	Rationales
Immunizations. Have you received the vaccine against *Human Papillomavirus (HPV)*? • When did you receive it? • Did you receive all three doses?	HPV is a risk factor for *cervical cancer*.
Sexual History • Have you ever had sex? • What type (vaginal, oral, or anal)? • Approximately how many sexual partners have you had? Male, female, or both? • Are you currently in a sexual relationship? Is it monogamous? • Have you ever experienced sexual abuse? • Do you experience any pain or bleeding with or after intercourse? • Do you experience urinary burning or infections related to intercourse?	Frank discussion opens opportunities for inquiry. Ascertaining a patient's experience is important to determine risks. Obtaining history not only opens discussion, but allows the nurse to conduct the examination with emotional support. Bleeding during intercourse may indicate an infection or possibly a *cervical polyp*. *Dysuria* or frequent urinary tract infections (UTIs) may be related to bladder trauma from intercourse.
Contraception • Do you use condoms or other barriers during sex? Sometimes or always? • Do you use contraception? • If so, what is currently used? • Have you ever used anything different? • Have you had any problems with any contraceptive forms?	Condoms provide some but not complete protection against STIs. The only 100% safe sex practice is abstinence.
Medications and Supplements • Are you taking any prescribed drugs?	Oral contraceptives, antidepressants, and antihypertensive agents can cause changes in

Key Questions	Rationales
• Are you taking any OTC medications? • Have you recently taken antibiotics?	menstrual cycles and libido. Certain antibiotics can strip normal vaginal flora, promoting *yeast infections*, and interfere with absorption of oral contraceptives.
STIs • Do you engage in unprotected sex? • Do you have multiple sexual partners? • Are you between 15 and 24 years of age? • Are you experiencing any pain within or discharge from the pelvic region?	See Table 19-1 at the end of this chapter.
Hormonal Contraceptive and Tobacco Use • Do you smoke? • Are you using hormonal contraceptives? • How old are you?	Tobacco is contraindicated for any patient 40 years or older who uses hormonal contraceptives. Combined use increases risk for vascular problems (see Chapter 13).

Health-Promotion Teaching

Women with a history of multiple partners are at risk for HPV and cervical cancer. Discuss this fact and recommend monogamy, abstinence, or consistent use of condoms with each act of intercourse.

Women currently using oral contraceptives are less likely to use barrier methods during sex. When counseling women, stress to them that oral contraceptives do not protect against STIs.

Incidence of cervical cancer has decreased in the past decades because of widespread use of Pap screening. The greatest risk factor for cervical cancer is infection with HPV. More than 100 types of HPV cause genital warts, some of which can lead to cervical cancer. Having unprotected sex increases the chance of contracting HPV. Not everyone infected with HPV develops cancer of the cervix. Other risk factors include tobacco use, infection with Chlamydia or HIV, poor diet, low income, and family history of cancer. HPV testing is a simple swabbing of the external and endocervical areas. This testing captures the types of HPV that cause high-grade cervical lesions that lead to cancer.

The HPV vaccine has been available and is recommended for females 9 through 26 years. Patients (and, in the case of minors, their parents) should be counseled regarding the availability.

Key Topics and Questions for Common Symptoms

Common Female Genital or Rectal Symptoms

- Pelvic pain
- Vaginal discharge, burning, or itching
- Menstrual disorders
- Structural problems
- Hemorrhoids

Questions on Common Symptoms	Rationale/Abnormal Findings
Pelvic Pain. Do you have any pain or discomfort? Provide details.	Many gynecological problems differ in the pain characteristics. Pelvic conditions increase in pain and intensity with exercise, intercourse, or prolonged standing. If the current problem is impairing functional ability, prioritize this.
Vaginal Burning, Discharge, or Itching • Have you ever been treated for an STI? • If you were, were your partner(s) also? • Did you have a follow-up examination to confirm treatment? • Are you aware of the different STIs? • Do you currently have vaginal discharge? If so, is there a color, odor, or consistency to it? • Do you have any itching or burning of your pubic hair, vulva, or vagina?	Differentiate itching between external and internal location. Vaginal discharge is a common symptom of STIs; however, a patient with an STI may have few or no symptoms. External itching can be caused by *pediculosis pubis* ("crabs"), *contact dermatitis, herpes simplex virus, condylomata acuminatum (external genital warts),* or *atrophic vulvitis.* See Tables 19-1 and 19-2.

Questions on Common Symptoms	Rationale/Abnormal Findings

Menstrual Disorders

- Have you experienced irregular menstrual cycles or skipped a cycle?
- Do you have cramps with menses?
- Do you take medication for cramps? How much? How often? Does it help?
- Do you experience preflow bloating, mood swings, headaches, or breast tenderness? Does it go away once your flow begins?
- Are there times other than your period when you have bleeding or spotting?
- Do you experience any bleeding or spotting following intercourse?
- Do menstrual conditions cause you to miss work, school, or activities?

Amenorrhea is the absence of menstrual periods. The most common causes of secondary amenorrhea are pregnancy and anovulation. **Dysmenorrhea** is pain with menses. *Premenstrual syndrome* is the emotional and physical symptoms that occur at the same time before menses each month. Intermenstrual bleeding or spotting or bleeding could indicate infection. Postintercourse bleeding or spotting could indicate an *STI* or *cervical polyp*.

Structural Problems

- Have you been treated for reproductive cancer, endometriosis, uterine fibroids, ovarian cyst, or abnormal bleeding?
- Have you noticed any change in the amount of hair in the vulva or around the abdomen or nipples?
- Have you gained weight especially in the midabdomen in the past 6 months?
- Have you noticed skin changes?

Endometriosis increases risk for infertility. Frequent ovarian cysts and menstrual irregularities warrant evaluation for *polycycstic ovarian syndrome (PCOS)*. Other symptoms of PCOS include obesity, acne, hirsutism, and *acanthosis nigricans* (hyperpigmentation around the back of the neck and under arms).

Hemorrhoids. Do you have hemorrhoids?

They are very common especially following childbirth.

Objective Data Collection

Equipment

Equipment for a full examination with cytological screening includes examination gown; sheet or drape; nonsterile examination gloves (latex and nonlatex); water-soluble vaginal lubricant; light unit (either goose neck or speculum attachment); wooden/plastic spatula; cervical brush (broom); endocervical brush; glass slide; slide fixative; liquid Pap base; culture tubes (DNA) for chlamydia and gonorrhea; sterile cotton swabs; large cotton swabs; small bottles with tops, one containing saline solution, one containing potassium hydroxide, and one containing acetic acid solution (white vinegar); and speculum (preferably warmed via heat source in examination drawer).

Technique and Normal Findings	Abnormal Findings
External Genitalia Inspect pubic hair for amount and distribution. Look for lice or nits. *Hair is evenly distributed and grows downward. No lice or nits are seen.*	Pediculosis pubis presents with itching (see Table 19-2 at the end of this chapter).
Inspect skin for redness, breakdown, papules, or vesicles. Bilaterally observe the inguinal area for erythema, fissures, or enlarged lymph nodes. Inspect the clitoris, noting size and shape. *The clitoris is 1 to 1.5 cm long.*	See Table 19-1 at the end of this chapter.
Inspect the labia majora for size and symmetry. Look for swelling or redness. Small inclusion cysts are common. Inspect the vaginal opening for swelling or redness (Fig. 19-1). *No protrusions are seen.*	See Table 19-1. Vulvar cancer is usually asymptomatic until the lesion becomes large enough that there may be itching, burning, pain, bleeding, or watery discharge. Any discharge or mucus requires a culture.

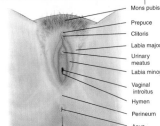

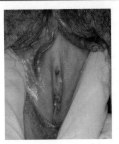

Figure 19.1 Inspecting the vaginal opening (introitus).

Inspect the vestibule for color, redness, swelling, odor, or discharge. Inspect the urethra for position and patency. *There is no discharge or redness.* Observe the Skene's glands at the 1 o'clock and 11 o'clock positions lateral to the urethra. *They are small, noninflamed, and occasionally not seen.*

Candidiasis is associated with vulvovaginal and rectal pruritus and dyspareunia (see Table 19-1).

Inspect the perineum. *The area between the introitus and anus is smooth with no lesions or tears. Any episiotomy scars are healed. The intact anus has no swelling, lacerations, or protrusions.*

Look for contact dermatitis and chancres of syphilis (see Table 19-1).

Internal Genitalia
Using the thumb and middle finger of a gloved hand, separate the inner labia minora. Insert the index finger approximately 1 cm and rotate it so that it faces upward. Gently press the index finger forward to assess the urethra and Skene's glands (Fig. 19-2).

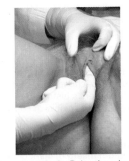

Figure 19.2 Palpating the Skene's glands and urethra.

(text continues on page 416)

Technique and Normal Findings	Abnormal Findings
With the index finger still inserted 1 cm, rotate the finger downward. Palpate with the index finger and thumb to feel the Bartholin's glands (Fig. 19-3). *No swelling or tenderness is noted on either side.*	Abnormal findings include an abscess of Bartholin's glands or urethral caruncle (Table 19-3). 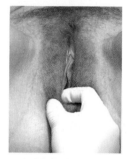 **Figure 19.3** Palpating the Bartholin's glands.
Locate the cervix. Explain to the patient what you are doing. This will help avoid inaccurate placement of the speculum later. While the index finger is still in place, ask the patient to squeeze the vaginal muscles around your finger to check vaginal tone. Ask the patient to then bear down slightly to assess for pelvic organ prolapse.	*Pelvic organ prolapse* is not limited to older women; many times obesity and gravity are factors. See Table 19-4.
Advanced Techniques *Speculum Examination.* The speculum is chosen based on the patient's history. See Box 19-1 for a review of correct use.	
Cervix and Os. With the speculum inserted, inspect the cervix and vaginal walls	Childbirth trauma may have torn the cervix, resulting in an irregular slit. Women who have

(text continues on page 418)

BOX 19.1 Tips For Using A Speculum

- Before use, make sure the speculum is warmed.
- Hold the speculum between the dominant index and middle fingers. The blades must stay together during insertion to avoid pinching the labia or vaginal walls.
- Place the thumb under the thumbscrew on the metal or the lever on the plastic type of speculum. The opposite hand will insert the index finger as done in the initial vaginal examination and place slight pressure downward.
- Do not use lubricants on the speculum because it can interfere with the cytology and culture readings.
- Insert the speculum in an oblique position along the top of the finger. A constant downward insertion prevents the anterior blade of the speculum from hitting the urethra or bladder and causing discomfort or pain. As the speculum moves in and downward, slowly remove the index finger. Have the patient exhale slowly as the speculum is inserted. This helps in relaxing the pubococcygeal muscles.
- Slowly rotate the speculum so that it is in a horizontal position with the bottom blade continuing to be pressed in a downward position at 45 degrees. Once the blade is completely inserted, slowly open the speculum blades while continually keeping a posterior pressure on the lower blade.
- Do not try to force the complete blade in if it causes the patient discomfort or pain.
- For most women the speculum most often used is the Pederson. The length is approximately 6 cm, which is the usual length of the vagina.
- Once the speculum is inserted fully the blades are opened slowly by pressing on the thumbpiece until the cervix comes into view at the end of the blades. As the cervix comes into view, the speculum is locked into place by tightening the screw on the thumb piece. Check with the patient at all steps to make sure she is comfortable.
- If the cervix is not visualized, the speculum may be too high. Repositioning with the blades pressed posterior may be necessary.
- The speculum should be removed in the reverse order of insertion, with careful attention given to keeping the blades open until the cervix is slid away from the blades. The thumb stays on the lever and is slowly released. As the speculum is rotated to an oblique position, the blades are slowly closed avoiding pinching the vaginal walls or labia or pulling the pubic hair.

Technique and Normal Findings	Abnormal Findings

(Fig. 19-4). *Cervix is smooth, pink, and midline. Position depends on uterine angle and may tilt anteriorly or posteriorly. The cervix of a nullipara woman has a small round os, while the parous woman has a horizontal or fish-mouth–looking slit.*

Inspect the surrounding area for increased discharge. *Clear secretions are normal.* If the woman has an intrauterine device, this is the time to check for the strings (two strings clear in color).

had vaginal births may have *nabothian cysts*, small benign nodules that resemble yellow pustules. Additional abnormal findings include *cervical polyps, DES syndrome, cervical dysplasia, carcinoma in situ,* and *cervical cancer* (Table 19-5).

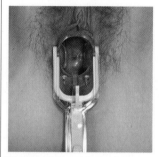

Figure 19.4 View of the normal cervix through the speculum.

Pap Smear and Cultures. The Pap smear screens for cervical cancer. An Ayre's spatula (wood or plastic) is used with an endocervical brush for glass slide examinations. A plastic cytology broom is used for a liquid Pap examination. See Box 19-2 for step-by-step instructions.

The Pap smear is used to evaluate cells from the cervix for precancerous or cancerous status.

Vaginal Wall. The vaginal walls are inspected during insertion and removal of the speculum for lesions, bleeding, erythema, or edema. Atrophic changes to the vaginal lining are common in older women.

Any secretion abnormal in amount, color, or odor is sampled for infection (see Table 19-1).

(text continues on page 420)

BOX 19.2 STEPS IN THE PAP SMEAR

1. The longer portion of the spatula is inserted into the cervical os and rotated 360 degrees as it is pressed against the cervix to gently scrape cells from the **squamocolumnar junction** of the cervix (Fig. A).
   This *transformation zone* includes the outer and inner areas of the endocervix and is the highest site of neoplastic involvement.
2. Secretions obtained from the spatula are then spread on a clear glass slide and a fixative spray is applied.
3. The endocervical brush is then inserted into the endocervix and rotated 720 degrees to ensure an adequate cell sample (Fig. B).
4. The endocervical brush is then gently rolled out on a clean glass slide, avoiding cell destruction. A spray fixative is applied and the slide labeled for cytology.
5. If a liquid base Pap is taken, the plastic broom is used. The tip of the broom is inserted into the endocervix and rotated 720 degrees.
6. The tip of the broom is removed and placed into the liquid solution (Fig. C).

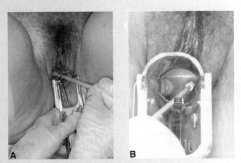

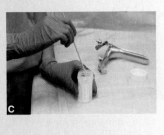

Technique and Normal Findings	Abnormal Findings
Bimanual Examination. Inform the patient that this part of the examination is to assess the ovaries and uterus by manually palpating from inside and outside.	See Tables 19-4 and 19-5.
At this time the examiner removes the gloves and places a new glove on the hand doing the internal examination. The index and second fingers are inserted in a downward fashion and slowly turned upward once the fingers reach the cervix. The thumb is kept upward or tucked in to keep it from pressing on the clitoris. The fingers rest internally at the posterior cervical area. The cervix is palpated for size, shape, and movement. The nonexamining hand is placed midway between the symphysis pubis and umbilicus (Fig. 19-5).	Preinvasive cancer of the cervix is often asymptomatic. In later stages, abnormal bleeding, especially after intercourse, is the first sign. 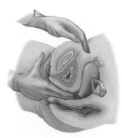 **Figure 19.5** Positioning of the hands in bimanual palpation of the cervix.
The uterus is now palpated between the pads of the fingertips. The uterus is moved upward so that the examining fingers can palpate between the top and back (Fig. 19-6). This position allows for evaluation	*Leiomyomas (fibroid tumors)* can cause abnormal uterine bleeding and back-age, abdominal pressure, constipation, incontinence, and dysmenorrhea if large. *Endometrial cancer* is the

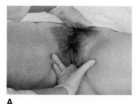
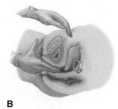

A   **B**

Figure 19.6 Bimanual palpation of the uterus. **(A)** External view. **(B)** Internal position of the hands.

Technique and Normal Findings	Abnormal Findings
of the size and shape of the uterus as well as its ability to move without tenderness or resistance. *Size is approximately 7 × 4 cm (occasionally larger in multigravidas). The uterus feels pear-shaped and smooth and moves freely.*	most common malignancy of the reproductive system and associated with abnormal uterine bleeding, uterine enlargement, or mass.
Once the uterus has been assessed, let the patient know that you are now going to check her ovaries. With the two fingers still deep in the vagina and facing upward, move to the lateral side of the uterus. If the right hand is examining, the fingers move first to the patient's right and the hand on the abdomen is placed medial to the anterior superior iliac spine. The two hands are brought together as close as possible. With a slow sweeping motion the fingers are moved down toward the introitus while allowing the adnexae to be palpated between them (Fig. 19-7). This is repeated on the patient's left side. *The ovary is often not felt, especially in older menopausal women. If palpated, it feels like a small almond.*	See Table 19-4.

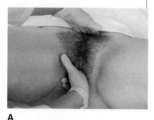
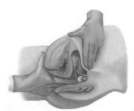

A **B**

Figure 19.7 Bimanual palpation of the ovaries.
(A) External view. **(B)** Internal position of the hands.

(text continues on page 422)

Technique and Normal Findings	Abnormal Findings

Rectovaginal Examination

After completing the vaginal examination, circumstances may warrant a rectovaginal examination (see Chapter 18). The examiner changes gloves and lubricates the index and middle fingers with water-based gel. He or she tells the patient that the examination will be slightly uncomfortable and may create pressure, but should not be painful.

Ask the patient to bear down slightly as the fingers are inserted. The index finger is inserted into the vagina and the middle finger is placed into the rectum (Fig. 19-8). *The septum feels smooth and intact. The posterior portion of the uterus may be felt and is smooth.*

This examination is used to evaluate any *rectocele* (bulging of rectum into the vagina) or *rectovaginal fistula* (opening between the vagina and the rectum allowing feces to enter the vagina).

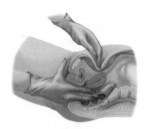

Figure 19.8 Rectovaginal examination.

Documentation of Normal Findings

External genitalia: Even hair distribution; no lesions present. Bartholin's glands, urethral glands, and Skene's glands (BUS): with no erythema, edema, or discharge. Vaginal introitus and walls: pink, moist with normal rugae, good anterior and posterior wall support, and no discharge present. Cervix: smooth round with no lesions and no tenderness upon movement. Uterus: normal size, shape, midposition, and freely mobile. Adnexa: No palpable masses and no tenderness to examination. Perineum: smooth. Anal area: pink, with no hemorrhoids, fissures, or bleeding. Rectal wall: smooth without masses or nodules, and good sphincter control.

♠ Lifespan Considerations

Pregnant Women
Assessment of the pregnant woman is discussed in detail in Chapter 27.

Newborns and Infants
On assessment of the newborn, it is not uncommon to see some pink discharge at the opening of the vagina. This is most often a result of maternal estrogen. In the female child the genitalia continues growing, except for the clitoris. Ambiguous genitalia is a congenital anomaly found in some newborns. This emergent condition requires referral for diagnostic evaluation.

Child and Adolescent
To conduct a genital examination on a young female child, allow the parent to hold her and have the child place her feet together like a frog. Allow the child to participate. Have the parent let the child know that it is OK to allow this examination, especially if she has been taught not to allow anyone to touch her genitals.

Age of onset of puberty in girls has continued to decline. Budding of the breast occurs first, followed by pubic hair, and finally onset of menses. Tanner's stages of female pubic hair are reviewed in Table 19-6.

Genital assessment of the adolescent is not required unless there has been initiation of sexual activity or there are genital tract problems. The opportunity for nurse education is greatest at this time, however. The adolescent is experiencing body changes, self-identity exploration, and relationship questions. The nurse should be direct and honest with the teen. Establishment of a trusting and confidential nurse–patient relationship is vital. Sexually active adolescent females should have an annual examination.

Older Adults
As women age, they experience many changes in the genitourinary tract related to limited or absent estrogen in the system. **Menopause** is 12 consecutive months without menses and usually occurs between 48 and 51 years. As estrogen levels decrease the uterus becomes smaller, the ovaries shrink, the normal vaginal rugae flatten, and the epithelium atrophies. These normal changes may lead to problems such as vaginal infections, urinary tract infections, **dyspareunia**, and

lowered libido. Older women are at increased risk for endometrial cancers and need education regarding abnormal signs and symptoms.

Common Nursing Diagnoses and Interventions

Diagnosis and Related Factors	Nursing Interventions
Ineffective sexuality patterns related to illness and altered body function	Gather sexual history. Determine the patient's and the partner's knowledge. Observe for stress, loss, or depression. Explore physical causes with chronic disease.
Risk for infection	Observe and report signs of infection. Use appropriate hand hygiene and follow standard precautions. Avoid use of indwelling catheters when possible.
Ineffective health maintenance related to deficient knowledge	Assess the patient's feelings about not following safe practices. Assess family patterns. Assist the patient to community groups. Assess access to health services.

Tables of Reference

Table 19.1 Common Infections

Condition and Presentation	Findings
Candidiasis 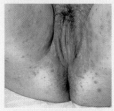	*Examination:* Vulvovaginal edema, erythema, and excoriation; thick white secretions, sometime only along inner vaginal walls *Wet Mount:* Pseudohyphae, occasional budding yeast
Bacterial Vaginosis 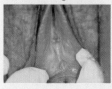	*Examination:* Creamy white to gray secretions that coat the vaginal walls with a strong "fishy" odor and vaginal itching or burning *Wet Mount:* Positive findings of clue cells on microscopy; possibly WBCs present as well
Chlamydia 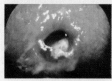	*Examination:* Changes in the cervical condition—reddened, mucopurulent from os, may bleed easily; possibly pain with pelvic examination *Wet Mount:* Increased WBCs and RBCs on slide
Herpes Simplex Type 2 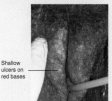 Shallow ulcers on red bases	*Examination:* Scattered vesicles along labia or matching vesicles on labia reflecting "kissing" lesions; surface ulcerations or crusted healing lesions; inguinal lymphadenopathy *Wet Mount:* >10 WBCs per high-powered microscopy

(table continues on page 426)

Condition and Presentation	Findings
Gonorrhea 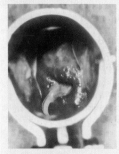	*Examination:* Yellow purulent discharge from the cervix; tenderness or pain with the pelvic examination *Wet Mount:* Gram stain shows intracellular diplococci
Trichomoniasis 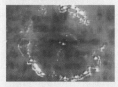	*Examination:* Purulent yellow to green frothy discharge with foul odor; pain on pelvic examination; cervical redness (strawberry-looking) and contact bleeding *Wet Mount:* Motile organisms >10 WBCs per high-powered microscopy
Condalomata Acuminatum 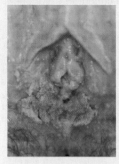	*Examination:* Fleshy pink or gray papilloma or wartlike projections at vulva, vagina, or anus *Wet Mount:* Direct visualization

Chancre

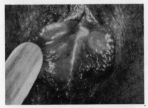

Seen in primary syphilis, this 1-cm buttonlike papule forms at the area of inoculation. This painless lesion with raised borders has a center of serous exudate. Present for 10–90 days.

Urethral Caruncle

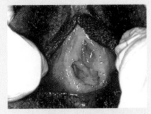

The patient usually has dysuria, hematuria, or frequently no response to antibiotics given for UTI. This condition is seen primarily in postmenopausal women. The caruncle develops from **ectropion** of the posterior urethral wall.

Contact Dermatitis

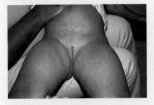

Acute symptoms are external itching or burning, which may extend to the inner thigh. The perineum may be erythematous and possibly excoriated. Occasionally, the perineum has localized wheals or vesicles with possible drainage.

Abscess of the Bartholin's Glands

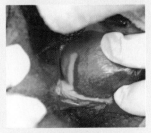

The patient has pain or tenderness in the Bartholin's area. Some abscesses develop gradually but usually very quickly within 2–3 days. They may rupture spontaneously or may need to be incised and drained.

(table continues on page 428)

Table 19.2 **Abnormalities of the External Genitalia** (*continued*)

Pediculosis Pubis (Crab lice)

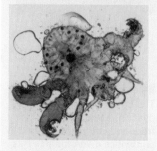

The patient presents with mild to severe itching, especially in the mons pubis and perineum. The external genitalia are excoriated. Tiny spots of blood and lice may be seen on the underwear. Nits (eggs) normally adhere to the pubic hair and can appear as small dark specks. The photo is an enlarged view of a single louse.

Table 19.3 **Pelvic Organ Prolapse Conditions**

Cystocele

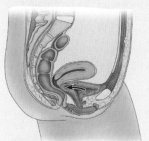

Rectocele

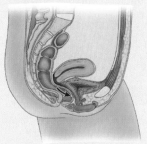

Protrusion of the bladder into the anterior vaginal canal and beyond usually results from weakening of supporting pelvic tissues. The patient may have stress incontinence, urge incontinence, and discomfort with intercourse.

Prolapse of the rectum into the posterior vaginal wall can be from a lack of pelvic tissue support, which commonly follows long vaginal births. The patient has difficulty with bowel movements, pain with intercourse, and rectal pressure.

Table 19.3   Pelvic Organ Prolapse Conditions (*continued*)

Uterine Prolapse

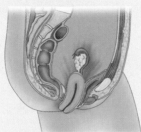

Descent of the uterus into the vagina and beyond results from pelvic relaxation and gradual weakening of uterine ligaments. It may be a consequence of multiple vaginal births or an enlarging uterus. The patient presents with low pressure, fecal impaction, and vaginal and uterine irritation.

Table 19.4   Abnormalities of the Cervix

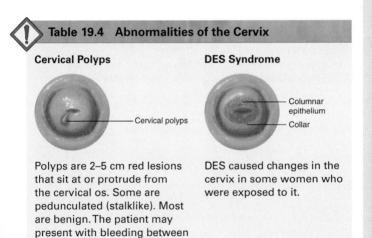

Cervical Polyps

Cervical polyps

Polyps are 2–5 cm red lesions that sit at or protrude from the cervical os. Some are pedunculated (stalklike). Most are benign. The patient may present with bleeding between menses or after intercourse.

DES Syndrome

Columnar epithelium

Collar

DES caused changes in the cervix in some women who were exposed to it.

(table continues on page 430)

Table 19.4   Abnormalities of the Cervix (*continued*)

Cervical Dysplasia, Carcinoma In Situ, and Cervical Cancer

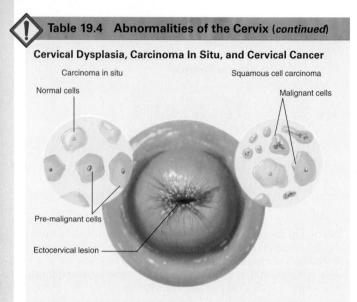

Carcinoma in situ

Squamous cell carcinoma

Normal cells

Malignant cells

Pre-malignant cells

Ectocervical lesion

- Cervical dysplasia is a neoplastic process that does not involve the basement membrane cells. It may also be referred to as cervical intraepithelial neoplasia.
- Carcinoma in situ involves the full thickness of the epithelium.
- Cervical cancer is when carcinoma in situ invades the basement membrane.

Table 19.5   Abnormalities of the Internal
             Reproductive Organs

Endometrosis

Endometrial tissue is found outside the uterus because of a retrograde flow of menstruation into the peritoneal cavity. This tissue adheres to other organs and causes pelvic pain, dyspareunia, dysmenorrhea, and, many times, infertility.

Fluctuant Ovarian Cyst

The ovarian follicle fails to rupture during the maturation phase. A fluid-filled cyst develops and either stays the same size or grows to be greater than the ovaries. The patient does not ovulate and has secondary amenorrhea (no menses). The cysts usually resolve spontaneously within two cycles. If the cyst enlarges, the patient presents with amenorrhea and low pelvic tenderness.

Ectopic Pregnancy

A fertilized ovum implants in a site other than the uterine endometrium. Risk factors include previous ectopic pregnancy, past pelvic infection, endometriosis, or tube abnormalities. The patient presents with symptoms of a normal pregnancy initially. As the ectopic pregnancy grows larger, there is internal hemorrhage and subsequent lower quadrant pain.

Leiomyoma: Uterine Fibroids

This benign condition appears as single or multiple tumors within the uterine wall. The patient presents with heavy flows, irregular bleeding, or pelvic pressure. Many women with fibroids are asymptomatic.

Solid Ovarian Mass

Benign cystic teratoma forms in the ovaries and contains structures such as bone, cartilage, or teeth. Many of the tissues come from dermoid derivatives such as skin, hair follicles, and sebum. This is why it is also known as a *dermoid cyst*. The second mass is a malignant ovarian neoplasm. Symptoms are so vague that many ovarian cancers are not found until advanced stages.

Acute Salpingitis

Salpingitis is also referred to as PID. Infection spreads throughout the uterus and up into the tubes, which swell and rupture. Scarring can occur even with treatment implemented; potential for infertility is high. *Chlamydia trachomatis* and *Neisseria gonorrhoeae* are the most common causative organisms.

Table 19.6 Tanner's Staging: Female Pubic Hair

Stage	Description
Stage 1: Preadolescent	The vellus over the pubes is not further developed than that over the anterior abdominal wall (ie, no pubic hair).
Stage 2 	Long, slightly pigmented, downy hair that is straight or only slightly curled appears chiefly along the labia.
Stage 3 	Hair is considerably darker, coarser, and more curled. It spreads sparsely over the junction of the mons pubis.
Stage 4 	Hair is now adult in type, but the area covered by it is still considerably smaller than in most adults. There is no spread to the medial surface of the thighs.
Stage 5 	Hair is adult in quantity and type, distributed as an inverse triangle of the classically feminine pattern. Spread is to the medial surface of the thighs, but not up the linea alba or elsewhere above the base of the inverse triangle.

Health Assessment Across the Lifespan

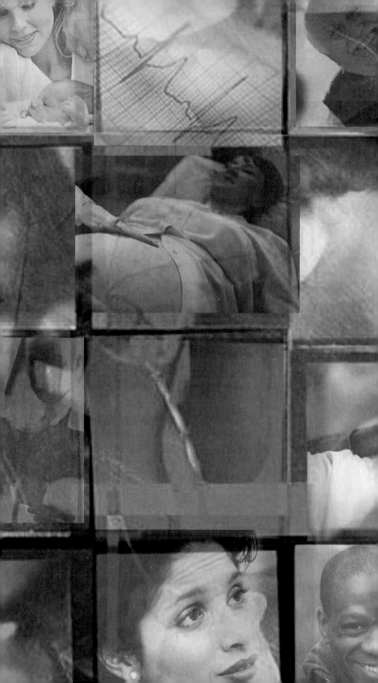

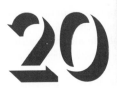

Adult Head-to-Toe Examination

Key Topics and Questions

History of Presenting Problem

Focus questions on issues and symptoms specific to the patient. Doing so, view the patient as a person with multiple issues. For each symptom, be sure to review the following:

- **Location**: "Where does it hurt?"
- **Duration**: "When did it start?" How long has it lasted?"
- **Intensity**: "On a scale of 1 to 10, how do you rate your problem, with 10 being worst?"
- **Quality**: "Tell me what it feels like?"
- **Alleviating/aggravating factors**: "What makes it better? Worse?"
- **Pain goal**: "What level of pain is acceptable to you?"
- **Functional goal**: "What would you like to be able to do if you were not in pain?

Past Health History

- **Assess for allergies**. Include iodine, shellfish, and latex. Assess the patient's reaction including rash, hives, anaphylaxis, uticaria, pruritis, GI upset, nausea, vomiting, or diarrhea. Validate answers against the chart.
- **Obtain past history of illness**. Include medical, surgical, and obstetric history.
- **Obtain list of medications**. Include over-the-counter drugs, herbals, and supplements.
- **Assess family history.** What was the condition? Who had it?
- **Assess childhood illnesses and immunizations**. Include influenza, pneumococcal, and purified protein derivative (PPD).

- **Obtain information on most recent screening assessments.** These include tuberculosis (TB), vision or hearing, and mammograms.
- **Evaluate mental health and psychiatric history.** Medications may provide clues (eg, antidepressants).

Review of Systems

- **General survey:** Fever, chills, weight loss, weight gain, fatigue.
- **Nutrition:** Nausea, loss of appetite, vomiting, indigestion, problems swallowing or chewing.
- **Skin, hair, and nails:** Rash, itch, lesions, nails, hygiene practices, hair loss.
- **Head and neck:** Headaches, dizziness, syncope, seizures, enlarged lymph nodes.
- **Eyes:** Glasses, contacts, blurry vision, double vision, loss of vision, swelling, tearing or dry eyes, and date of last vision examination.
- **Ears:** Hearing loss, pressure, earache.
- **Nose, mouth, and throat:** Congestion, sore throat, voice change, usual dental care, last dental visit.
- **Thorax and lungs:** Shortness of breath, wheezing, cough.
- **Heart:** Fast or slow pulse, heart murmur, chest pain, pounding or fluttering in chest, swelling in feet, rings tighter than usual.
- **Peripheral vascular:** Cramping, pain, numbness in extremities.
- **Breast:** Pain, tenderness, discharge, lump, date of last self-breast examination.
- **Abdominal/gastrointestinal:** Frequency of bowel movements and description, bloody stool, diarrhea, constipation, soiling of clothes, hemorrhoids.
- **Abdominal/genitourinary:** Frequency and description of urine, difficulty or burning with urination, blood in urine, urination at night, urgency, increased frequency, wetting of clothes, feeling of incomplete emptying or dribbling.
- **Musculoskeletal:** Mobility, pain, stiffness, spasm, tremor, gait, impaired balance, foreign bodies, or implants.
- **Neurological:** Headache, one-sided weakness, memory loss, confusion.
- **Genitalia, female:** Vaginal discharge, pain with menstruation, excessive bleeding with menstruation, last menstrual period (LMP), pain with sexual intercourse.
- **Genitalia, male:** Discharge, pain, swelling, lumps, trauma, erectile dysfunction.

- **Endocrine:** Excessive thirst, increased urination, hair loss, skin changes, hot flashes.
- **Mental health:** Anxiety, depression, abnormal thoughts, difficulty sleeping.
- **Summary:** How would you say that your health is in general?

Objective Data Collection

Equipment

Equipment for a comprehensive adult head-to-toe physical assessment includes cotton swabs, drapes, gown, examining gloves, nasal speculum, ophthalmoscope/otoscope, reflex hammer, blood-pressure cuff, scale with height measure, stethoscope, thermometer, tongue blade, watch with second hand, and vision charts. If specimens are needed, additional tools include vaginal speculum, lubricant, culture media, glass slides, KOH, Hemoccult testing cards and solution, and Pap smear spatula.

Technique and Normal Findings	Abnormal Findings
Wash hands or use gel. Wipe stethoscope.	
Vital Signs Obtain temperature. *35.8°C to 37.3°C*	Hypothermia, hyperthermia
Obtain pulse. *60 to 100 bpm*	Tachycardia, bradycardia, irregular rate. If irregular, take apical pulse.
Obtain respirations. *12 to 20/min*	Bradypnea, tachypnea, hyperventilation, Cheyne-Stokes, apnea.
Obtain blood pressure. *Systolic 100 to 12; diastolic 60 to 80 mm Hg*	Hypertension, hypotension, auscultatory gap. Perform orthostatic BP and P if indicated.
Obtain oxygen saturation level. *92% to 100%*	Less than 92%.

(text continues on page 438)

Technique and Normal Findings	Abnormal Findings
General Survey Inspect overall skin color. *Pink*	Pallor, jaundice, flushing, cyanosis, erythema, ruddy, mottled
Evaluate breathing effort. *No dyspnea*	Dyspnea, head of bed elevated, tripod position
Observe appearance. *Appears stated age*	Appears older than stated age
Assess mood. *The patient is calm, pleasant, and cooperative. Appropriate affect.*	Flat or inappropriate affect, depression, elation, euphoria, anxiety, irritable, labile.
Observe nutritional status. *Appears well-nourished.*	Appears poorly nourished, overweight, or obese.
Evaluate personal hygiene. *Good personal hygiene.*	Poor personal hygiene
Assess posture. *Posture erect.*	Slouching, bent to one side
Observe for physical deformities. *No obvious physical deformities.*	Obvious physical deformity present
Perform safety check. *Call bell within reach; bedside stand positioned; ID band correct; IVs, medications, tubes, and drains intact.*	Unsafe environment, medications or IVs not verified.
Skin Inspect skin with each corresponding body area. Inspect color; check for rashes and lesions. *Skin pink, no cyanosis. No telangiectasia, erythema, or papules.*	Changes in skin pigmentation. If there are lesions or rashes, identify configuration. Note any infections or infestations.
Palpate for moisture, temperature, texture, turgor, and edema. *Skin warm, slightly dry, and intact. Good turgor on upper extremities; no edema, lesions, or tenderness.*	Growths or tumors are abnormal. Describe any wounds or incisions including size, depth, color, exudate, and wound borders.
Head Evaluate facial structures. *Symmetrical structures without edema, deformities, or lesions. Patent nares.*	Asymmetry, edema, deformities, ptosis, lesions. Absence of "sniff," deviated septum, polyps, drainage.

Technique and Normal Findings	Abnormal Findings
Observe facial expression. *Appropriate to situation.*	Anxious, facial grimace; facial droop, asymmetry.
Inspect hair and scalp. *Straight hair with normal distribution. Hair supple and thick. Scalp pink and smooth without pests, flaking, lesions, or tenderness.* Palpate cranium, temporal artery, and temporomandibular joint (TMJ). *Normocephalic, head midline. Temporal artery 2 to 3+ bilaterally, nontender. TMJ moves freely; no crepitus or tenderness.*	Facial asymmetry may indicate damage to CN VII or *stroke*. Enlarged bones or tissues are associated with *acromegaly*. A puffy "moon" face is associated with *Cushing's syndrome*. Increased facial hair in females may be a sign of *Cushing's syndrome* or *endocrinopathy*. Periorbital edema is seen with *congestive heart failure* and *hypothyroidism* (*myxedema*).
Assess cranial nerve V, motor strength and light touch, three facial branches. *Strong contraction of muscles and senses light touch on forehead, cheek, and chin.*	Decreased or dulled sensation, weakness, or asymmetric movements.
Assess cranial nerve V and VII: squeeze eyes shut, wrinkle forehead, clench teeth, smile, puff cheeks. *Facial movements are strong and symmetrical.*	A weak blink from facial weakness may result from paralysis of CN V or VII.
Inspect lids, lashes, and brows. *No ptosis, lid lag, discharge, or crusting. Even lash distribution. Brows with hair loss on outer third.*	Depressed or absent corneal response is common in contact lens wearers.
Mouth and Throat Inspect mouth with light and tongue blade. Inspect inside lips, buccal mucosa, gums, teeth, hard/soft palates, uvula, tonsils, pharynx, tongue, and floor of mouth (APRN may use light from otoscope). *Lips, mucosa, gums, and palates are pink and smooth. Floor of mouth intact, moist, smooth. Pharynx pink, intact. Tongue pink and rough. No lesions or tenderness. Teeth white, intact with good occlusion.*	Lesions, sponginess, or edema; bleeding gums; missing or discolored teeth; malocclusion; inflammation or tenderness of ducts.

(text continues on page 440)

Technique and Normal Findings	Abnormal Findings
Grade tonsils. *Tonsils 0 to 2+. Pink with no discharge or lesions.*	Swollen glands or tonsils (3+ to 4+).
Note mobility of uvula when patient says "ahh." *Uvula midline and symmetrical.*	Uvula asymmetrical or enlarged.
Assess cranial nerve XII; look for symmetry of tongue when extended. *Tongue midline; extends symmetrically.*	A tongue that deviates to one side is common with *stroke*.
Eyes	
Assess near and distant vision. *Reads newsprint accurately. Snellen test 20/20.*	Less than 20/20 corrected. Vision blurred. Note use of glasses, contact lenses, or assistive devices.
Inspect conjunctiva and sclera. *Pink, moist conjunctiva; white sclera.*	Sclera yellow with *jaundice*. Conjunctiva pink with *inflammation*.
Inspect cornea, iris, and anterior chamber. *Cornea and lens are clear.* Assess cranial nerves III, IV, and VI and extraocular movements (EOMs). *EOMs intact, no nystagmus.* Assess visual fields, peripheral vision. *Visual fields equal to examiner's.*	A narrow angle indicates *glaucoma*. Cloudiness of the lens can indicate *cataract*.
Darken room. Obtain light. Assess cranial nerve II. *Pupils equal, round, and reactive to light and accommodation (PERRLA L 6-4, R 6-4).*	Asymmetry, pinpoint, or "blown" pupils; describe measure of pupil and response to light.
With an ophthalmoscope, check red reflex, disc, vessels, and macula. *Red reflex symmetric. Discs cream-colored with sharp margins. Retina pink. No hemorrhages or exudates; no arteriolar narrowing. Macula yellow.*	(Advance practice)

Technique and Normal Findings	Abnormal Findings
Ears Turn on lights. Inspect ear alignment. *Ears aligned properly.* Palpate auricle, lobe, and tragus. *Ears are without lesions, crusting, masses, or tenderness.*	Microtia, macrotia, edema, cartilage pseudomonas infection, carcinoma on auricle, cyst, and frost bite are abnormal findings.
Change to otoscope head. Perform otoscope examination of canal and tympanic membrane. Move to opposite side of patient. *Canals with small amount of moist yellow cerumen. Tympanic membranes intact, gray, and translucent; light reflex and body landmarks present.*	Redness, external swelling, and discharge indicate *external otitis.* Obstructed canal can be by either foreign body or cerumen.
Assess cranial nerve VIII hearing. *Whispered words heard bilaterally.*	Unable to repeat whispered words.
Obtain tuning fork. Perform Rinne test (on mastoid) if the patient has hearing loss. *Air conduction longer than bone conduction.*	Bone conduction longer or the same as air conduction is evidence of *conductive hearing loss.*
Perform Weber test (at midline of skull) if the patient has hearing loss. *No lateralization.*	Unilateral identification of the sound indicates *sensorineural loss* in the ear that the patient did not hear the sound or had reduced perception.
Nose and Sinuses Inspect external nose. *Midline, no flaring or crusting.*	Asymmetry, swelling, or bruising from trauma or with lesions or growths.
Assess nostril patency. *Patent bilaterally.*	Unable to sniff because of *deviated septum* or *obstructed nares.*
Perform otoscopic examination of mucosa, turbinates, and septum. *Nasal mucosa pink, intact; no polyps. No drainage. Turbinates and septum intact and symmetrical.*	Infection, inflammation of nasal mucosa may be present with *viral, bacterial, or allergic rhinitis.*

(text continues on page 442)

Technique and Normal Findings	Abnormal Findings
Palpate frontal and maxillary sinuses. *No frontal or maxillary sinus tenderness.*	Redness and swelling over the sinuses may represent *acute infection, abscess, or mucocele.*
Neck Inspect symmetry. *Neck symmetrical, moves freely without crepitus.*	Neck asymmetrical or with crepitus
Test flexion, extension, lateral bending, rotation, range of motion (ROM), and strength. *Full ROM, strength 4 to 5+ bilaterally.*	Reduced neck ROM is less than 4+.
Palpate tracheal position midline. *Trachea at midline.*	Deviated trachea.
Palpate carotid pulse. *Carotid pulse 2 to 3+ bilaterally.*	Carotid pulses may be reduced from *carotid stenosis.*
Inspect jugular veins. *No jugular venous distention.*	Jugular veins may be either flat or distended.
Palpate preauricular, post-auricular, occipital, posterior cervical, tonsillar, submandibular, submental, anterior cervical, and supraclavicular nodes. *They are not palpable or tender.*	Lymph nodes are not freely movable or are tender.
Neurological Assess mental status and level of consciousness. *The patient is alert. Eyes open spontaneously.*	Agitated, asleep, lethargic, obtunded, restless, stuporous. Use coma scale if reduced. Does not respond to stimuli or pain; decorticate rigidity, decerebrate rigidity, or no response to pain.
Assess orientation. *Oriented × 3.*	A&O × 2 (person and place). A&O × 1 (person). Disoriented × 3.
Assess ability to follow commands. *Follows directions.*	Unable to follow commands, such as squeeze my hand or sit up.
Evaluate short- and long-term memory. *Immediate, recent, and distant memory intact.*	Immediate, recent, or distant memory impaired; describe specific details.

Technique and Normal Findings	Abnormal Findings
Assess speech. *Speech clear.*	Speech difficult to understand.
Assess hearing. *Hears voices and responds appropriately.*	Difficulty understanding spoken words. Hard of hearing. Note hearing aids or assistive devices.

Upper Extremities

Evaluate circulation, movement, and sensation (CMS). Assess hands and joints. Evaluate nails on upper extremities. *CMS intact. Nails smooth without clubbing. Joints without swelling or deformity.*	Decreased CMS, including color, temperature; capillary refill greater than 3 seconds, pulses, decreased movement, decreased sensation, and paresthesia. Nails are breakable, cracking, inflamed, jagged, bitten, and clubbing.
Perform hand grasp for ROM and muscle strength. *4 to 5+ muscle strength symmetrical.*	Decreased ROM, swelling, or nodules in joints. Muscle strength asymmetrical or 0 to 3+
Musculoskeletal and Neurological. Perform finger-to-nose test if indicated. *Smooth and intact.*	*Ataxia* is an unsteady, wavering movement with inability to touch the target. During rapid alternating movements, lack of coordination is *adiadochokinesia.*
Test rapid alternating movements if indicated. *Smooth and intact.*	Inability to identify objects correctly (*astereognosis*) may result from damage to the sensory cortex caused by *stroke.*
Test stereognosis if indicated. *The patient identifies key or other object.*	Cortical sensory function may be compromised following a *stroke.*
Test graphesthesia if indicated. *The patient identifies the number 8 or another number.*	

Anterior Thorax

Assess breathing effort, rate, rhythm, and pattern; position to breathe. *Breathes easily, with symmetrical expansion and contraction.*	Dyspnea, orthopnea, paroxysmal nocturnal dyspnea. Rhythm regular, sitting straight upright, or using tripod position to breathe.

(text continues on page 444)

Technique and Normal Findings	Abnormal Findings
Inspect chest shape and skin. *AP to transverse ratio 1:2 symmetrical. Skin intact.* If patient is on an examination table, inspect costovertebral angle, configuration, and pulsations. *No pulsations visible. No dyspnea, retractions, or accessory muscle use.*	Barrel chest, funnel chest, pigeon chest, thoracic kyphoscoliosis.
Auscultate breath sounds. *Bronchovesicular sounds midline, vesicular in lung periphery. Lung sounds clear.*	Diminished or absent breath sounds, bronchial or bronchovesicular sounds in lung periphery. Describe adventitious sounds (crackles, gurgles, wheezes, stridor, pleural rub). Are they inspiratory or expiratory? Do they clear with coughing? Where specifically do you hear them?
Assess for cough, inspect sputum. *No cough or sputum.*	Cough (brassy, harsh, loose, productive) present. Sputum (color, consistency, amount) present.
Inspect precordium. *Point of maximal impulse (PMI) may be visible or absent.*	PMI lateral to midclavicular line; heaves or thrills.
Assess heart rate, rhythm, murmurs, and extra sounds. *Heart rate and rhythm regular. No gallops, murmurs, or rubs.*	Tachycardia, bradycardia, irregular rhythm, murmurs (systolic versus diastolic), extra sounds (S3, S4, friction rub).
Auscultate heart with bell at apex and left sternal border with the patient lying down. Auscultate heart with diaphragm in aortic, pulmonic, left sternal border, tricuspid, and mitral, with patient on left side. *Heart rate and rhythm regular; no murmurs, gallops, or rubs.*	If rhythm is irregular, identify if the irregularity has a pattern or is totally irregular. For example, every third beat missed would be a regular irregular rhythm. No detectable pattern is characteristic of *atrial fibrillation*, common in older adults. Murmurs, rubs, or gallops are abnormal in adults.
Palpate chest for fremitus, thrill, heaves, and point of maximal impulse. *Tactile fremitus symmetrical; no thrill, heave, or lift. Cardiac impulse nonpalpable.*	Asymmetrical fremitus may occur with unilateral disease (eg, lung tumor). Thrills, heaves, and lifts indicate turbulence over a valve and are abnormal.

Technique and Normal Findings	Abnormal Findings
Percuss anterior chest from apex to base and sides. *Lung fields resonant with dullness over heart area.*	Dull lung percussion indicates increased consolidation as with *pneumonia*.
Auscultate carotid artery. *No bruit.*	Bruits over the carotid indicate *carotid artery stenosis*.
Breasts	
Inspect the breasts. Have the patient raise arms overhead, press hands together, and lean forward. *No retraction or dimpling; symmetrical movement.*	Retraction, dimpling, or discharge may indicate *breast cancer*.
Palpate breasts and nipple for discharge. *No lesions or masses; no discharge. Nontender.*	
Palpate axillary nodes. *Axillary nodes not palpable, nontender.*	Positive nodes may indicate *breast cancer*, especially if immovable or tender.
Abdomen	
Inspect abdomen. *Abdomen symmetrical, rounded, or flat. Smooth, intact skin without lesions or rashes. Peristalsis and pulsations evident in thin patients. Flat, round umbilicus.*	Scars, striae, ecchymosis, lesions, prominent dilated veins, rashes, marked pulsation. Red, everted, enlarged, or tender umbilicus.
Auscultate bowel sounds. *Bowel sounds present in all quadrants.*	Hypoactive, hyperactive, or absent bowel sounds.
Auscultate aorta, renal, and femoral arteries with bell. *No bruit.*	Venous hum, friction rub, and bruits are abnormal arterial sounds.
Percuss abdomen in all quadrants and for gastric bubble.	Abdomen tympanic in all quadrants. Gastric bubble percussed 6th left ICS at midclavicular line (MCL).
Percuss liver margin at right MCL.	Liver border above ribs at right MCL.
Percuss spleen.	Spleen percussed in 10th left ICS posterior to midaxillary line.

(text continues on page 446)

Technique and Normal Findings	Abnormal Findings
Palpate abdominal tenderness, distention in all quadrants. *Nontender, soft.* Palpate liver, spleen, and kidneys. *Liver lower border less than one finger below costal border at right MCL. Spleen and kidneys nonpalpable.*	Large masses, hard, tenderness with guarding or rigidity, rebound tenderness. Liver palpable more than one finger below costal border at right MCL.
Palpate aorta, femoral pulses, and inguinal lymph nodes or hernias. *Aorta palpable, smooth. Femoral pulses 2 to 3+. No inguinal nodes or hernias.*	An enlarged aorta (>3 cm) or one with lateral pulsations that are palpable can indicate *abdominal aortic aneurysm.*
Evaluate swallowing, chewing, aspiration risk, special diet. *Eats more than 75% of meal without difficulty.*	Dysphagia, impaired chewing, impaired swallowing, medically prescribed diet, tube feedings, significant weight gain/loss.
Ask about nausea, vomiting, constipation, diarrhea. *No N/V/D.*	Nausea, vomiting, constipation, or diarrhea. Describe characteristics of emesis (eg, coffee grounds, blood).
Inspect stool; record last bowel movement. Ask about passing flatus. *Last BM within patient's normal, soft and brown. Passing flatus.*	Dark stool may indicate blood in it. If hemorrhoids are present, the stool may be normal but has bright red blood coating it.
Inspect urine color, character, and amount with voiding. *Urine clear, yellow, and greater than 30 mL/hr.*	Urine dark, bloody, red, with sediment, cloudy, or less than 30 mL/hr.
Lower Extremities Inspect skin and nails for symmetry, edema, veins, and lesions. *Toenails white and smooth. Skin intact, slightly pale, and symmetrical, without edema, varicose veins, or lesions.*	Note areas of pressure on heels and if they blanch with pressure. Lesions, ulcers, varicosities, edema. Mottled, ruddy, reddened, or flaky skin. Note indurations with infection or inflammation.
Palpate dorsalis pedis pulses bilaterally. Palpate popliteal pulse and posterior tibial pulse. *Pulses 2 to 3+.*	Diminished or absent pulses. If present, obtain Doppler for assessment. Bounding (4+) pulses are also abnormal.

Technique and Normal Findings	Abnormal Findings
Assess capillary refill on both feet. *Brisk capillary refill less than 3 seconds.*	Capillary refill greater than 3 seconds.
Inspect and palpate edema on ankle, shin. *No edema.*	1+ barely perceptible (2 mm) 2+ moderate (4 mm) 3+ moderate (6 mm) 4+ severe (>8 mm)
Palpate for tenderness and temperature. *Feet warm, no tenderness.*	Tenderness to palpation, feet cool or cold.
Palpate lower extremities and joints from hips to toes. *No tenderness or swelling.*	
Observe ROM of joints. *Full joint ROM.*	Limited or reduced ROM.
Test muscle strength on feet, observe for symmetry. Test muscle strength in hips, knees, and ankles. *Strength 4 to 5+.*	Strength 0 to 3+
Test sensation. *Appropriately identifies when touched.*	Loss of sensation
Obtain reflex hammer. Perform deep tendon reflexes—patellar, Achilles, and Babinski. *Patellar, Achilles DTRs 2+; Babinski negative.*	If reflexes are 3 to 4+ they are brisker than normal. If they are 0 to 1+, they are diminished or absent. A positive Babinski indicates a poor neurological outcome.
Posterior Thorax Move behind the patient. Palpate thyroid. *Thyroid borders palpable, no masses, nodules, or enlargement noted.*	Thyroid enlargement or masses can be seen more easily when the patient swallows and while illuminating the neck with a tangential light.
Inspect skin, symmetry, configuration, and observe respirations. *Chest oval, symmetrical, without barrel chest. AP: transverse ratio 1:2. Respirations 20 without dyspnea.*	In barrel chest, which can accompany chronic obstructive pulmonary disease (*COPD*), the transverse: AP ratio approximates 1:1, giving the chest a round appearance.
Palpate spine and scapulae. *Spine straight, without scoliosis, kyphosis, or lordosis. Scapulae symmetrical.*	Scoliosis and kyphosis can limit respiratory excursion. Asymmetry and paradoxical respirations occur in *flail chest*.

(text continues on page 448)

Technique and Normal Findings	Abnormal Findings
Assess tactile fremitus. *Tactile fremitus symmetrical.*	Increased tactile fremitus over an area indicates increased consolidation.
Percuss posterior chest from apex to base to sides. *Lung fields resonant.*	Dullness occurs with increased consolidation; hyperresonance occurs with hyperinflation as in *COPD*.
Test flank tenderness (kidney). *No tenderness to indirect percussion.*	Kidney tenderness is present with *urinary tract infection*.
Auscultate breath sounds. *Breath sounds clear.*	Coarse breath sounds are abnormal. Crackles, gurgles (ronchii), and wheezing are abnormal adventitious sounds.
Inspect lower back, buttocks (redness, symmetry). *No redness, breakdown.* Inspect spine. *Spine straight, skin intact.*	Any redness, especially over pressure areas, is a concern. Scoliosis, lordosis, and kyphosis are abnormal spine findings.

Gait and Balance/Fall Risk

Evaluate fall risk: history of falling, secondary diagnosis, ambulatory aid, IV therapy, gait, and mental status. *Scores at low risk on fall scale.*	Gait abnormalities include hesitancy, unsteadiness, staggering, reaching for external support, high stepping, foot scraping, inability to completely raise the foot off the floor, persistent toe or heel walking, excessive pointing of toes, asymmetry of step height or length, limping, stooping, wavering, shuffling, waddling, excessive swinging of pelvis or shoulders, and slow or rapid speed.

Musculoskeletal and Neurological

Perform heel-to-shin test for coordination. *Smooth, coordinated movement.* Have the patient stand. Note muscle strength and coordination when moving. *Moves easily in the environment.*	The dominant side usually has slightly better coordination. Poor coordination may be from pain, injury, deformity, or *cerebellar disorders*.

Technique and Normal Findings	Abnormal Findings
Observe spinal alignment, hip level, gluteal and knee folds. *Spine straight, posture erect.* Assess spine flexion, extension, lateral bending, and rotation. *Full ROM in spine.*	*Scoliosis* or low back pain may cause the patient to lean forward or to the side when standing or sitting.
Ask the patient to walk on heels and then toes, and then to stand on one foot and then the other. *Good balance and coordination.*	
Skin Breakdown Evaluate risk for skin breakdown: sensory perception, moisture, activity, mobility, nutrition, friction, and shear. *Scores at low risk for skin breakdown.*	High scores on the Braden scale place the patient at high risk.
Wounds, Drains, and Devices Assess intravenous, drainage, catheter, suction. *Wound healing, drains intact, catheter draining well, suction on. IV site clean, dry intact without erythema or tenderness.*	Pressure ulcers may be deep tissue, Stage I, Stage II, Stage III, Stage IV, or unstagable. Wound drainage is classified as serous (clear), sanguineous (bloody), serosanguineous (mixed), fibrinous (sticky yellow), or purulent (pus). Note any signs or symptoms of infection.
Male Genitalia Obtain gloves and Hemoccult card. *No redness, discharge skin intact.* Palpate the scrotum. *No tenderness, lumps, or masses.*	Abnormal findings are no hair, patchy growth, or distribution in a female or triangular pattern; infestations; inflammation; lesions, or dermatitis.
Assess for inguinal hernia. *No hernia.*	
Female Genitalia Obtain gloves, speculum, gel, and hemoccult card. Inspect perineal and perianal areas. *No redness or tenderness, skin intact.*	Vulvar or vaginal pain, flu-like symptoms (eg, chills, fever), sores on the vulva or genital region, scattered vesicles along the labia, matching vesicles on the labia reflecting "kissing" lesions, surface ulcerations or crusted healing lesions, and inguinal lymphadenopathy.

(text continues on page 450)

Technique and Normal Findings	Abnormal Findings
Insert speculum. Inspect cervix and vaginal walls. *Vaginal walls pink, no lesions. Cervix pink, round, with no discharge.* Obtain specimens. Remove speculum. *No infections, Pap test negative.*	(For advanced practice)
Perform bimanual examination of cervix, uterus, and adnexa. *No pain when moving cervix, uterus midline; no enlargement, masses or tenderness. Adnexa and ovaries smooth, no masses or tenderness.*	(For advanced practice)

Rectum

Inspect perianal area. *No redness or tenderness; skin intact.*	Look for thrombosed hemorrhoids, rectal fissures, or hard stool.
With lubricated finger, palpate rectal wall (and prostate in male). *No hemorrhoids, fissures, lesions, masses, or tenderness. Rectal wall intact. Male: prostate smooth and round.* Obtain stool sample for occult blood. *Stool soft and brown.*	(For advanced practice)

Closure

Summarize findings for patient. "Does this sound accurate?" • Assess room for safety (bedside table, lights, call light, toileting). "Do you have any concerns?" • Assess for questions or further needs. "Is there anything else I can do?" • Wash hands or use hand gel when leaving.	Summarizing findings provides closure and ensures accurate conclusions. Asking an open-ended question allows the patient to add any other information that might have been overlooked. Assessing for safety is of primary importance. Always assess the patient and environment for risks. Follow up on care planning and interventions for the next visit.

21

Pregnant Women

Subjective Data Collection

Key Topics and Questions for Health Promotion

Key Questions	Rationales/Abnormal Findings
Family History. Do you have a family history of diabetes, hypertension, twins, or genetic illnesses?	Positive family history of these findings may increase the patient's risk for them.
Age. What is your date of birth? What is your age?	Pregnant teens have increased nutritional requirements and are at increased risk for complications, especially preeclampsia. Mothers who will be 35 years or older at the time of birth are at increased risk for miscarriage and genetic anomalies and may have increased preexisting health problems.
Culture. With what ethnicity you identify? Do you have a religious preference?	Some cultures or religions have important childbirth rituals or norms. Some genetic diseases or pregnancy complications (eg, gestational diabetes, hypertension) are more prevalent in certain ethnic groups.
Pregnancy History. What previous miscarriages, terminations, or pregnancies have you had?	Document each by date, length of gestation, length of labor, type of delivery, type of anesthesia and any adverse reaction, sex and weight of the infant, and complications. Past patterns can suggest possible current issues.

(text continues on page 452)

Key Questions	Rationales/Abnormal Findings
Pap Smears. Have you had any abnormal Pap smears in the past?	Patients with past abnormalities may have a recurrence with pregnancy.
Sexually Transmitted Infections (STIs). Have you had any past STIs?	Verify that prior STIs were treated according to protocol. Assess risk of reexposure, because many STIs are potentially harmful to the fetus.
Breast History. Have you had any breast reductions or implants? Any abnormal mammogram results?	Document surgeries and whether an attempt was made to preserve the ability to breast-feed. Document any other breast health issues, type of nipple (everted, flat, inverted), and past difficulties with nursing.
Infertility. Have you had any problems with infertility?	If conception or pregnancy was difficult, fully document her history, including any medication or type of assisted reproduction used.
Psychological Issues. Do you have depression, anxiety, or eating disorders?	Pregnant women with a history of these psychiatric conditions are at risk for exacerbations.
Headaches. Have you had headaches or migraines?	Patients with frequent headaches may need to change their medication, especially in the third trimester. Those with frequent migraines are at increased risk for postpartum stroke. Severe headaches may signify *preeclampsia*.
Allergies. Do you have any allergies? What is your reaction?	Some conditions common in pregnancy (ie, urinary tract infections [UTIs], positive Group B Strep status) are treated with antibiotics, to which a patient may be allergic.
Violence. Do you have a history of physical abuse, sexual abuse, or exposure to violence?	Pregnancy and labor can elicit painful memories or cause overprotective behavior. Also, pregnancy is a time when domestic violence increases.

Key Questions	Rationales/Abnormal Findings
Contraception. What type of contraception have you used? When did you last use it?	It may be difficult to establish ovulation and likely date of childbirth in patients who were using hormonal contraceptives prior to pregnancy. If conception date is unclear, ultrasound dating in the first trimester can be offered.
Support System. What type of support system do you have?	Patients without a stable support system are at risk for poor nutrition, domestic violence, poor housing, and increased stress.
Personal Habits. Do you use tobacco, alcohol, or other drugs?	Provide support and cessation resources to patients who want them.
Recent Immigration. How long have you lived in this country?	Immigrants are at risk for infections and cephalopelvic disproportion. Another consideration is female circumcision, which reduces the size of the introitus.
Access to Care. Do you have any financial concerns? Are you able to come to appointments?	Patients with no access to medical care before pregnancy are less likely to have had a preconception visit.

Key Topics and Questions for Common Symptoms

Common Symptoms in Pregnancy

- Morning sickness
- Growing pains
- Increased vaginal discharge
- Increased urination
- Breast tenderness or discharge
- Periumbilical pain in the second trimester
- Fetal hiccups
- Braxton Hicks contractions

For each symptom, be sure to review location, characteristics, duration, aggravating factors, alleviating factors, accompanying symptoms, treatment, and the patient's view of the problem.

Key Questions	Rationales/Abnormal Findings
Morning Sickness. Have you been experiencing nausea, vomiting, or other physical symptoms with this pregnancy? • Is there a particular time you have symptoms? • Does anything relieve symptoms? • Does anything make symptoms worse?	Morning sickness is thought to be associated with high estrogen levels, diet, and emotions. Usually, morning sickness can be managed on an outpatient basis if the woman increases B vitamins and fluid intake and uses methods of relaxation. For most patients, nausea and vomiting are a self-limiting condition that does not require medical intervention.

△ *SAFETY ALERT 21-1*
With hyperemesis gravidarum, women cannot keep anything in their stomach long enough to digest. They lose weight and experience fluid and electrolyte imbalances. They may require IV fluids or even hospitalization.

Growing Pains • Have you experienced pains or other sensations in your lower abdomen? • Describe how they feel and how long they last. • Does movement or activity trigger the pains? • How often do they occur?	In the first trimester, stretching of the round and broad ligaments that support the growing uterus cause sharp, short pains with a stabbing quality.
Discharge • Have you noticed any increase in vaginal discharge? • Describe the quantity and quality. • Does it have an odor or color? • Do you have any itching, burning, or discomfort associated with it?	Pregnant women have increased clear vaginal discharge from increased estrogen production. Patients describe this discharge as just like normal discharge, except that there is more of it. Discharge like nasal mucus or cottage-cheese, any color other than clear, or with a foul odor, may be from vaginal infection or *STI*.
Increased Urination • Have you noticed a need to urinate more frequently? • How much water are you drinking every day?	Increased urination results from increased progesterone. This is one reason why it is important for the woman to drink 2 L/day of water. If urinary frequency is

Key Questions	Rationales/Abnormal Findings
• How often do you urinate? • Is urination accompanied by any pain or pressure? • Any blood in urine?	accompanied by suprapubic pressure, dysuria (painful urination), hematuria (blood in the urine), or flank pain, she may have an *UTI*.
Breast Tenderness and Discharge • Have you noticed any change in the size of your breasts? • Have you experienced any breast pain or feelings of fullness? • Have you noticed any nipple discharge? If so, please describe it.	Some patients feel breast changes even before the pregnancy test is positive. Rapid growth of alveoli, addition of a fat layer, and construction of the duct system for breast-feeding can result in feelings of fullness or even pain. A supportive, properly fitted bra and acetaminophen if necessary can help relieve pain. Later in pregnancy, the patient may notice nipple discharge, which is almost always colostrum leaking in preparation for birth. The provider should verify that discharge is not from infection or a tumor.
Periumbilical Pain • Have you experienced any pain or pressure around your umbilicus? • If so, does any movement or activity trigger the pain?	About halfway through pregnancy, women commonly feel a stretching pain all around the umbilicus, resulting from ligaments stretching as the uterus accommodates the growing fetus.
Fetal Hiccups and Other Spasms • Do you notice any regular fetal movements? • Do you think the fetus is having hiccups or sucking the thumb?	Fetal hiccups result from spasms of the fetal diaphragm triggered by an immature neurological system. Mothers sometimes report that it feels as if the fetus is having a seizure. Rarely, this is true. Such symptoms tend to resolve near term.
Braxton Hicks Contractions • Have you experienced any irregular contractions with this pregnancy?	Braxton Hicks contractions prepare the body for labor. They are usually irregular, with fewer than five in 1 hour. They are also

(text continues on page 456)

Key Questions	Rationales/Abnormal Findings
• How often and how long do they last? • How painful are these contractions? • Does anything resolve the contractions?	short (<30 seconds) but may be painful. They may begin as early as the second trimester, especially for patients who have had babies before, but are more common in the third trimester. They are to be differentiated from preterm labor contractions, which are regular, do not resolve, occur more frequently than four in 1 hour, get longer and stronger over time, and result in cervical change.

Objective Data Collection

Assessment During the Initial Visit

Technique and Normal Findings	Abnormal Findings
General Survey/Vital Signs. Document weight, blood pressure, other vital signs, and pain level (Fig. 21-1). Obtain a urine sample. Test urine for glucose and protein.	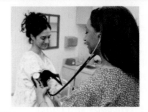 **Figure 21.1** Assessing the patient's blood pressure.
Nutrition. Most women gain little weight in the first trimester. A simple rule of thumb for a woman of normal prepregnant weight is that she will gain about 10 lbs by 20 weeks and about 1 lb/week for the remaining 20 weeks, for a total of 25 to 30 lbs.	Call excessive (or not enough) weight gain to the attention of the provider.
Nutritional requirements in pregnancy are to increase intake by 300 cal/day in the second and	Women who fail to meet these nutritional requirements risk *low birth weight* or *intrauterine*

Technique and Normal Findings	Abnormal Findings
third trimesters, complete protein intake to 60 g/day, elemental iron intake by 27 mg/day, and vitamin intake. A good resource for women to check dietary adequacy is www.mypyramid.gov	*growth restricted babies* and increased difficulties with breast-feeding.
Skin. Inspect the skin. Increased melanization may lead to **linea nigra** (hyperpigmented line from symphysis pubis to top of the fundus) and **chloasma** (blotchy areas on the cheeks, nose, and forehead).	
Abdomen. Smooth muscles (ie, intestines and kidneys) relax and dilate as a result of increased circulating progesterone levels.	Stasis can result, causing *constipation* and *UTIs*.
By 10 to 12 weeks, it is common to be able to hear the fetal heartbeat with a Doppler (Fig. 21-2). Place ultrasonic gel on the Doppler's transducer and then apply the device to the woman's abdomen. In the first trimester, the fetal heartbeat usually is audible just above the symphysis pubis. If the uterus is palpable superior to the pubic bone, the heartbeat may be heard higher in the abdomen as well.	For overweight women, it may take until 14 weeks to hear the heartbeat with a Doppler. Morbidly obese women may need serial ultrasounds to monitor fetal well-being.

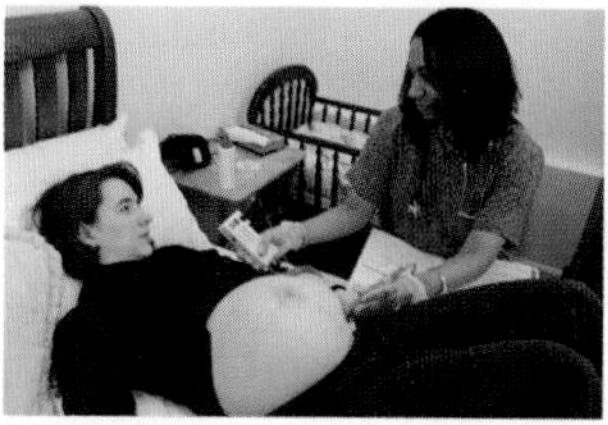

Figure 21.2 Use of Doppler ultrasound.

(text continues on page 458)

Technique and Normal Findings	Abnormal Findings
As pregnancy progresses, the experienced RN can palpate the fetal back, which feels firm and smooth. Usually, it is easiest to hear the fetal heart by placing the Doppler on the fetal back, because the bony skeleton transmits sound well.	
By the end of pregnancy, the uterus would have stretched and grown by more than 15-fold (Fig. 21-3).	Stretching of supporting ligaments can lead to sharp round pain as soon as the first trimester.

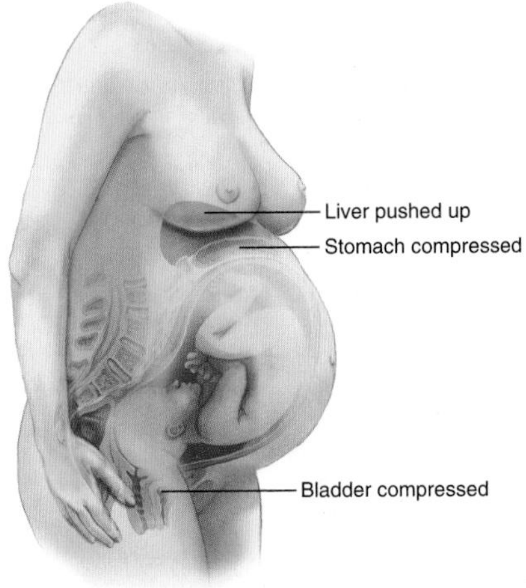

Liver pushed up
Stomach compressed
Bladder compressed

Figure 21.3 Growth of the uterus near term.

Breasts. First-trimester changes include increased breast size and more fullness and sensitivity. Areolae may darken and Montgomery glands may become more prominent. Nipples may be more erectile.	Breast changes may result in upper backache. Some women notice growth of accessory breast tissue, often near the axillae.
Genitalia. The woman may notice frequent urination and increased normal vaginal secretions.	

Assessment During Routine Pregnancy Visits

Technique and Normal Findings	Abnormal Findings
General Survey/Vital Signs. Ask the patient how she is doing. Elicit a description of and chart any problems.	Counsel patients who feel dizzy to sit down. Check for postural hypotension. Other possible causes of dizziness include dehydration, anemia, edema of the inner ear, and hypoglycemia.
Checking the urine, including specific gravity to ensure hydration. Draw blood, if ordered, to check for low blood glucose level or anemia.	Proteinuria 1+ or greater may indicate *preeclampsia*. Other signs of preeclampsia include significantly increased blood pressure; sudden edema, especially of the face; persistent headache; and malaise.
Skin. Changes over pregnancy are primarily attributable to the increasing fetus, uterus, and amniotic fluid volume (Fig. 21-4). The woman may get **striae gravidarum** ("stretch marks") on the abdomen, thighs, and breasts. Linea nigra may darken, and terminal hairs may appear on the abdomen.	

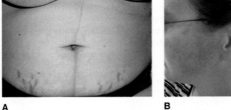

A   **B**

Figure 21.4 **(A)** Linea nigra and striae. **(B)** Melasma.

Technique and Normal Findings	Abnormal Findings
Nose, Mouth, and Throat. Capillaries with lax walls proliferate from increased production of progesterone by the placenta.	Epistaxis (nosebleed) is common. Some women have cervical spotting when a capillary breaks.
Thorax and Lungs. Respirations increase. The growing fetus limits the ability of the lungs to expand.	Toward the end of the second trimester, women may experience dyspnea with exertion.

(text continues on page 460)

Technique and Normal Findings	Abnormal Findings
Although respiratory rate changes little during pregnancy, tidal volume and minute ventilation increase dramatically.	The mother may experience this change as shortness of breath.
Heart. Blood volume and cardiac output increase. Increased work for the heart leads to a 10- to 15-beat increase in maternal heart rate.	The pregnant woman may subsequently experience palpitations.
Cardiac output decreases when the woman is supine, because the weight of the fetus impedes venous return and increases when she is lateral. Sitting and standing also decrease venous return from the extremities.	*Dependent edema* may result. In the arms, it may lead to *carpal tunnel syndrome*. In the legs, standing for long periods can result in *varicosities*. Help prevent these problems by teaching ways to promote venous return. See Box 21-1.
In the third trimester, rate of iron transfer from mother to fetus increases. FDA-approved prenatal vitamins provide the extra iron required to maintain health during pregnancy.	Women whose initial iron stores are low or who do not obtain sufficient iron during pregnancy become anemic. Women with anemia at the time of childbirth are at increased risk for transfusion.
Peripheral Vascular. Decreased peripheral vascular resistance results in a somewhat lower blood pressure during the second trimester. Optimal circulation to the placenta (and fetus) is achieved in the left lateral position.	As blood volume increases and the growing fetus impedes venous return, pressure on valves in the lower extremities can result in their failure. *Varicose veins* form or worsen. Spider veins may appear.

BOX 21.1 PATIENT TEACHING: SLEEPING AND POSITIONING IN PREGNANCY

*A*dvise pregnant women to sleep on their sides during the third trimester. Help alleviate discomfort by teaching about strategic placement of pillows. In addition to the pillow under her head, the woman can put a thick pillow between the legs, which raises the upper leg until it is parallel with the mattress and relieves strain on the abdominal muscles and ligaments. Wedging another pillow behind the woman's back allows her to lie at a 45-degree angle with her back supported, without impeding venous return. A pillow under the abdomen further supports the suspensory ligaments.

Technique and Normal Findings	Abnormal Findings
Breasts. The Montgomery tubercles (sebaceous glands) on the areola may enlarge. Nipples may darken, enlarge, and begin to discharge colostrum.	
Abdomen. By 20 weeks' gestation, the uterus is at about the umbilicus; by 36 weeks, it nears the bottom of the sternum (Fig. 21-5). Muscles of the abdominal wall may separate (**diastasis recti**) and not return to normal until several weeks after childbirth.	*Gastric reflux (heartburn)* is common as sphincter tone decreases and gastric pressures increase from displacement of the stomach. Antacids can usually relieve infrequent heartburn; however, frequent use causes a rebound effect, meaning that the woman needs more over time for less relief. Use of H2 blockers (eg, ranitidine) is both safe in pregnancy and more efficacious.

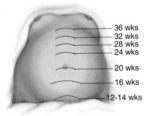

— 36 wks
— 32 wks
— 28 wks
— 24 wks
— 20 wks
— 16 wks
— 12-14 wks

Figure 21.5 Growth in fundal height over pregnancy.

Technique and Normal Findings	Abnormal Findings
The gallbladder does not contract as well as usual.	Retained bile salts can increase risk of gallstones and ***pruritus gravidarum*** (a rash with intense itching along the striae of the abdomen).
During the third trimester, the growing uterus mechanically displaces the intestines.	Pregnant women are at risk for constipation. Straining during bowel movements can also cause painful or itchy hemorrhoids.
Musculoskeletal System. With fetal growth, the maternal center of gravity changes and risk for falls increases. Pregnant women should not lift anything weighing more than 20 lbs. They should use good body mechanics when lifting anything.	Backaches are common.

(text continues on page 462)

Technique and Normal Findings	Abnormal Findings
The musculoskeletal system changes noticeably at the end of pregnancy. The modest increase in the pelvic diameter that results from relaxation of the cartilage allows the fetus to "drop," "lighten," or "engage" in the pelvis.	Increased weight from the fetus and breast tissue and the change in the center of gravity place strain on the abdominal muscles. Exercises to strengthen abdominal muscles ("cat stretch" and pelvic tilts against a wall), may provide some relief. Hormonal changes near term, especially increased relaxin, loosen the cartilage between the pelvic bones. Women complain that they waddle like a duck when they try to walk.

Leopold's Maneuvers

Leopold's Maneuvers are designed to estimate fetal position. Registered nurses usually only need to do the first and second maneuvers to locate the fetal heart rate and verify that the presenting part is the head.

1. Palpate the uterine fundus to determine whether it contains the head or buttocks. The head moves independently of the torso, but the buttocks do not (Fig. 21-6A).
2. Locate the fetal back by holding the fetus firmly on one side while palpating the other side. Then reverse the procedure. The back feels firm and smooth; the opposite side contains "small parts" (arms and legs) that feel irregular (Fig. 21-6B).
3. Palpate just above the symphysis pubis to identify the presenting part. It should be the part opposite that found in the fundus (Fig. 21-6C).
4. Finally, palpate the fetal head to determine whether it is flexed or deflexed. If it is properly flexed, a protrusion (the brow) will be palpated on the opposite side as the fetal back. If the head is deflexed, the protrusion (the occiput) will be palpated on the same side as the back (Fig. 21-6D).

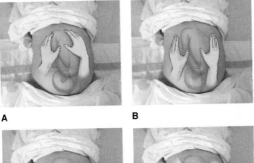

A   **B**

C   **D**

Figure 21.6 **A–D:** Leopold's maneuvers.

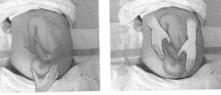

Common Nursing Diagnoses and Interventions Associated with Pregnancy

Diagnosis and Related Factors	Nursing Interventions
Health-seeking behaviors related to pregnancy diagnosis	Educate on nutrition and overeating, develop exercise plan, teach stress management techniques. Instruct in smoking cessation, provide health screening.
Readiness for enhanced parenting	Use family centered care, encourage positive parenting, provide mother-to-infant skin contact, allow the parent to assist in newborn's bath.
Readiness for enhanced family coping due to new role	Assess the structure, resources, and coping abilities of families. Encourage caregivers to become involved in support groups. Acknowledge cultural influences.

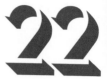

Children: Newborns Through Adolescents

Key Topics and Questions for Health Promotion

Key Questions	Rationales
Current Problems. What brings you here today? • When was the last time the child was well? • How and when did the problem begin? What was health like immediately before? • How has the illness progressed? • What symptoms are there? In what order did they appear? • Does anything make the symptoms better or worse? • What treatments or medications have you given? • Has the child received medical attention for this illness before?	This question elicits the presenting issue in the parent's own words. These questions help identify how long any illness has been present and establish normal state of health. This line of questioning is designed to understand the course and progress of the present illness.
Family History. Tell me a little bit about your family and home.	This helps clarify socioeconomic situation, living conditions, other family members, and background and education of the parents.
Does anyone in your family have diabetes; hypertension; heart disease; elevated cholesterol level; asthma; allergies; cancer; liver, kidney, or gastrointestinal problems; arthritis; or learning problems?	A positive response to any of these increases the child's risk as well and may signal a need for additional testing.

Key Questions	Rationales
Has anyone in the family died before age 50 years?	Family history provides information about the seriousness of diseases.
How is the health of the mother? Father? Siblings?	Illness in an immediate family member can cause changes in family functioning and dynamics.

Pregnancy and Birth History
* Were there unusual circumstances or health problems during pregnancy?
* What was the duration of pregnancy, type of labor and birth, and type of anesthesia used for labor?
* What was the Apgar score? Did the child require any resuscitation?
* What was the birth weight?
* Did the child go home with the mother or spend time in the neonatal intensive care unit (NICU)?
* Have there been infections, serious illnesses, hospitalizations, or surgeries since birth?
* Well-child checkups?

These questions help elicit the obstetric and birth history to identify risk factors.

Medications/Supplements. What medications are being taking? Are immunizations current?

This is to determine past medical history.

Developmental History. For older children, find out if development is within expected parameters and age at sitting, standing, walking, speech, and toilet training.

Development history may provide clues about any current delays or issues.

Risk Factors
Infant Injury Prevention
* Does your child sleep on the back?
* Does the child sleep with a bottle?
* Have you childproofed your home for choking hazards and secured poisons?

This is to identify risk factors and promote health. Once risk factors are assessed, patient teaching can be performed.

(text continues on page 466)

Key Questions	Rationales
• Have you learned CPR?	
• Has the infant had any accidents or injuries?	
Lead Risk	
• Does your child live in or regularly visit a house or child-care facility built before 1950?	"Yes" to any of these three questions requires health care providers to take a blood level on children 0 to 72 months old (and possibly beyond if at risk).
• Does your child live in or regularly visit a house or child-care facility built before 1978 that is being or has recently (within the last 6 months) been renovated or remodeled?	
• Does your child have a sibling or playmate who has or had lead poisoning?	
Tuberculosis (TB) Screening	
• Does the child have HIV?	"Yes" to any of these questions requires the administration of a purified protein derivative tuberculin test to the patient.
• Is the child in close contact with people known or suspected to have TB?	
• Is the child or those in close contact known to be alcohol dependent or intravenous drug users or to reside in a long-term care facility, correctional or mental institution, nursing home/facility, or other long-term residential facility?	
• Is the child foreign-born and from a country with high TB prevalence?	
• Is the child from a medically underserved low-income population, including a high-risk racial or ethnic minority population?	

Health-Promotion Teaching

Safe Sleep Habits. To prevent sudden infant death syndrome (SIDS), infants should always be placed on their backs to sleep. The mattress should be firm. Pillows, soft toys, excessive blankets, and bedding should not be in the crib. The infant should not sleep in the same bed with a sleeping adult. It is too easy for the tiny face to be covered inadvertently and for the infant to be smothered.

Choking Prevention. Parents should remain vigilant about the environment and remove hazards. Advise parents to get down on their hands and knees and survey the environment from the infant's perspective. Any small object within the infant's reach is a possible hazard. Anything that can fit in the infant's mouth and be inhaled should be removed from reach: balloons, toys with small parts, safety pins, small balls, broken crayons, coins, and so on. Firm or round foods (eg, hot dogs, seeds, grapes, raw carrots, apples) should be cooked or chopped into tiny pieces before serving to an infant or very young child.

Immunizations. Newborns and infants need vaccines against diseases with serious consequences. The Centers for Disease Control (CDC), the American Academy of Pediatrics (AAP), and the American Academy of Family Physicians collaborate to provide a schedule of recommended immunizations. Inform parents that it is important for children to receive vaccines at the ages and times recommended to ensure the highest level of protection. If a child misses an immunization or gets behind schedule, a catch-up schedule is available on the AAP Web site.

Car Seats. Ask parents how children are secured when riding in the car. Anytime an infant or a child younger than 4 years is in the car, the child should be restrained in a car seat for safety. More detailed recommendations are listed on the AAP Web site.

CPR Training. Inquire if the parents know CPR. Traditionally, NICUs teach parents infant CPR before discharge because these infants are at higher risk than are healthy infants for respiratory and cardiac arrest. Nevertheless, it is important for all parents and babysitters to know CPR. Many communities offer classes for nominal fees. A newer resource is *Infant CPR Anytime.* This self-directed learning kit, developed by the AAP in coordination with the AHA, contains a manikin for practicing CPR and a video demonstrating CPR that the learner can view and review, as needed.

Poison Control. Ask parents how they have secured medications, cleaning compounds, and other chemicals at home. Explain that safety locks should be placed on cabinets close to the floor, and to put medication and other toxic chemicals in high, locked cabinets. Teach the precaution of ordering all prescription medications with childproof lids.

Breast-feeding/Iron-rich Foods. For families with infants, ask the mother if she is breast-feeding. If she is, determine how long she plans to continue. Breast milk is the best food for the growing infant. For the first 4 to 6 months, it is the only food that the infant needs. Ideally, every baby should be breast-fed for the 1st year of life. Iron-fortified infant formula is an acceptable alternative for mothers who cannot or choose not to breast-feed. Whole cow's milk is not an appropriate food for children younger than 1 year.

As long as the woman has adequate iron stores, iron supplementation for exclusively breast-fed infants is not necessary during the first 6 months. After 6 months, the parents may introduce meats or other iron-rich food sources to the infant's diet.

Preventing Tooth Decay. Inquire about the child's daily intake of sugar, especially sugary drinks. Assess if infants or small children are ever allowed to go to sleep with a bottle of milk, formula, juice, or other sugary drink. This practice can lead to *baby bottle tooth decay*, in which sugar sticks to and coats the primary teeth. Bacteria in the mouth break down the sugars for food and produce acids that cause decay. Some parents may not understand why primary teeth are important. Baby bottle tooth decay is most pronounced on the upper front teeth and is highly visible while the child's self-image is forming. In addition, if the primary teeth experience significant decay, they may require extraction. Because the primary teeth serve as placeholders, if they are lost too early, the secondary teeth may come in excessively crooked.

Preventing Drunk Driving. Discuss this topic with adolescents by providing scenarios in which they have alternatives to riding with impaired drivers. Encourage the use of a designated driver if the teen is in a situation in which he or she anticipates drinking or drug use.

Fire Safety. Children have a larger skin surface area than body weight. Burns on them make up a larger percentage of their surface area than for adults; therefore, burns are much more serious for children in terms of fluid replacement and potential for infection. Children and adolescents require protection against fire and must be taught the dangers of and significant respect for fire. The family should establish and discuss a family fire plan and escape routes.

Water Safety. Once near a pool the young child unable to swim should always wear a life jacket. Around lake and murky water the necessity of a life jacket may continue until the adolescent can demonstrate strong swimming skills. Encourage children to learn to swim and take swimming lessons to develop the ability to at least save themselves in water over their head.

Safe Street Crossing. Assess if the child walks to school, parks, or playgrounds. The safest route and safe street rules should be discussed with the child. Discuss walking facing traffic and crossing the street.

Helmet Use. Most states require helmets for riders of motorized vehicles on state roads. A child on an all-terrain motorized vehicle is encouraged to always wear a helmet. Helmets should also be worn during high-risk sports, such as football, hockey, baseball, skiing, and snowboarding. Head trauma secondary to accidents is a common childhood injury with long-term sequelae. Wearing a bicycle helmets reduces the incidence of brain injury in children.

Sunscreen. All children, no matter what their skin type or color, should apply sunscreen with SPF of at least 15 when exposing the skin to the sun or be completely covered with clothing and a large brimmed hat to prevent skin damage and skin cancer. Sunglasses that block both UVA and UVB light are also recommended to prevent the development of cataracts.

Drug and Alcohol Prevention. Continue to answer questions and counsel pediatric patients about the dangers of alcohol and drugs, emphasizing immediate over long-term risks. Assess for mental health issues, because drug-seeking behaviors are often ways in which people self-medicate for other problems. A potentially effective way to prevent young people from using substances is to explain how they interfere with the accomplishment of developmental tasks, which are difficult if the child or teen is impaired.

Obesity Prevention. Discuss the child's BMI according to sex and age. Nutritional and activity information early is important if the BMI is at or above the 85th percentile. The family should receive nutrition information from the **My Pyramid** guidelines (see Chapter 4). Children 2 years and older should consume daily at least two servings of fruit; three servings of vegetables, with at least one-third being dark green or orange; and six servings of grain products, with at least three being whole grains. Children 2 years and older should consume daily less than 10% of calories from saturated fat, no more than 30% of calories from total fat, and 2,400 mg or less of sodium; they also need to meet dietary recommendations for calcium. Educate families about multivitamins with iron for high-risk individuals, as well as about food choices at school.

Children and caregivers also need explanations about vigorous physical activity and assessment of their engagement in such activity. Young people need to exercise for at least 3 days/week for at least 20 minutes, with examples of appropriate activities.

Mental Health Issues. Discuss actions to deal with threats at school, conflict resolution, and school resources available. Intervene immediately if a parent or child admits to concerns about hurting self or others. A patient or family member who describes a plan to complete suicide requires hospital admission for mental health concerns.

Contraception and Prevention of Sexually Transmitted Infections (STIs). Discuss abstinence, safe-sex practices, and avoidance of high-risk behaviors with sexually active adolescents. Answer questions of all patients regarding sexuality and sexual health. Encourage group activities and normalize the decision not to engage in sexual activity. For those adolescents who choose to continue sexual activity, encourage use of condoms. Also teach about the signs, symptoms, and consequences of untreated STIs. Urge immediate screening and treatment for symptoms and yearly examinations for sexually active adolescents even if they are asymptomatic.

Objective Data Collection

Newborn and Infant Examination

The following sections focus first on those assessments conducted as part of the initial newborn screening. Then the content focuses on a head-to-toe assessment of the infant, emphasizing techniques, findings, or abnormalities specific to this age group. For more information, refer also to the "Lifespan Considerations" in earlier chapters.

Technique and Normal Findings	Abnormal Findings
Newborn: Apgar Score. The Apgar score gives important clues about how well the newborn is adapting to life. The newborn receives a score of 0 to 2 in each of five areas for a possible total of 10. The score is calculated at 1 minute and again at 5 minutes of life. *A score of 7 to 10 indicates a vigorous newborn adapting well to the extrauterine environment.*	If the 5-minute score is less than 7, continue to score every 5 minutes until the score is above 7, and the newborn is intubated or is transferred to the nursery. See Table 22-1.
Newborn: Gestational Age During pregnancy, gestational age is calculated from the date of the last menstrual period or by results of an early sonogram. After birth physical characteristics and neuromuscular assessment are used to evaluate gestational age.	
Reflexes. Evaluation of newborn reflexes gives information about neurologic status. See Table 22-2 at the end of this chapter.	Diminished reflexes indicate the possibility of neurological or developmental deficits.
General Survey. Keep in mind the age of the infant in months and the correlated expected development. Collect data through observation during the visit. Notice interactions between the infant and the parent. *The infant has good muscle tone, a symmetrical appearance, and appears well. Respirations are unlabored. The parent picks up on cues from the infant, who is alert and engaged, unless sleeping. A normal variant is stranger anxiety that begins around 9 months.*	The infant is listless and uninterested in interaction. The parent pays little attention and does not pick up on cues. *Phenylketonuria, maple syrup urine disease,* and *diabetic acidosis* have characteristic odors. Poor hygiene or inappropriate dress for the weather should alert the nurse to watch for other signs of neglect.

(text continues on page 472)

Technique and Normal Findings	Abnormal Findings
Vital Signs. Axillary temperature measurement is appropriate for the newborn. After 1 month of age, axillary or tympanic temperatures are appropriate. *Range of normal is 97.7°F to 98.6°F (36.5°C to 37°C).*	Both elevated and decreased temperatures can signal infection in the newborn because regulatory mechanisms are not fully mature.
Measure apical pulse and respiratory rate for a full minute each with the infant at rest. *Pulse range for the newborn is 110 to 160 bpm, decreasing to 80 to 140 for infants older than 1 month. Respiratory rate is 30 to 60 breaths/min for newborns and 22 to 35 for infants.*	Tachycardia, bradycardia, tachypnea, and bradypnea are abnormal findings at rest. These terms are defined as falling above or below the ranges listed.
Blood pressures are not measured routinely in the infant. *If taken, systolic pressures are 50 to 70 for newborns and 70 to 100 for infants older than 1 month.*	A difference between upper and lower extremity blood pressures may indicate *coarctation of the aorta.*
Measurements. Place a protective covering on an infant scale. Zero the scale and position the infant with your hands just above, but not touching, to prevent a fall (Fig. 22-1). 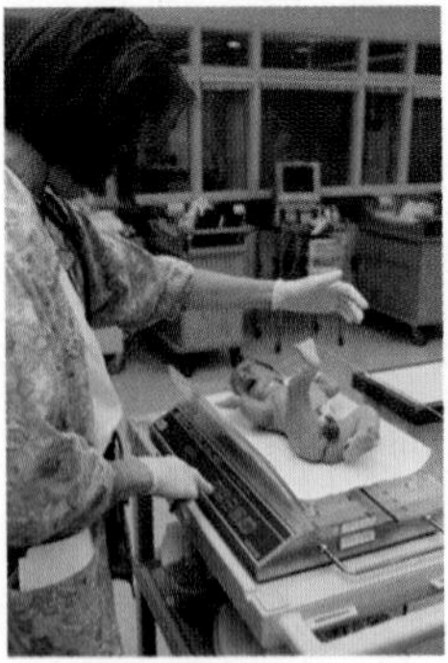	Length varies with heredity. A small head may indicate *microcephaly*, while a large head may be from *hydrocephalus* or *increased intracranial pressure.* A small chest circumference may be from prematurity.

Figure 22.1 Weighing the infant.

Technique and Normal Findings	Abnormal Findings

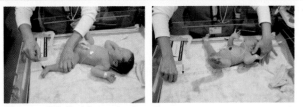

Figure 22.2 Measuring length.

Technique and Normal Findings	Abnormal Findings
Use a tape measure to carefully measure from the crown of the head to the heel. It may be helpful to place the infant on the examination table; then use a pencil to place a mark at the crown and another mark at the heel. Use the tape measure to measure the length between the two markings (Fig. 22-2). Measure head and chest circumferences (Fig. 22-3). Plot measurements. *Measurements are above the 10th and below the 90th percentile. Compare with previous visits. The infant is gaining height and weight at a steady pace.*	

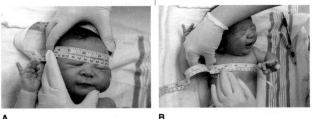

A **B**
Figure 22.3 (A) Measuring head circumference.
(B) Measuring chest circumference.

Technique and Normal Findings	Abnormal Findings
Nutrition. Inspect general condition of the skin, hair, and nails. *A well-nourished infant has soft, supple skin and shiny hair.*	Indications that the infant is not eating enough are parental reports of fussing, crying, and not seeming satisfied after feeding;

(text continues on page 474)

Technique and Normal Findings	Abnormal Findings
Ask about urination and bowel movements. *The infant getting enough to eat wets a diaper 4 to 6 times per day and has regular soft and formed bowel movements.*	sallow skin tones with poor turgor; dry brittle hair and nails; weight loss; and consuming less than 100 kcal/kg/day.
If the infant is bottle-feeding, ask how many ounces per feeding and how many feedings per day. *The infant is consuming approximately 100 kcal/kg/day.* If the parent is having difficulty determining intake and there is a question as to adequacy, ask the parent to keep a diary of the infant's intake for the next 3 days and report back.	Failure to thrive is described as weight that falls below the 5th percentile for the child's age. Causes to further evaluate include inadequate calorie intake, inadequate absorption, increased metabolism, or defective use of food sources.
Mental Status. Observe sleep states and behavior. *An alert 1-month-old infant engages with the eyes when face-to-face and responds to voices by turning toward the sound or tracking with the eyes. An older infant reaches for an object the parent or examiner offers. During the 1st month or 2, crying is a normal response to handling and undressing. Crying should stop with gentle rocking in the arms or while holding the infant against the shoulder. As the infant matures, the infant may smile and interact, as long as movements are not sudden or threatening and the voice stays calm and reassuring.*	Abnormal findings are when interaction between the infant and the parent is not synergistic and the older infant is excessively clingy or does not warm up to the examiner after a period of interaction. Excessive irritability and inconsolable crying may be early signs of a change in mental status. Later signs may be a high-pitched cry, or lethargy and listlessness.
Violence. Assess the parent for signs of domestic violence because children living in violent situations are much more likely to suffer abuse than children in households uncomplicated by violence. *Parental*	Signs that should raise suspicion of child abuse and neglect are listed in Table 22-3 at the end of this chapter.

Technique and Normal Findings	Abnormal Findings

findings include a relaxed, confident demeanor with appropriate affect, good grooming, and appropriate interaction with and concern for the infant.

Skin, Hair, and Nails. Inspect. *Healthy infant's skin is soft, not excessively dry, and supple. It is free of rashes, lesions, bruising, and edema. Normal skin variants are illustrated in Table 22-4. Hair is soft and shiny. Nails are soft, of an appropriate length, and not growing inward.*

Note if any rashes or lesions are macular, patchy, petechial, or vesicular. Is there excoriation from scratching? Are any nails lifting off the nail bed? Are nails dry and brittle? Areas of inflammation around nails with nails poking into the skin suggest *ingrown nails.* Poor elasticity and tenting of the skin when lightly pinched are associated with *dehydration.* Pallor or pale mucous membranes may indicate *anemia.* Yellow, jaundiced skin tones require further investigation, because elevated bilirubin levels are toxic to the growing brain. Periorbital edema has various causes. Dependent edema may occur with renal or cardiac disease.

Head and Neck. Assess head size and shape. Check for symmetry. Palpate anterior and posterior fontanels and sutures (Fig. 22-4). Trace along each suture line with the tips of the fingers to ensure they have not fused prematurely. *The posterior fontanel usually is palpable until 3 months of age, although it may be closed at birth. The anterior fontanel does not close until 9 to 18 months. The anterior fontanel is flat, not sunken or bulging, with the infant at rest and sitting. Sometimes pulsations correlating with the infant's pulse can be felt. The fontanel may bulge*

A head flattened from the back or one side may indicate positional ***plagiocephaly*** or ***brachycephaly***. Differentiate positional plagiocephaly from plagiocephaly caused by ***craniosynostosis***, premature closure of the cranial sutures. This condition can lead to impaired brain development if several sutures are involved and corrective surgery is not done in a timely fashion. Bulging fontanels at rest are a sign of increased cranial pressure or ***hydrocephalus***. Sunken fontanels are associated most commonly with acute dehydration.

(text continues on page 476)

Technique and Normal Findings	Abnormal Findings

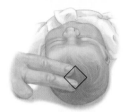

Figure 22.4 Assessing the fontanels and sutures.

slightly when the infant cries. Suture lines are easily palpable. **Craniotabes**, *soft areas on the skull felt along the suture line, are normal, particularly in premature infants.*

Observe the infant's face. Look for symmetry of movement.

Asymmetrical movements may indicate *Bell's palsy* or a more serious heart condition.

Check range of motion (ROM) by rotating the head toward the right shoulder and then the left, and then bending the neck so that the right ear moves toward the right shoulder and the left ear toward the left shoulder. *The neck has full ROM. Head lag and head control correlate with expected development.*

Persistence of head lag beyond the 4th month is a sign of developmental delay. Limited ROM of the neck is associated with *meningeal irritation.* Webbing on the sides of the neck may indicate a congenital anomaly. An enlarged thyroid gland with a bruit is a sign of *thyrotoxicosis.*

Inspect and palpate the trachea. *It is midline with no swelling or masses.* Auscultate for any bruits. *No bruits are present.* Palpate the clavicles. *They are smooth with no pain or crepitus.* Palpate the preauricular, suboccipital, parotid, submaxillary, submental, anterior and posterior cervical, epitrochlear, and inguinal lymph nodes. *Any palpable lymph nodes are small, mobile, and nontender.*

Deviated trachea should be reported to the primary care provider. Crepitation over the clavicles in a newborn immediately after birth may indicate a *fracture.* By 3 weeks of age a small lump may be felt on the bone following a clavicle fracture. Treatment usually is not indicated.

Technique and Normal Findings	Abnormal Findings
Eyes. Look for symmetry. Assess spacing. Inspect the lids for proper placement. Observe the general slant of the palpebral fissures. Inspect the inside lining of lids (palpebral conjunctiva), bulbar conjunctiva, sclera, and cornea. *Eyes are parallel and centered. Ptosis is absent. Sclerae are clear and white.*	Upward or downward slanting or small palpebral fissures are associated with some congenital conditions (eg, *fetal alcohol syndrome*). Eyes too close together, too far apart, or asymmetrical can occur with chromosomal abnormalities or illnesses. Exophthalmos may indicate *thyrotoxicosis.* An eyelid that droops (ptosis) may indicate *oculomotor nerve (cranial nerve III) impairment.*
Assess ocular alignment to detect strabismus using the corneal light reflex test or cover test. *Some strabismus is normal in the first few months of life.* Assess pupils for shape, size, and movement. *They are round, equal, and clear.* Test their reaction to light. Quickly shine a light source toward the eye and then remove it. *The pupils are equal and reactive to light.*	Abnormal pupils are asymmetrical, respond sluggishly, are "blown," or are pinpoint.
Use an ophthalmoscope to obtain the red reflex. Ensure that you have a +1 or =2 D lens. With the infant lying on the examination table or sitting in the parent's lap, approach from the side while looking into the ophthalmoscope. Shine the light from approximately 15 to 26 in away. If you do not visualize a red/orange reflection from the eye, make small adjustments with the instrument until you see the red reflex. Repeat in the opposite eye. *A red reflex is present.*	If the red reflex cannot be elicited in the newborn, the infant needs a complete eye examination by a specialist. Absence of the red reflex in newborns is associated with *congenital cataracts* and *neuroblastoma.*

(text continues on page 478)

Technique and Normal Findings	Abnormal Findings
Observe the infant for light perception and ability to fix on and follow a target. *Newborns are sensitive to light and often keep their eyes closed for long periods. They have a limited ability to focus, but by 3 months they can follow objects.* An infant with any abnormal findings should be referred to an advanced practitioner for further testing.	At birth, the visual system is the least mature of the sensory systems. Development progresses rapidly over the first 6 months and reaches adult level by 4 to 5 years.
Ears. Assess ear placement. *Ears are symmetrical. The top of the pinna lies just above an imaginary line from the inner canthus of the eye through the outer canthus and continuing past the ear.* Skin tags are a normal finding.	Ears below the imaginary line are low-set and may indicate *chromosomal abnormalities*. One ear that is significantly smaller than the other or extra ridges and pits may be associated with middle ear abnormalities or congenital kidney disorders.
At the end of the examination, use the pneumatic otoscope to visualize the tympanic membranes and to check the eardrums. Test the pneumatic otoscope before each use to ensure there are no leaks. Squeeze the bulb, then place the tip against your fingertip and release the bulb. Suction on the fingertip confirms the integrity of the system.	*Otitis media* is common in infants. Early diagnosis and intervention result in the best outcomes.
Position the infant. Ask the parent to hold him or her with the body facing the parent. Then the parent should wrap one arm around the infant to draw the body close and pin down the arms. The other arm should hold the infant's head against the parent's chest. Hold the bulb in one hand and then use that hand to pull the pinna up and back. Gently insert the otoscope	Always brace the hand holding the otoscope against the infant's face, so that if the infant moves the otoscope moves with him or her to avoid injuring the tympanic membrane.

Technique and Normal Findings	Abnormal Findings

approximately ¼ in into the ear canal. Visualize the tympanic membrane and light reflex. *The tympanic membrane is convex, intact, and translucent and allows visualization of the short process of the malleus. The cone of light is visible in the anterior inferior quadrant.*

Gently squeeze the bulb to blow a puff of air into the ear canal. *The tympanic membrane responds by moving.*

If there is no or diminished movement, suspect *otitis media*. Other conditions that can cause diminished movement include perforation or tympanosclerosis. See also Chapter 9.

Screening for hearing acuity includes evaluation of developmental milestones, such as the Moro reflex in neonates.

Abnormal findings include lack of Moro reflex, inability to localize sound, or lack of understandable language by 24 months.

Nose, Mouth, and Throat. Inspect the nose. *It is fully formed, in the midline of the face, with symmetrical nares and nasolabial folds.* The best way to check patency is to hold a small mirror or specimen slide that has been chilled under the nose. *Condensation on the glass is evidence of patency.*

Nasal flaring is a sign of respiratory distress. A flattened nasal bridge and macroglossia (enlarged tongue) are associated with *chromosomal abnormalities*. A flat philtrum and thin upper lip are associated with fetal alcohol syndrome (*FAS*). A deviated uvula or a uvula with a cleft (rare), and red, inflamed tonsils should be noted.

Inspect the lips, mouth, and throat. Defer throat examination to the end, unless the infant cries. The uvula can easily be visualized when the infant is crying. *Lips are symmetrical and fully formed. Young infants may have a white nodule on the upper lip. Sometimes referred to as a sucking blister, this is harmless. The tongue does not get in the way of feeding. The mucous membranes of the mouth, nose, and throat are moist and pink.*

(text continues on page 480)

Technique and Normal Findings	Abnormal Findings
Thorax and Lungs. Observe the infant's breathing pattern. *The thorax is symmetrical. Chest expansion is equal bilaterally. There are no signs of distress or use of accessory muscles.* Auscultate all lung lobes from the front, back, and under both arms. *Breath sounds are equal bilaterally and typically louder and more bronchial than in adults. Inspiration is slightly longer than expiration.*	An asymmetrical chest wall or an expanded anterior-posterior diameter (pigeon breast) or funnel shape (depressed sternum) should not be present. Retractions anywhere are a sign of respiratory distress. Wheezes, crackles, and grunting are always abnormal, as are absent or diminished breath sounds.
Assess oxygenation. *Pink nail beds with crisp capillary refill time and pink mucous membranes and tongue are all signs of adequate oxygenation. Blueness surrounding the mouth (**circumoral cyanosis**) can be normal, especially when the infant is crying, as long as the lips and tongue remain pink.*	
Heart and Neck Vessels. Palpate the point of maximum impulse (PMI). Auscultate the heart; inspect and auscultate the neck vessels. *The PMI may be difficult to palpate. Heart rhythm is regular with a single S_1 and a split S_2. Some murmurs are nonpathologic—typically they are soft and nonspecific in character (Box 22-1). Neck vessels are nondistended without bruits.*	Tachycardia at rest, persistent bradycardia, and clubbing are abnormal, as are a single S_2, ejection clicks, and loud, harsh murmurs. If central cyanosis is present, evaluation of preductal and postductal oxygenation saturation is in order. Measure and compare readings in both upper extremities and one lower extremity. Oxygen saturation lower than 90% is abnormal. Infants with central cyanosis need a full cardiac evaluation by a cardiologist.
Peripheral Vascular. Note character and quality of the brachial and femoral pulses. Compare left to right and upper with lower. *All pulses are equal; pulse rate matches apical heart rate.*	Weak, thready pulses indicate low cardiac output. Bounding pulses are associated with conditions characterized by right to left shunts (eg, *patent ductus arteriosus*).

BOX 22.1 CHARACTERISTICS OF INNOCENT AND ABNORMAL HEART MURMURS

Innocent Murmurs

Innocent murmurs are associated with normal first and second heart sounds (S1 and S2). They occur in systole (except for the venous hum). They are usually very brief, well localized, and heard near the left sternal border. On a scale from 1 to 6, these usually are graded 1 or 2 without a thrill. The intensity changes with position, usually decreasing when standing. Innocent murmurs that may be auscultated in children are as follows:

- *Still's murmur*: a vibratory functional murmur, louder in the supine position
- *Pulmonary flow murmur*: increased flow, louder in the supine position, accentuated by exercise, fever, excitement
- *Venous hum*: continuous, loudest when sitting

Abnormal Murmurs

A murmur that sounds like a breath sound or is harsh or blowing (of any degree of intensity) signifies regurgitation of blood and pathology. Factors that increase the likelihood of an abnormal murmur include the following:

- Symptoms such as chest pain, squatting, fainting, tiring quickly, shortness of breath, or failure to thrive
- Family history of Marfan's syndrome or sudden death in young (<50 years) family members
- Other congenital anomaly or syndrome (eg, Down's syndrome)
- Increased precordial activity
- Decreased femoral pulses
- Abnormal S2
- Clicks
- Loud or harsh murmur (>Grade II)
- Increased intensity of murmur when the patient stands

Technique and Normal Findings	Abnormal Findings
	Palpable pulses in the upper extremities in correlation with diminished pulses in the lower extremities may indicate *coarctation of the aorta* or an *interrupted aortic arch*.

(text continues on page 482)

Technique and Normal Findings	Abnormal Findings
Breasts. Observe the nipples. *Areolae are full and the nipple bud is well formed. Both male and female newborns may have swollen breasts that even leak a watery fluid from the lingering effects of maternal hormones.*	Check for any supernumerary (extra) nipples below the normal nipples. See Chapter 14.
Abdomen. Inspect. *It is cylindrical, protrudes slightly, and moves in synchrony with the diaphragm. Superficial veins may be visible in fair-skinned infants. The umbilicus is clean with no discharge, bulging, or scarring.* Auscultate bowel sounds. *They are heard in all four quadrants and may be softer immediately after eating.* Percuss the abdomen. *Dullness in the right upper quadrant helps outline the lower edges of the liver. Tympany is normal over an air-filled stomach and bowel.*	A dull sound when percussing above the symphysis pubis may indicate a distended bladder. If abdominal distention is present, evaluate for a fluid wave. Note size, shape, position, and mobility of any masses. Palpable kidneys should prompt further investigation. Loud, grumbling sounds may indicate hunger. Bowel sounds heard in the chest can indicate a diaphragmatic hernia.
Palpate the abdomen. *It is soft, without rigidity, tenderness, or masses. The lower liver margins can be palpated from 1 to 2 cm below the right costal margin. The tip of the spleen may be palpable in the left upper quadrant.* Try to locate the kidneys using deep palpation in both upper quadrants. Be sure to palpate for hernias in the umbilical and inguinal regions. *The kidneys cannot be palpated; no hernias are present.*	The abdomen may be distended and firm with genitourinary masses or malformation. Gastrointestinal obstruction and imperforate anus are also causes of a firm abdomen.
Musculoskeletal. Note shape and appearance of the hands, palms, fingers, feet, and toes. *Ankles have full ROM. Feet return to a neutral position without assistance. Feet are flat before the infant begins walking.*	Throughout examination, note any asymmetrical movements. Crepitus with joint movement or any limitation of movement is abnormal. In *talipes varus (club foot)*, one or both feet are plantar-flexed and turn abnormally

Technique and Normal Findings	Abnormal Findings

| | inward. In *talipes valgus*, seen less commonly, the foot or feet turn outward. |

Ortolani's Maneuver. Position the infant supine on the examining table. With the baby's legs together, flex the knees and hips 90 degrees. With your middle fingers over the greater trochanters and thumbs on the inner thighs, abduct the hips while applying upward pressure (Fig. 22-5A). *No clicking or clunking sounds are heard.*

Signs of congenital hip dislocation include positive Ortolani's and Barlow's maneuvers and asymmetrical thigh and gluteal folds. Infants with talipes varus, talipes valgus, or hip dislocation should be referred to an orthopedist for evaluation and treatment.

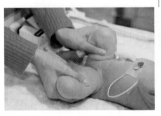
A

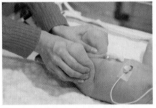
B

Figure 22.5 **(A)** Ortolani's maneuver. **(B)** Barlow's maneuver.

Barlow's Maneuver. Maintain your hold and the 90-degrees flexion; apply downward pressure while adducting the hips (Fig. 22-5B). *The head of the femur remains in the acetabulum.*

Neurological. Assessments made throughout give clues about the nervous system and cranial nerve function. *The infant blinks when a bright light is shined in the eyes and when a loud noise, such as a clap, is produced close by.*

Signs of neurological dysfunction include persistence of newborn reflexes past the time they normally disappear, involuntary movements, and abnormal posturing. Failure to blink when a bright light is shined in the eyes may indicate blindness.

(text continues on page 484)

Technique and Normal Findings	Abnormal Findings
Inspect, then palpate along the length of the spine. *There are no dimples or tufts of hair.*	Absence of a blink upon production of a loud noise may denote deafness. Dimpling or tufts of hair on the spine may indicate *spina bifida occulta*.
Female Genitalia. Gently part the labia and observe the structures of the vestibule. Visualize the vaginal opening. *The labia majora cover the vestibule. For the first few weeks after birth, the newborn may have an enlarged clitoris and labia from lingering effects of maternal hormones. The genital area is clean and free of foul odors.*	Redness, swelling, bleeding, or torn tissue may indicate sexual abuse. The law mandates the reporting of signs of abuse to child protective services. A hymen that completely covers the vagina (*imperforate hymen*) requires minor surgery before puberty to allow exit of menstrual flow. Other abnormal findings include *labial adhesions/ fusion, lesions,* and foul-smelling discharge.
Male Genitalia. Inspect the penis. Note cleanliness and placement of the urethral meatus. *It is at the top of the glans penis and midline.* For the uncircumcised penis, partially retract the foreskin to observe the meatus. Evaluate the scrotum for size, color, and symmetry. *Testes are descended bilaterally; the area is free of edema, masses, and lesions.*	*Meatal stenosis,* an inadequate urethral opening, *hypospadias,* or *epispadias,* should be referred to a pediatric urologist. Note if the testes remain undescended. This condition requires evaluation if it persists into the toddler stage. See also Chapter 18.
Anus and Rectum. Inspect the anus. Use a gloved little finger to palpate it. *It is well formed with no redness or bleeding. The muscle contracts with light pressure.* Rectal examination is not done unless there is evidence of irritation, bleeding, or other symptoms.	Investigate redness, bleeding, or other signs of irritation for possible cause (eg, sexual abuse, fissures). Small white worms indicate a *pinworm infection*.

Older Children and Adolescents

The following presentations focus on those areas of examination, normal findings, or abnormal concerns that are significantly different from those with adults. For additional information, see also the "Lifespan Considerations" in earlier chapters of this book.

Technique and Normal Findings	Abnormal Findings
Vital Signs. Take height, weight, heart rate, respiratory rate, temperature, and blood pressure. Plot height and weight on appropriate growth charts; calculate BMI. Routine blood pressures begin at 3 years if blood pressure at birth was within normal limits. *Charts for blood pressure are available at the National Heart, Lung and Blood Institute's Web sites.*	Any blood pressure over the 90th percentile is considered borderline hypertensive and deserves follow-up.
General Survey. Observe the child's demeanor. Look for signs of distress, discomfort, or anxiety. Note attentiveness and affect. Listen for speech difficulties. *By 2 years, the child uses two-word sentences; by 3 years, 75% or more of speech should be understandable.*	Flat affect, no eye contact, and clinging to the caregiver may need further evaluation to assess for *autism* and other psychiatric concerns.
Observe for ROM, coordination, and musculoskeletal symmetry. *ROM is full with 4–5+/5 strength symmetrically.*	Asymmetry of movement and lack of coordination should be further evaluated.
Skin, Hair, and Nails. Inspect and palpate. *Skin is smooth and dry. Hair is evenly distributed. Nails are smooth and without clubbing.* Eccrine (sweat) glands become fully functional at adolescence. Apocrine (sex) glands do not become active until puberty.	Dimpling, ripples, or discoloration in nails can be signs of *trauma* or *fungus*. Note *acne* during adolescence. With a gloved hand, feel any rash or skin complaints for elevation and size of papules, nodules, or cysts.

(text continues on page 486)

Technique and Normal Findings	Abnormal Findings
Head and Neck. Inspect and palpate. Observe neck ROM. *Head and neck are symmetrical; neck ROM is full. Anterior and posterior cervical nodes may be palpable but not enlarged or tender. No nodules are noted.*	Limited neck ROM requires further evaluation for *meningitis* or *torticolis.* Tender swollen lymph nodes may indicate infection. Tonsils frequently look large at this time but will appear smaller as the head and neck grow.
Eyes and Vision. Inspect. *The eyes are PERRLA. EOMs are at 180 degrees. Corneal light reflexes are equal. There is no deviation during the cover and alternate cover tests. Fundoscopic examination reveals a distinct disk with no vessel nicking.*	Unequal and nonreactive pupils may signify *increased intracranial pressure.* Unequal EOMs or CLR may indicate *esotropia* or *exotropia* (see Chapter 8). Deviation with the cover test demonstrates an *esophoria* or *exophoria.* All these findings require further evaluation.
Assess distance vision using a screening test based on developmental stage. *Visual acuity in toddlers is 20/200 bilaterally; in preschoolers it is 20/40, improving to 20/30 or better by 4 years. By 5 to 6 years old, visual acuity should approximate that of adults (20/20 in both eyes).*	
Screen for color blindness in patients 4 to 8 years old.	
Ears and Hearing. Inspect the ears. *They have a formed pinna, the top of which touches an imaginary straight line through both pupils.*	Ear deformities are connected to kidney problems, cognitive deficits, and learning problems.
As head shape changes, visualization of the tympanic membrane requires alterations in technique. From 1 to 2 years, pull straight back on the pinna to straighten the ear canal for visualization of the tympanic membrane. After 2 to 3 years of age pull up and back on the top of the pinna. Once visualized,	Infection is suspected if the tympanic membrane is erythematous or yellow, there is drainage in the canal, or there is limited mobility. See Chapter 9.

Technique and Normal Findings	Abnormal Findings
use the pneumatic bulb to test for movement of the tympanic membrane. *The tympanic membrane is gray, nonerythematous with the light reflex and landmarks visualized.*	
Mobility is demonstrated with pneumoscopy. Palpate the pinna for tenderness and nodules. *The tympanic membrane is mobile; no tenderness or nodules are on the pinna.*	Tenderness with manipulation of the pinna may indicate *otitis externa*. Swollen, erythematous turbinates may indicate infection. Pale swollen turbinates may indicate *allergic rhinitis*.
Screening for hearing acuity includes evaluation of developmental milestones. If there is a developmental lag or caregivers are concerned, a pediatric audiologist should perform a formal evaluation.	Abnormal findings include inability to localize sound or lack of understandable language by 24 months.
Nose, Mouth, and Throat. Inspect. *The nose is midline, nares are patent, and turbinates are pink with unrestricted air passage.* Note the number of deciduous and permanent teeth. *No caries are present.* In the mouth, tonsils are present and +1 to +4 (see Chapter 10). *There is no erythema or exudate.*	*Dental caries* are the most common infectious disease in childhood. Poor dental health is associated with poor physical health. Note any missing teeth. Erythema and exudate may be an infectious process.
Thorax and Lungs. Inspect. *There are no increased work of breathing and retractions.* Palpate the thorax. *There is no tenderness along intercostal spaces.* Percuss. *The lungs are resonant.* Auscultate the thorax and lungs. *Breath sounds are clear in all lobes. No crackles, gurgles, or wheezes are noted.*	Pain along ribs may be indicative of injury or viral infection such as costochondritis.
Heart and Neck Vessels. Inspect for visible pulses on the thorax. Palpate and auscultate the PMI. *The PMI is at the midclavicular*	A visible PMI may signify increased cardiac load and increased oxygen requirements.

(text continues on page 488)

Technique and Normal Findings	Abnormal Findings
line (MCL) in infancy and moves slightly laterally with age to the 4th intercostal space (ICS) just to the left of the MCL in children younger than 7 years and then to the 5th ICS in children older than 7 years. There is no bounding PMI.	
If heart enlargement is suspected percussion can assist in determining size. Auscultate the heart in all six designated areas on the chest and in the back. Assess with the child in two positions: lying and/or sitting and/or standing. *Closure of the tricuspid and mitral valves (S1) and the pulmonic and aortic (S2) valves is clear, crisp, and single. There are no murmurs, rubs, or gallops.* Observe the jugular venous pulsations. *The neck vessels are not distended or flat.*	If a murmur is detected description of the murmur should include the intensity (Grades 1 through 6), timing, duration, quality, pitch, PMI, and if and to where it radiates (see Chapter 12). Characteristics of **innocent heart murmurs** and abnormal murmurs are noted in Box 22-1.
Peripheral Vascular. Inspect. *Color is pink in all extremities and mucous membranes.* Palpate peripheral pulses. *Pulses are equal in all extremities; there are no differences between upper-extremity and lower-extremity pulses.* Assess blood pressure in each extremity. *If there are slight differences, they are less than 10 mmHg.*	Outside of the immediate newborn period, cyanosis requires immediate intervention. *Coarctation of the aorta* can present with unequal pulses between the upper and lower extremities. After the aorta leaves the heart, if there is a narrowing of the vessel then the lower extremities are not well oxygenated and pressure increases on the left side of the heart.
Breasts. Inspect the breasts. Refer to Chapter 14 for sexual maturity and Tanner's staging.	Onset of pubertal changes before 8 years in girls and 9 years in boys may be too early and needs further evaluation.
Abdomen. Inspect, palpate, and percuss the abdomen. *No distension is noted. A protuberate abdomen is common in toddlers. There are no masses or tenderness. The abdomen has a*	With distension, assess for tenderness and ascites. Palpation for abdominal masses is important, because **Wilms' tumors** of the kidney occur in toddlers and early school-age children.

Technique and Normal Findings	Abnormal Findings
normal hollow or tympanic sound. The liver is at the lower right costal margin.	Significant abdominal tenderness requires further evaluation for *appendicitis*, *Crohn's disease*, *ulcerative colitis*, *gastroenteritis*, or other illnesses. Percussion can assist in determining the size of a palpable mass.
Musculoskeletal. Inspect muscles and joints. Evaluation of scoliosis is a focused part of the examination just prior to and during puberty (see Chapter 16). Observe ROM in all joints. Palpate muscles and joints. *Spine is straight. No joint tenderness is noted. ROM is full and symmetrical.*	Limited ROM in any joint requires further evaluation. Joint tenderness with palpation should be further evaluated for trauma and infection.
Neurological. Assess orientation. Observe for symmetry. Test deep tendon reflexes and evaluate for equality. Ensure active movement and full strength in all extremities. *Older children are oriented to time and place. Movements are symmetrical; DTRs 2+. Strength 4 to 5+.*	Any noted asymmetry of gait, facial features, or movement needs further evaluation.
Assess developmental progress for age. The Denver Developmental Screening Test is used for children 1 month to 6 years. For children older than 6 years, academic performance is noted. *Scores are within norms for the age.*	Confusion, unusual behaviors, delayed development progress, and poor academic performance need further assessment.
Genitalia. Inspect the genitalia. Refer to Chapters 18 and 19 for sexual maturity and **Tanner's staging**.	Onset of pubertal changes before 8 years in girls and 9 years in boys needs further evaluation. Visualization of the genitalia is recommended in a complete examination to detect early infections, trauma, or developmental concerns. *(text continues on page 490)*

Technique and Normal Findings	Abnormal Findings
Note if the male is circumcised or uncircumcised with the urethra midline at the end of the glans. Palpate the scrotum. *The testes are in the scrotal sac and are smooth with no nodules noted.*	The testes descend into the scrotal sac by age 6 months. If surgical repair is required, it should ideally happen before 2 years of age to prevent decreased fertility. **Hypospadias** requires intervention (see Chapter 18). Adolescent boys should be assessed for testicular nodules; if found, they must be evaluated to rule out testicular cancer. Other testicular abnormalities (eg, hydrocele, varicocele, spermatocele) can be detected with testicular palpation.
Inspect the anus and rectum. *Skin is without irritation, erythema, or fissures.*	Irritation or fissures require evaluation for constipation, worms, or sexual abuse.

Tables of Reference

Table 22.1   Apgar Scoring System

	0	1	2
Heart rate	Absent	Slow below 100 beats/min	More than 100 beats/min
Respiratory effort	Absent	Slow or irregular	Good crying
Muscle tone	Limp	Some flexion of extremities	Active motion
Reflex irritability (response to catheter in nostril)	No response	Grimace, frown	Cough or sneeze
Color	Blue or pale	Body pink, extremities blue	Completely pink

⚠ **Table 22.2   Newborn Reflexes**

Rooting

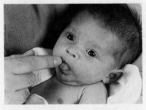

Suck

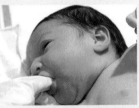

Gently stroke the cheek. The newborn turns toward the stimulus and opens the mouth. This reflex disappears at 3–4 months.

Place a gloved finger in the newborn's mouth. He or she should vigorously suck. The reflex may persist during infancy.

(table continues on page 492)

Moro (Startle)

Galant's (Trunk Incurvation)

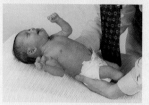

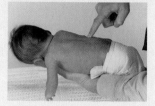

Moro occurs when the infant is startled or feels like he or she is falling. Bring the infant to sit. Support the upper body and head with one hand; flex the chest. Suddenly let the head and shoulders drop a few inches while releasing the arms. The arms and legs extend symmetrically. The arms return toward midline with the hand open and the thumb and index finger forming a "C." Moro disappears by 4–6 months of age.

Place the newborn in ventral suspension. Stroke the skin on one side of the back. The trunk and hips should swing toward the side of the stimulus. Galant's reflex is normally present for the first 4–8 weeks of life.

Stepping

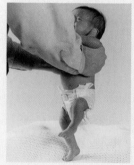

Hold the infant upright. Allow the soles to touch a flat surface. The legs flex and extend in a walking pattern. This reflex exists for the first 4–8 weeks of life and persists with neurological conditions.

Tonic Neck

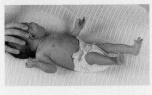

Turn the head of the supine infant to one side. The arm and leg extend on the side to which the face is pointed. The contralateral arm and leg flex, forming the classic fencer position. Repeat by turning the head to the other side—the position will reverse. This reflex is strongest at 2 months and disappears by 6 months.

Palmar Grasp

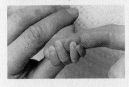

Babinski

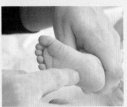

Stroke one side of the infant's foot upward from the heel and across the ball of the foot. The infant responds by hyperextending the toes: the great toe flexes toward the top of the foot and the other toes fan outward. This reflex lasts until the child is walking well.

Place your finger in the newborn's palm; the infant's fingers will firmly grasp your finger. This reflex is strongest between 1 and 2 months.

⚠ Table 22.3   Red Flags for Child Abuse

Category	Details
Reported history of the injury	The story keeps changing or is inconsistent between partners or over time. Details of the trauma do not correlate with the type or extent of injury. No history of trauma is given.

(table continues on page 494)

Table 22.3 Red Flags for Child Abuse (continued)

Category	Details
Delay in treatment	A significant delay elapses between the time of injury and when the parent seeks treatment.
"Doctor shopping"	The parent changes physicians, health care facilities, or both frequently.
Injuries consistent with abuse	Bruises appear on infants before they walk. Bruising or other injuries are in varied stages of healing. Multiple types of injuries appear. Injuries resemble an object, such as cigarette burns, burns in the shape of an iron, or loop marks. Grab or slap marks or human bite marks are visible. Evidence exists of immersion burns—these are usually well demarcated and bilateral (eg, both hands or feet) or occur on the buttocks and feet.
Fractured bone	Any fracture in an infant who is not walking should raise the index of suspicion for abuse, unless there is a verifiable cause.
Types of fractures associated with physical abuse	These include multiple fractures, fractured ribs, fractured humerus, and skull fracture.
Pattern of injury consistent with shaken baby syndrome	Signs include subdural hematoma, retinal hemorrhages, rib fractures, and bilateral bruising in the rib cage.

Table 22.3 Red Flags for Child Abuse (*continued*)

Category	Details
Injuries consistent with sexual abuse	Any of the following in the genital area, anus, or both indicates sexual abuse: • Bleeding • Bruising • Redness
Signs of neglect	Examples include poor hygiene, clothes inappropriate for the weather, evidence of tissue wasting, signs of poor nutrition, failure to gain weight, and untreated illness.

Table 22.4 Normal Skin Variants in Newborns and Infants

Mongolian Spots

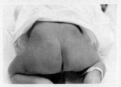

These bluish pigmented areas on the lower back or buttocks are common in infants of Asian, African, or Hispanic descent.

Spider Nevus

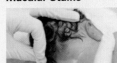

Macular Stains

Also known as "stork bites," these capillary malformations appear on the eyelid(s), between the eyebrows, or on the nape of the neck. They tend to fade within 1–2 years.

This benign lesion has a central arteriole from which thin-walled vessels radiate outward like spider legs. The lesion blanches when compressed.

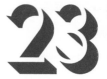

Older Adults

Key Topics and Questions for Health Promotion —

Key Questions	Rationales/Abnormal Findings
Current Problem. Ask, "Tell me why you came to the clinic today" or "What brought you to the hospital?"	If the reply is a medical diagnosis such as "heart attack," encourage the patient to describe symptoms.
Family History. Ask about the health of close family members to help identify and teach about diseases for which the patient may be at risk.	Note *high blood pressure, coronary artery disease, high cholesterol, stroke, cancer, diabetes, obesity, alcohol or drug addiction,* or *mental illness.*
Mobility Level and Functional Ability. When assessing an older adult returning to or living in the community, identify his or her ability to manage instrumental activities of daily living (Box 23-1).	Many older adults define health as ability to perform self-care. Some older adults require complete assistance, while others are completely functionally independent.
Abilities measured by the Lawton IADL scale include use of the telephone, finance management, shopping, laundry, housekeeping, food preparation, and use of transportation. Older adults who can manage these tasks are more likely to be able to live independently.	Hospital discharge planners or community health nurses use the Lawton IADL instrument to identify appropriate matches of supportive services and family assistance that might allow an older adult to maintain independence in the community. Because the tool relies on accurate self-report, information can be misleading with elders who lack insight into their functional losses (eg, *Alzheimer's disease*).

BOX 23.1   Lawton Instrumental Activities of Daily Living (IADL)

Instructions: Ask the patient to describe her/his functioning in each category; then complement the description with specific questions as needed.

Ability to Telephone

1. Operates telephone on own initiative: looks up and dials number, etc.
2. Answers telephone and dials a few well-known numbers.
3. Answers telephone but does not dial.
4. Does not use telephone at all.

Shopping

1. Takes care of all shopping needs independently.
2. Shops independently for small purchases.
3. Needs to be accompanied on any shopping trip.
4. Completely unable to shop.

Food Preparation

1. Plans, prepares, and serves adequate meals independently.
2. Prepares adequate meals if supplied with ingredients.
3. Heats and serves prepared meals, or prepares meals but does not maintain adequate diet.
4. Needs to have meals prepared and served.

Housekeeping

1. Maintains house alone or with occasional assistance (eg, heavy work done by domestic help).
2. Performs light daily tasks such as dishwashing and bed making.
3. Performs light daily tasks but cannot maintain acceptable level of cleanliness.
4. Needs help with all home maintenance tasks.
5. Does not participate in any housekeeping tasks.

(box continues on page 498)

Laundry

1. Does personal laundry completely
2. Launders small items; rinses socks, stockings, and so on.
3. All laundry must be done by others.

Mode of Transportation

1. Travels independently on public transportation, or drives own car.
2. Arranges own travel via taxi, but does not otherwise use public transportation.
3. Travels on public transportation when assisted or accompanied by another.
4. Travel limited to taxi, automobile, or ambulette, with assistance.
5. Does not travel at all.

Ability to Handle Finances

1. Manages financial matters independently (budgets, writes checks, pays rent and bills, goes to bank); collects and keeps track of income.
2. Manages day-to-day purchases but need help with banking, major purchases, controlled spending, and so on.
3. Incapable of handling money.

Scoring: Circle one number for each domain. Total the numbers circled. The lower the score, the more independent the older adult is. Scores are only good for individual patients. It is useful to see the score comparison over time.

Key Questions	Rationales/Abnormal Findings
Risk for Falls. Ask the patient, "Have you ever fallen? Do you have any dizziness?" Several fall risk assessment instruments are available to assist health care providers in identifying those older adults most at risk.	Serious injuries related to falls increase with age.

Key Questions	Rationales/Abnormal Findings

Medications/Polypharmacy

- "What medications are you taking?
- What is the dose?
- What is the schedule for medications?
- Do you understand why you take each medication?"

Older adults take more than 30% of prescription medications in the United States.

Ask the patient to bring in a bag of all medications at home and to identify those currently being taken. If this is not possible, phrase questions based on body system. For example, "Do you take any medications for your heart or blood pressure?" This approach is also useful when asking about over-the-counter (OTC) medications. Be sure to specifically ask how frequently the patient takes each OTC medication or supplement.

While examining each drug label, determine whether the patient is taking it as prescribed and if there are medications that should not be used together. Identify accuracy by calculating how many days are between today and the refill date, noting how many pills the pharmacist included and counting out the number of tablets left in the container to obtain an estimate of pills taken.

Ask about herbal or nutritional supplements and if any alternative health care providers have recommended other treatments.

Ask, "Do you take any medications belonging to others, including medications prescribed to a spouse, caregiver, friend, or neighbor?"

It is not unusual for elders living in retirement communities to share medications.

Identify how often and when the patient takes each drug:

- "Do you follow the prescription on the bottle? If not, why not?"
- "Are you experiencing side effects? If so, what kinds?"
- "Do you take medications with food, water, or alcohol?"

This important information allows the nurse to identify how frequently the patient is missing doses or overdosing.

(text continues on page 500)

Key Questions	Rationales/Abnormal Findings
Skin Breakdown. Identify risk for skin breakdown, especially for hospitalized and inactive patients. Many health care facilities use the Braden scale, with interventions based on the total score. See Chapter 6.	A score of 14 to 18 on Braden indicates a high risk for pressure ulcers.

Health-Promotion Teaching

Skin Care. Skin cancers increase with age and life-long sun exposure. Especially observe for skin cancer changes in older adults with the following risk factors: fair, freckling skin; light-colored eyes, red or blond hair, tendency to burn easily with sun exposure, male gender, and history of cigarette smoking. Teach patients to wear sunscreen at all times. Recommend hats and clothing that covers the skin. Teach patients to do a skin assessment and observe for cancers. See also Chapter 6.

Nutrition. Older adults need added vitamin D, because aging and smoking tend to impair vitamin D synthesis. Groups at risk for folate deficiency include patients with alcoholism, those who follow "fad" diets, and people of low socio-economic status. Older adults may compensate for diminished taste of sweet and salty foods by adding sugar and salt to their diet at a time when they are at increased risk for diabetes, hypertension, and heart disease. Their basal metabolic rate is declining concurrently with reductions in physical activity. When this occurs, caloric needs are significantly reduced. Older adults are also at increased risk for malnutrition as a result of social isolation. Eating alone is particularly problematic for people with reduced mobility, receiving social assistance, or both. Poor dentition may detract from enjoying meals. Community programs such as Meals on Wheels offer food services to people with disabilities or chronic illnesses who live in social isolation.

Safety. Assess for any signs of elder abuse and safety in the home. The older adult may have stairs that are a risk for falling, cooking surfaces that can be a fire hazard, or cords that can easily be tripped over. Focus teaching on keeping cooking surfaces clean and having cords out of walking areas. Rooms should be well lit. For hospitalized patients, a bed alarm may be helpful.

Key Topics and Questions for Common Symptoms

For each symptom, be sure to review location, characteristics, duration, aggravating factors, alleviating factors, accompanying symptoms, treatment, and the patient's view of the problem.

Common Symptoms in Older Adults

- Incontinence
- Sleep deprivation
- Pain
- Cognitive changes
- Depression
- Elder abuse

Questions to Assess Symptoms	Rationales/Abnormal Findings
Incontinence. Have you ever leaked urine or lost bladder control?	Incontinence is common among hospitalized patients and those in long term care. Risks include increasing age, caffeine intake, limited mobility, impaired cognition, diabetes, the use of medications, obesity, Parkinson's disease, stroke, and prostate problems.
Sleep Deprivation • What time do you turn off the lights? • How many awakenings do you have in a night? • Do you feel rested on arising?	Insomnia may be acute or chronic. It may affect falling asleep, staying asleep, or early morning wakening. Risk factors include female gender, increased age, and medical or psychiatric illness.
Pain • Do you have pain or discomfort? • Has pain affected your ability to function normally? For example, has it affected diet, sleep, or mood?	Chronic illness may increase pain in the older adult. The patient may be hesitant to report pain because of fear of dependence or wanting to be a "good patient." Pain may affect normal functions.

(text continues on page 502)

Questions to Assess Symptoms	Rationales/Abnormal Findings
Cognitive Status. Some specific tips for using this examination in older adults are found in Box 23-2. See also Chapter 5.	
Depression. Although older adults are at risk for depression, the illness is not a normal or inevitable part of aging (Box 23-3). To assess for depression, ask: • "Do you struggle with depression? • Have you ever suffered from depression?"	Depression is more common in people with multiple chronic health problems or who have recently suffered the loss of a spouse, friend, family member, or pet. Decisions about moving out of a family home because of increasing care needs may also lead to depressive symptoms.

BOX 23.2 ASSESSMENT OF COGNITIVE STATUS

- Introduce the test. State "I am going to conduct a test of your thinking skills. This is a screening test and I want you to do your best."
- If a family member is present, it is wise to let him or her know that he or she is not allowed to answer for the older adult. Patients with mild dementia may look to a spouse or child to assist them with questions.
- If you detect that the patient is somewhat suspicious of your questions based on previous interactions, start with questions under the language section of the examination (ie, "What is this?" point to your watch, and have him or her identify watch). Usually these questions offer the patient some success in responses and allow you to complete more of the screening.
- Do not provide clues to answers. For example, when asking the orientation questions, simply say, "Can you tell me what month this is?" Do not say, "Well, we recently had our Thanksgiving break." If the patient is uncertain, simply restate the question. "Can you tell me the month?"
- Allow enough time for the patient to respond to the question that you have asked.
- Reassure the patient if he or she worries that the response might be incorrect. "It's OK if some of these are difficult for you." However, don't falsely tell patients that they are doing fine. Identify that this is simply a screening test and will help you better understand how to provide care for this patient.

BOX 23.3 Geriatric Depression Scale: Short Form

Choose the best answer for how you have felt over the past week:
1. Are you basically satisfied with your life? YES/**NO**
2. Have you dropped many of your activities and interests? **YES**/NO
3. Do you feel that your life is empty? **YES**/NO
4. Do you often get bored? **YES**/NO
5. Are you in good spirits most of the time? YES/**NO**
6. Are you afraid that something bad is going to happen to you? **YES**/NO
7. Do you feel happy most of the time? YES/**NO**
8. Do you often feel helpless? **YES**/NO
9. Do you prefer to stay at home, rather than going out and doing new things? **YES**/NO
10. Do you feel you have more problems with memory than most? **YES**/NO
11. Do you think it is wonderful to be alive now? YES/**NO**
12. Do you feel pretty worthless the way you are now? **YES**/NO
13. Do you feel full of energy? YES/**NO**
14. Do you feel that your situation is hopeless? **YES**/NO
15. Do you think that most people are better off than you are? **YES**/NO

Answers in **bold** indicate depression. Score 1 point for each bolded answer.

A score >5 points is suggestive of depression. A score >10 points is almost always indicative of depression. A score >5 points should warrant a follow-up comprehensive assessment.

Source: Yesavage, J. A., Brink, T. L., Rose, T. L., et al. (1982). Development and validation of a geriatric depression screening scale: A preliminary report. *Journal of Psychiatric Research*, 17, 37–49.

Questions to Assess Symptoms	Rationales/Abnormal Findings
If the screening examination reveals risk for or actual depression, assess for potential suicide risk. Mentally healthy older adults report that thoughts about death and suicide ideation are relatively rare.	Factors that contribute to suicide in older adults include mental disorders (especially depression), physical illness, personality traits such as hostility, hopelessness, inability to verbally express psychological pain and dependency on others, and recent life events and losses.

(text continues on page 504)

Questions to Assess Symptoms	Rationales/Abnormal Findings
Elder Abuse. Older adults are vulnerable to abuse by family members. Continued abuse may be compounded because of nondetection by professionals, in part because elderly patients often do not report violence.	Many victims are isolated; some are ashamed and embarrassed or feel guilt and self-blame. In addition, some elders experience fear of reprisal, retribution from caregivers, or losing their home or independence. Others are pressured by relatives not to report.

Objective Data Collection

Equipment

- Stethoscope
- Thermometer and BP cuff or electronic vital signs monitor
- Watch or clock with a second hand
- Otoscope
- Ophthalmoscope

Technique and Normal Findings	Abnormal Findings
General Survey Observe age-related changes. Assess for any decreasing functional abilities and self-care. Note changes in mental status. *By the eighth or ninth decade, body contours are sharper and facial features more angular. Posture tends to have a general flexion. Gait has a wider base of support. Steps are shorter and uneven. The patient may need to use the arms to help aid in balance.*	Poor hygiene and inappropriate dress may be from decreased functional ability, medications, infection, dehydration, or malnutrition. Inappropriate affect, inattentiveness, impaired memory, and inability to perform ADLs may indicate *dementia*, medications, dehydration, poor nutrition, underlying infection, or hypoxia.
Height and Weight If possible, measure height with the person standing erect against a wall without shoes.	⚠ *SAFETY ALERT 23-1* *Do not attempt to determine height when a frail older adult is standing on the weight scale. This creates a risk of falling.*

Technique and Normal Findings	Abnormal Findings
Calculate Body Mass Index. *BMI is 25 to 29, slightly higher than the recommended BMI for younger adults.*	BMI is above 29 or below 25.

Vital Signs

Temperature. Assess temperature. *Mean body temperature is 36°C to 36.8°C (96.9°F to 98.3°F).*

Aging adults are less likely to develop fever, but more likely to succumb to *hypothermia.*

Pulse. Assess apical pulse for 1 minute. *Normal range is 60 to 100 bpm.*

Variation in rhythm may develop. The radial artery may stiffen from *peripheral vascular disease.*

Pulse rate takes longer to rise to meet sudden increases in demand and longer to return to resting state. Resting heart rate tends to be lower than for younger adults.

Heart sounds may be more difficult to assess and PMI more difficult to palpate because of increased air space in the lungs, which increases the anterior-posterior diameter of the chest.

Respirations. Assess respirations. *Decreased vital capacity and inspiratory volume can cause respirations to be shallower and more rapid (16 to 24 breaths/min).*

Respiratory rates greater than 24 are not normal and should be followed with further examination for cyanosis of the nail beds or the perioral area.

Pulse Oximetry. Assess pulse oximetry. *Oxygen saturation is greater than 92%.*

Peripheral vascular disease, decreased carbon dioxide levels, cold-induced vasoconstriction, and anemia may complicate assessment of oxygen saturation on the fingers.

Skin, Hair, and Nails

Examine skin carefully for breakdown, especially in the perineal area of older adults who are incontinent, and in any area at risk for pressure ulcers. Seborrheic keratoses are extremely common. These dark brown, pigmented lesions are waxy appearing areas

Bruising in various stages of healing might indicate abuse. *Pressure ulcers* should be staged and interventions begun immediately. Patchy white scaly areas on the scalp indicate *seborrhea*, common with *Parkinson's disease.* Very thick yellow over grown toenails are usually

(text continues on page 506)

that appear on sun-exposed areas of the body. Photoaging findings include coarse wrinkles over sun-exposed areas, solar lentigines (age or liver spots), and actinic keratosis. *Wrinkling is increased; skin is coarse in sun-exposed areas. Scalp hair is thinned. Skin is less elastic and may be dry (although dryness is more often linked to poor hydration). It is common to note thinning of the epidermal layer, more pronounced in the 8th and 9th decades. Nail beds may have ridges. Toenails may become thickened.*

a sign of *onychomycosis* (tinea unguium). *Stasis dermatitis* is common in older adults with a history of varicosities, phlebitis, and trauma. Lower extremities have a reddish-brown ruddy appearance and are usually edematous, but not inflamed or infected. *Herpes zoster* (shingles) is a red painful vesicular or pustular rash that follows the distribution of a dermatome along the trunk or even into the legs. Older adults have a less vigorous immune response and are at risk for developing this rash especially during times of illness or hospitalization.

Head and Neck

Inspect the head and neck. *Appearance is symmetrical. Facial expression is appropriate to situation.* Palpate the skull and hair. *Skull is smooth; there is no pain or mass. Hair is thin and gray.* Palpate the sternocleidomastoid and trapezius muscles. *There is no pain or masses.* Palpate the thyroid. *Thyroid is not enlarged.*

Downward gaze with little eye contact, flat affect, or facial tension may be a sign of *depression* or *anxiety*. Swelling, masses, tumors, or *goiter* are abnormal. An extremely thin patient may have sunken facial hollows. A patient with extremely thick structures may have thyroid problems. Clicking or crepitus in the temporomandibular joint is associated with jaw or neck pain. Note limitations in movement in the neck.

Eyes and Vision

Inspect the eyes. *Senile ptosis (sagging of the upper lid down across the eye), dry eyes that appear irritated and red, and a decreased corneal reflex may be present.*

Ectropian (turning of the lid outward) or entropian (turning of the lid inward) may be observed. Reduced visual fields, especially unilaterally, can be a sign of a *stroke* or central neurological lesion. Loss of vision can significantly affect daily functioning including dressing, grooming, and ambulating safely.

Technique and Normal Findings	Abnormal Findings
Test vision, pupillary reflex, and extraocular movements. *Older adults may have difficulty with focusing properly (presbyopia), glare, and accommodation. A smaller pupil size is normal. Upward gaze is reduced because of muscle changes and laxity. Also common is a grayish yellow ring around the iris (arcus senilus). Visual fields may be slightly diminished with confrontation but should not show unilateral differences. On ophthalmoscopic examination, retinal margins may be less distinct; drusen (yellow spots) may be on the macula.*	

Ears and Hearing

Inspect for lesions or changes to the auricle. *No pain, masses, or lesions are present.*	Ulcerated lesions in older men with a history of sun exposure may be *squamous cell carcinoma.*
Perform the otoscopic examination. *There may be a gray tympanic membrane or narrowed or wax-occluded ear canal. On the Weber test, conductive hearing loss causes lateralization of hearing to the ear occluded with wax. Bone conduction may be longer than air conduction in the ear occluded with wax on the Rinne test.*	High-frequency sounds are lost most commonly. Early treatment of the causes of conductive hearing loss or information on assistive devices is important.

Nose, Mouth, and Throat

Inspect the nose, mouth, and throat. Test nasal patency. *Septal deviation is common.* Make note of the color and	Pale mucosal membranes can indicate *anemia* or *malnutrition.* Malodorous breath may indicate dental disease, poor hygiene,

(text continues on page 508)

Technique and Normal Findings	Abnormal Findings

moisture of the mucosal membranes of the nose and oral cavity. *These are pink to pinkish red and moist. The tongue is pinkish red, moist, and has no fissures. A slightly dry oral mucosa is common; a fissured tongue is a sign of dehydration. Varicosities under the tongue are common. The gag reflex is intact, although it may mildly diminish.*

or underlying disease. Poor dentition can markedly influence nutritional intake. A bright red tongue can indicate *vitamin C or B1 deficiency*. Overgrowth of white patchy plaque on the tongue may be from poor dental hygiene or a **fungal or yeast infection** (*oral candidiasis*). Poor oral care may indicate cognitive impairment. Absent or markedly diminished gag reflex is associated with *stroke, alcoholism,* or *neurological disorders*. Patients with diminished or absent gag reflexes are at risk for aspiration pneumonia.

Thorax and Lungs
Inspect the chest. *The patient may have an increased anterior-posterior diameter related to rigidity of the chest wall.* Test for tactile fremitus. Percuss the lungs. *Chest wall is free of pain, swelling, or masses. Tactile fremitus is not increased; percussion is resonant.* Auscultate breath sounds. *Older adults who can take good breaths should have normal breath sounds. Harsh rhonchi are sometimes found because of the difficulty of clearing materials. Have the patient cough and then listen again. It is common for older adults to have scattered rales at the lung bases.*

Increased fremitus or dullness with percussion, especially at the lung bases, can indicate fluid accumulation. Older adults with chronic lung disease have hyperresonance on examination. Older women may have kyphosis that affects audibility of lung sounds at the bases. Listen for breath sounds at the lateral sides of the posterior wall. Lung sounds may be difficult to hear with advanced lung disease or may sound diminished and tight. Listening after a nebulizer treatment may give a clearer picture.

Heart and Neck Vessels
Auscultate heart sounds. *Pulse rates of 50 to 60 beats/min are common and often related to cardiac medications. Heart rate*

Loud (grade 3 or greater) or harsh holosystolic murmurs suggest valvular (usually aortic) stenosis and can sometimes be

Technique and Normal Findings	Abnormal Findings

*and rhythm are regular with
no murmurs, rubs, or gallops.
As older adults reach their 80s
and 90s, murmurs are com-
mon, especially grade 2 systolic.* Observe neck vessels.
*No jugular venous distention
is present.*

heard radiating up to the neck.
Loud murmurs radiating from
the apex to around the side
of the chest wall are usually
mitral. Consider findings from
the whole examination when
a patient has a loud murmur.
Specifically look for edema,
abdominal distension, other
signs of fluid retention, and
respiratory findings to identify
congestive heart failure. Arryth-
mias, especially *atrial fibrillation,*
are common but abnormal. Note
whether this is an irregularly
irregular rhythm; be concerned
if the rate is greater than 100.
Abdominal aortic pulsations that
extend over a wide area indicate
an *aortic aneurysm.*

Peripheral Vascular
Palpate peripheral pulses.
*Pulses are 2 to 3 on a 4-point
scale and symmetrical.*

Note absent pulses; contact the
primary provider if this finding
is new. It can seriously interfere
with wound healing. Vascular
disease may be venous or
arterial (see Chapter 13).

Breasts
Palpate. Because breast tissue
loses density with age, masses
or nodules are easier to feel. *No
masses or nodules are present.*

Mastectomy scars should be
noted and palpated.

Abdomen
and Elimination
Inspect, auscultate, palpate, and
percuss the abdomen. Perform
the rectal examination. *Take
extra time to listen for bowel
sounds. Finding a mass of stool
in the lower left quadrant is
common. A flaccid or soft,*

A distended abdomen can
signify gas, stool, or fluid.
Asymmetry or masses may
be signs of *severe constipation* or *cancer.* Perform a rectal
check for anyone with a lower
abdominal mass. Patients with

(text continues on page 510)

Technique and Normal Findings	Abnormal Findings
distended abdomen can be related to deconditioning and loss of muscle control. Bowel sounds may be slow, but are easy to hear. Rectal examination may show external hemorrhoids.	large amounts of abdominal ascites usually have *liver disease* or *cancerous involvement of the liver*. Internal or external hemorrhoids should not be painful, fiery red, or inflamed. Fecal *incontinence* or involuntary passage of stool is abnormal. See Chapter 15.

Musculoskeletal System

Obtain height. *Loss of up to 6 inches can occur by 70 to 80 years.* Perform focused assessments of the bones, muscles, and joints as indicated. *Neck flexion and hyperextension are somewhat reduced. Likelihood of spinal kyphosis is increased (more common in women). There may be a generalized decrease in strength and mildly decreased ROM. Older adults with arthritis may have enlarged joints, especially at the knees and in the hands.* When possible, test the patient's ability to stand from a seated position, walk a short distance, and turn around. *Patients should be able to do this smoothly, without balance problems, stumbling, or assistance.*

Examination of ROM of the upper extremities is important, especially for hospitalized older adults. Limited shoulder abduction can be addressed immediately to prevent "frozen shoulder," a common condition during or after hospitalization. Pain on spinal palpation after a fall should raise concerns about possible *compression fracture*. Large nodules in the distal interphalangeal joints are *Heberden nodes*, while enlargements of the proximal interphalangeal joints are *Bouchard nodes*, common with *arthritis* (see Chapter 17). Contractures of the hips and knees are abnormal but common in patients who regularly use a wheelchair. These contractures change gait and balance and place the patient at risk for further immobility.

Neurological

Cranial Nerves. Test cranial nerves. *Common findings include decreased upward gaze.*

Older adults who appear to have a blank or blunted affect may have *depression, dementia,* or *Parkinson's disease.*

Technique and Normal Findings	Abnormal Findings
Balance and Coordination. Test balance and coordination. *There may be slowing of psychomotor finger-nose testing, or finger-to-finger testing. Heal-to-toe walking may be impaired. Gait with or without an assistive device shows smooth steps that may be wide based.*	See Chapters 16 and 17 for a thorough review of abnormal gaits.

⚠ SAFETY ALERT 23-2

Do the Romberg test only when a chair is directly behind the patient and the examiner is at the patient's side to assist.

Test sensation. *Peripheral sensation and proprioceptive (position) sense may diminish slightly.*	**Clinical Significance 23-1** Unilateral findings on neurological examination may be evidence of a cerebrovascular accident.
Reflexes and Muscle Strength. Test reflexes and muscle strength. *Reflexes normally diminish; muscle strength against resistance may be slightly diminished in those with musculoskeletal conditions.*	*Parkinson's disease* has a resting, usually unilateral tremor that does not include the head and neck. Tremor of the hand or neck, that is heard in changes in the voice or occurs in the hand only when the person is initiating an action is intentional. Diminished grip strength or unilateral loss of strength against resistance is abnormal. Severely diminished or absent sensation or proprioception indicates *peripheral neuropathy*.
Male and Female Genitourinary Inspect genitals. *Thinning of genital hair and testicular or penile atrophy are common. Vaginal skin may be thinned.*	A full bladder after recently voiding is a sign of *urinary retention.* Underwear smelling of urine, staining of urine, or leaking urine indicates incontinence.

Common Nursing Diagnoses and Interventions for Older Adults

Diagnosis and Related Factors	Nursing Interventions
Adult failure to thrive related to depression	Assess for depression. Complete mini-mental exam. Provide cues in the environment for food intake. Provide reality orientation. Encourage patients to reminisce and share life histories.
Disturbed sensory perception: visual or auditory, related to aging process	Provide adequate lighting. Keep background noise low, such as turning off the TV when talking. Make sure that patient has devices such as glasses or hearing aid.
Imbalanced nutrition, less than body requirements relating to isolation	Note laboratory tests such as total protein, albumin and prealbumin. Weigh patient daily. Monitor food intake and record the percentage of meal eaten.

ILLUSTRATION CREDIT LIST

(3rd ed.). Philadelphia: Lippincott Williams & Wilkins; *Lipoma:* Image provided by Steadman's.

Table 6.5: *Stage I, Stage II, Stage III, Stage IV:* Nettina, S. M., MSN, RN, CS, ANP. (2001). *The Lippincott manual of nursing practice* (7th ed.). Lippincott Williams & Wilkins.

Table 6.7: *Longitudinal Ridging, Onycholysis, Pitted Nails, Yellow Nails, Half-and-half Nails, Dark Longitudinal Streaks:* Goodheart, H. P., MD. (2009). *Goodheart's photoguide to common skin disorders* (3rd ed.). Philadelphia: Lippincott Williams & Wilkins; *Koilonychia, Clubbing, Splinter Hemorrhages:* Image provided by Steadman's; *Beau's Lines:* Bickley, L. S. (2009). *Bates' guide to physical examination and history taking* (10th ed.). Philadelphia: Lippincott Williams & Wilkins.

Table 6.8: *Alopecia Areata, Traction Alopecia, Trichotillomania:* Goodheart, H. P., MD. (2009). *Goodheart's photoguide to common skin disorders* (3rd ed.). Philadelphia: Lippincott Williams & Wilkins; *Hirsutism:* Image provided by Steadman's.

CHAPTER 7

Table 7.1: *Hydrocephalus, Fetal Alcohol Syndrome:* Gold, D. H., MD, & Weingeist, T. A., MD, PhD. (2001). *Color atlas of the eye in systemic disease.* Baltimore: Lippincott Williams & Wilkins; *Cretinism (Congenital Hypothyroidism):* Centers for Disease Control and Prevention Public Health Image Library.

Table 7.2: *Acromegaly:* Willis, M. C., CMA-AC. (2002). *Medical terminology: A programmed learning approach to the language*

of health care. Baltimore: Lippincott Williams & Wilkins; *Bell's Palsy, Cerebral Vascular Accident (Stroke), Myxedema:* Dr. P. Marazzi/Photo Researchers, Inc.; *Cushing's Syndrome:* Ostler, H. B., Maibach, H. I., Hoke, A. W., & Schwab, I. R. (2004). *Diseases of the eye and skin: A color atlas.* Philadelphia: Lippincott Williams & Wilkins; *Scleroderma:* Gold, D. H., MD, & Weingeist, T. A., MD, PhD. (2001). *Color atlas of the eye in systemic disease.* Baltimore: Lippincott Williams & Wilkins; *Goiter:* Scott Camazine/Photo Researchers, Inc.

CHAPTER 8

Figures 8.7, 8.10, 8.16, and 8.17: Tasman, W., & Jaeger, E. (2001). *The Wills Eye Hospital atlas of clinical ophthalmology* (2nd ed.). Lippincott Williams & Wilkins.

Figure 8.9: Gold, D. H., MD, & Weingeist, T. A., MD, PhD. (2001). *Color atlas of the eye in systemic disease.* Baltimore: Lippincott Williams & Wilkins.

Figure 8.11: Courtesy of Terri Young, MD

Figures 8.12, 8.13, and Box 8.1: Bickley, L. S. (2009). *Bates' guide to physical examination and history taking* (10th ed.). Philadelphia: Lippincott Williams & Wilkins.

Table 8.2: *Jaundice, Cataract:* Rubin, E., M. D., & Farber, J. L., MD. (1999). *Pathology* (3rd ed.). Philadelphia: Lippincott Williams & Wilkins; *Iris Nevus, Blepharitis, Bacterial Conjunctivitis, Glaucoma, Amblyopia, Hordeolum (Stye):* Tasman, W, & Jaeger, E. (2001). *The Wills Eye Hospital atlas of clinical ophthalmology*

(2nd ed.). Lippincott Williams & Wilkins; *Hyphema, Allergic Conjunctivitis:* Fleisher, G. R., MD, Ludwig, S., MD, Baskin, M. N., MD. (2004). *Atlas of pediatric emergency medicine.* Philadelphia: Lippincott Williams & Wilkins; *Chalazion:* Bickley, L. S. (2009). *Bates' guide to physical examination and history taking* (10th ed.). Philadelphia: Lippincott Williams & Wilkins; *Exophthalmos:* Goodheart, H. P., MD. (2009). *Goodheart's photoguide to common skin disorders* (3rd ed.). Philadelphia: Lippincott Williams & Wilkins; *Osteogenesis Imperfecta:* Ostler, H. B., Maibach, H. I., Hoke, A. W., & Schwab, I. R. (2004). *Diseases of the eye and skin: A color atlas.* Philadelphia: Lippincott Williams & Wilkins.

Table 8.3: *Horner's Syndrome, Adie's Pupil, Mydriasis (Dilated Fixed Pupil), Oculomotor (CN III) Nerve Damage:* Tasman, W., & Jaeger, E. (2001). *The Wills Eye Hospital atlas of clinical ophthalmology* (2nd ed.). Lippincott Williams & Wilkins; *Key Hole Pupil (Coloboma):* Courtesy of Brian Forbes, MD; *Miosis (Small Fixed Pupil):* Gold, D. H., MD, & Weingeist, T. A., MD, PhD. (2001). *Color atlas of the eye in systemic disease.* Baltimore: Lippincott Williams & Wilkins.

Table 8.4: *AMD, Retinopathy, Retinitis Pigmentosa:* Tasman, W., & Jaeger, E. (2001). *The Wills Eye Hospital atlas of clinical ophthalmology* (2nd ed.). Lippincott Williams & Wilkins; *Copper Wiring:* McConnell, T. H. (2007). *The nature of disease pathology for the health professions.* Philadelphia: Lippincott Williams & Wilkins.

CHAPTER 9

Figure 9.5B: Moore, K. L., PhD, FRSM, FIAC, & Dalley, A. F., II, PhD. (1999). *Clinically oriented anatomy* (4th ed.). Baltimore: Lippincott Williams & Wilkins.

Table 9.1: *Microtia:* Biophoto Associates/Photo Researchers, Inc.; *Macrotia:* Saturn Stills/Photo Researchers, Inc.; *Edematous Ears, Cartilage* Staphyloccous *or* Pseudomonas *Infection:* Ostler, H. B., Maibach, H. I., Hoke, A. W., & Schwab, I. R. (2004). *Diseases of the eye and skin: A color atlas.* Philadelphia: Lippincott Williams & Wilkins; *Carcinoma on Auricle:* Goodheart, H. P., MD. (2009). *Goodheart's photoguide to common skin disorders* (3rd ed.). Philadelphia: Lippincott Williams & Wilkins; *Cyst:* Young, E. M. Jr, Newcomer, V. D., Kligman, A. M. (1993). *Geriatric dermatology: Color atlas and practitioner's guide.* Philadelphia: Lea & Febiger; *Tophi:* SPL/Photo Researchers, Inc.

Table 9.2: *TM Rupture:* Courtesy of Michael Hawke, MD, Toronto, Canada; *Acute Otitis Media:* Moore, K. L., PhD, FRSM, FIAC, & Dalley, A. F., II, PhD. (1999). *Clinically oriented anatomy* (4th ed.). Baltimore: Lippincott Williams & Wilkins; *Scarred TM:* Weber, J. RN, EdD, & Kelley, J. RN, PhD. (2003). *Health assessment in nursing* (2nd ed.). Philadelphia: Lippincott Williams & Wilkins; *Foreign Body*: Dr. P. Marazzi/Photo Researchers, Inc.

CHAPTER 10

Table 10.1: *Epistaxis (Nosebleed):* Ian Boddy/Photo Researchers, Inc.; *Nasal Polyps:* Handler, S. D.,

Myer, C. M. (1998). *Atlas of ear, nose and throat disorders in children* (p. 59). Ontario, Canada: BC Decker; *Deviated Septum:* Moore, K. L., PhD, FRSM, FIAC, & Dalley, A. F., II, PhD. (2008). *Clinically oriented anatomy* (6th ed.). Baltimore: Lippincott Williams & Wilkins; *Perforated Septum, Foreign Body:* Dr. P. Marazzi/Photo Researchers, Inc.

Table 10.2: *Cleft Lip/Palate:* Rubin, E. MD, & Farber, J. L., MD. (1999). *Pathology* (3rd ed.). Philadelphia: Lippincott Williams & Wilkins; *Bifid Uvula:* Courtesy of Paul S. Matz, MD; *Acute Tonsillitis or Pharyngitis:* BSIP/Photo Researchers, Inc.; *Strep Throat:* Centers for Disease Control and Prevention Public Health Image Library.

Table 10.3: *Herpes Simplex Virus, Candidasis, Leukoplakia, Black Hairy Tongue, Carcinoma:* Goodheart, H. P., MD. (2009). *Goodheart's photoguide to common skin disorders* (3rd ed.). Philadelphia: Lippincott Williams & Wilkins.

Table 10.4: *Baby Bottle Tooth Decay:* Fleisher, G. R., MD, Ludwig, S., MD, & Baskin, M. N., MD. (2004). *Atlas of pediatric emergency medicine*. Philadelphia: Lippincott Williams & Wilkins; *Dental Caries:* Langlais, R. P., & Miller, C. S. (1992). *Color atlas of common oral diseases*. Philadelphia: Lea & Febiger. Used with permission; *Gingival Hyperplasia:* Courtesy of Dr. James Cottone; *Ankyloglossia (Tongue Tie):* Courtesy of Paul S. Matz, MD.

CHAPTER 11
Figures 11.1, 11.2, 11.3, and 11.4A,B: Photos by B. Proud.

Figure 11.5A, B: Moore, K. L., PhD, FRSM, FIAC, & Dalley, A. F., II, PhD. (2008). *Clinically Oriented Anatomy* (6th ed.). Baltimore: Lippincott Williams & Wilkins.

CHAPTER 12
Figure 12.4: Bickley, L. S. (2009). *Bates' guide to physical examination and history taking* (10th ed.). Philadelphia: Lippincott Williams & Wilkins.

CHAPTER 13
Table 13.2: *Acute Arterial Occlusion:* Nettina, S. M., MSN, RN, CS, ANP. (2001). *The Lippincott manual of nursing practice* (7th ed.). Lippincott Williams & Wilkins; *Abdominal Aortic Aneurysm:* Moore, K. L., PhD, FRSM, FIAC, & Dalley, A. F., II, PhD. (2008). *Clinically oriented anatomy* (6th ed.). Baltimore: Lippincott Williams & Wilkins; *Raynaud's Phenomenon and Raynaud's Disease:* Marks, R. (1987). *Skin disease in old age*. Philadelphia: JB Lippincott.

Table 13.3: *Chronic Venous Insufficiency, Neuropathy:* Marks, R. (1987). *Skin disease in old age*. Philadelphia: JB Lippincott; *Deep Vein Thrombosis:* Dr. P. Marazzi/Photo Researchers, Inc.; *Thrombophlebitis:* Biophoto Associates/Photo Researchers, Inc.; *Lymphedema:* Rubin, E. MD, & Farber, J. L., MD. (1999). *Pathology* (3rd ed.). Philadelphia: Lippincott Williams & Wilkins.

CHAPTER 14
Figures 14.1, 14.3A–D, 14.6, 14.7, and 14.8: Photo by B. Proud.
Figures 14.4 and 14.9: Mulholland, M. W., Maier, R. V., et al. (2006).

Greenfield's surgery scientific principles and practice (4th ed.). Philadelphia: Lippincott Williams & Wilkins.

Table 14.2: *Carcinoma 1, Carcinoma 2:* Mulholland, M. W., Maier, R. V., et al. (2006). *Greenfield's surgery scientific principles and practice* (4th ed.). Philadelphia: Lippincott Williams & Wilkins; ***Paget Disease, Mastitis:*** Sweet, R. L., Gibbs, R. S. (2005). *Atlas of infectious diseases of the female genital tract*. Philadelphia: Lippincott Williams & Wilkins; ***Mastectomy:*** Steve Percival/Photo Researchers, Inc.; ***Gynecomastia:*** Courtesy of Christine Finck, MD.

CHAPTER 15

Figures 15.3, 15.4, and 15.5: Photo by B. Proud.

CHAPTER 16

Figures 16.11 and 16.13A–C: Photo by B. Proud.

Figure 16.12: Bickley, L. S. (2009). *Bates' guide to physical examination and history taking* (10th ed.). Philadelphia: Lippincott Williams & Wilkins.

Figures 16.14A,B and 16.15A,B: Moore, K. L., PhD, FRSM, FIAC, & Dalley, A. F., II, PhD. (2008). *Clinically oriented anatomy* (6th ed.). Baltimore: Lippincott Williams & Wilkins.

Table 16.4: *Atrophy, Joint Effusions, Epicondylitis:* Bickley, L. S. (2009). *Bates' guide to physical examination and history taking* (10th ed.). Philadelphia: Lippincott Williams & Wilkins; ***Joint Dislocation, Polydactyly, Swan Neck and Boutonniere Deformity, Syndactyly, Ulnar Deviation:*** Strickland, J. W., &

Graham, T. J. (2005). *Master techniques in orthopeadic surgery: The hand* (2nd ed.). Philadelphia: Lippincott Williams & Wilkins; ***Rheumatoid Arthritis:*** Gold, D. H., MD, & Weingeist, T. A., MD, PhD. (2001). *Color atlas of the eye in systemic disease*. Baltimore: Lippincott Williams & Wilkins; ***Rotator Cuff Tear, Bursitis, Ganglion Cyst, Dupuytren's Contracture, Heberden's and Bouchard's Nodes, Carpal Tunnel Syndrome:*** Berg, D., & Worzala, K. (2006). *Atlas of adult physical diagnosis*. Philadelphia: Lippincott Williams & Wilkins; ***Genu Valgum:*** Courtesy of Bettina Gyr, MD; ***Congenital Hip Dislocation:*** Bucholz, R. W., MD, Heckman, J. D., MD. (2001). *Rockwood & Green's fractures in adults* (5th ed.). Lippincott Williams & Wilkins; ***Herniated Nucleus Pulposus:*** Daffner, R. H. (2007). *Clinical radiology the essentials* (3rd ed.) Philadelphia: Lippincott Williams & Wilkins; ***Talipes Equinovarus:*** Courtesy of J. Adams; ***Acute Rheumatoid Arthritis:*** Image provided by Stedman's; ***Ankylosing Spondylitis:*** McConnell, T. H. (2007). *The nature of disease pathology for the health professions*. Philadelphia: Lippincott Williams & Wilkins.

CHAPTER 17

Figures 17.1, 17.7, and 17.10: Bickley, L. S. (2009). *Bates' guide to physical examination and history taking* (10th ed.). Philadelphia: Lippincott Williams & Wilkins.

Figure 17.6: Photo by B. Proud.

Table 17.2: *Paralysis:* Centers for Disease Control and Prevention Public Image Library; ***Dystonia:*** Fleisher, G. R., MD, Ludwig,

W., MD, & Baskin, M. N., MD. (2004). *Atlas of pediatric emergency medicine*. Philadelphia: Lippincott Williams & Wilkins.

CHAPTER 18

Figures 18.2, 18.3, 18.4, and 18.5: Photos by B. Proud.

Table 18.1: *Phimosis, Paraphimosis, Hypospadias:* Courtesy of T. Ernesto Figueroa; *Balanitis:* Fleisher, G. R., MD, Ludwig, S., MD, & Baskin, M. N., MD. (2004). *Atlas of pediatric emergency medicine*. Philadelphia: Lippincott Williams & Wilkins; *Epispadias:* MacDonald, M. G., Seshia, M. M. K., et al. (2005). *Avery's neonatology pathophysiology & management of the newborn* (6th ed.). Philadelphia: Lippincott Williams & Wilkins.

Table 18.2: *Scabies Infection, Syphilis:* Goodheart, H. P., MD. (2009). *Goodheart's photoguide to common skin disorders* (3rd ed.). Philadelphia: Lippincott Williams & Wilkins; *Chlamydia:* Image from Rubin, E. MD, & Farber, J. L., MD. (1999). *Pathology* (3rd ed.). Philadelphia: Lippincott Williams & Wilkins; *Gonorrhea:* Sanders, C. V., & Nesbitt, L. T. (1995). *The skin and infection*. Baltimore: Williams & Wilkins.

Table 18.3: *Testicular Torsion, Varicocele:* Courtesy of T. Ernesto Figueroa, MD.

Table 18.4: *Rectal Polyp, Carcinoma of the Rectum and Anus:* Mulholland, M. W., Maier, R. V., et al. (2006). *Greenfield's surgery: Scientific principles and practice* (4th ed.). Philadelphia: Lippincott Williams & Wilkins; *Rectal Prolapse:* Courtesy of Mary L. Brandt, MD; *Prostatitis:* Image from Rubin, E. MD, & Farber, J. L., MD. (1999). *Pathology* (3rd ed.). Philadelphia: Lippincott Williams & Wilkins.

CHAPTER 19

Figures 19.1B, 19.2, 19.4, 19.6A, and 19.7A: Photo by B. Proud.

Figures 19.3 and Box 19.2A,B: Berg, D., & Worzala, K. (2006). *Atlas of adult physical diagnosis*. Philadelphia: Lippincott Williams & Wilkins.

Table 19.1: *Candidiasis:* Goodheart, H. P., MD. (2009). *Goodheart's photoguide to common skin disorders* (3rd ed.). Philadelphia: Lippincott Williams & Wilkins; *Bacterial Vaginosis, Chlamydia, Gonorrhea, Trichomoniasis, Condylomata Acuminatum:* Sweet, R. L., & Gibbs, R. S. (2005). *Atlas of infectious diseases of the female genital tract*. Philadelphia: Lippincott Williams & Wilkins.

Table 19.2: *Pediculosis, Chancre, Abscess of the Bartholin's Gland:* Sweet, R. L., & Gibbs, R. S. (2005). *Atlas of infectious diseases of the female genital tract*. Philadelphia: Lippincott Williams & Wilkins; *Urethral Caruncle:* Courtesy of Allan R. De Jong, MD; *Contact Dermatitis:* Courtesy of George A. Datto, III, MD.

CHAPTER 21

Figure 21.4A: Goodheart H. P., MD. (2009). *Goodheart's photoguide to common skin disorders* (3rd ed.). Philadelphia: Lippincott Williams & Wilkins

INDEX

Page numbers followed by b indicate boxes; those followed by f indicate figures; those followed by t indicate tables.